SLEEP, DREAMING, & SLEEP DISORDERS

An Introduction

Second Edition

William H. Moorcroft
Luther College

UNIVERSITY PRESS OF AMERICA

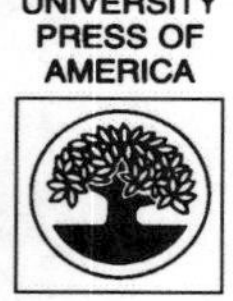

Lanham • New York • London

University Press of America®, Inc.
4720 Boston Way
Lanham, Maryland 20706

3 Henrietta Street
London WC2E 8LU England

Printed in the United States of America
British Cataloging in Publication Information Available

Library of Congress Cataloging-in-Publication Data

Moorcroft, William H.
Sleep, dreaming, and sleep disorders : an introduction /
William H. Moorcroft. — 2nd ed.
p. cm.
Includes bibliographical references and index.
1. Sleep. 2. Dreams. 3. Sleep disorders. I. Title.
QP425.M66 1993 612.8'21—dc20 93–5259 CIP

ISBN 0–8191–9250–3 (cloth : alk. paper)
ISBN 0–8191–9251–1 (pbk. : alk. paper)

The paper used in this publication meets the minimum requirements of American National Standard for Information Sciences—Permanence of Paper for Printed Library Materials, ANSI Z39.48–1984.

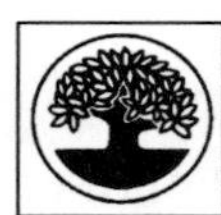

This book is dedicated to my sleeping partner

CHRISTINA PERRIN MOORCROFT

and

our three dreams, MARCY, DREW, and PAT.

TABLE OF CONTENTS

Preface

We can imagine that in the distant past some early human was unable to continue an enjoyable endeavor because of their body's demand for sleep. That individual may have been the first to ask, "Why do I have to sleep?" and "What happens during sleep?" Surprisingly, these and similar questions, which must have been repeated uncountable times over the centuries of human existence, have only begun to be answered in the last 45 years!

We also know that dreaming has been an age-old source of human wonderment. In this case, humans have had answers - or so they thought - since the time of the earliest written records and probably long before. Yet again, it is only within the last 45 years that we are getting closer to discovering the true meaning and function of dreaming.

Similarly, the problems of sleep - or at least the more obvious ones such as insomnia, being over sleepy, and snoring - have long plagued humans and resulted in much speculation (as well as numerous strange and wondrous "cures"). And yet again, it is only within the last few decades that we have really begun to investigate, understand, and adequately treat these and other previously unsuspected sleep problems.

For it was in 1953 that Aserinsky and Kleitman, while studying the brain waves of a sleeper, were surprised to notice that eye movements occurred periodically in their subject who was, by all indicators, completely asleep. Four years later, Bill Dement - then a student of Kleitman - discovered the connection between these eye movements during sleep and dreaming (Dement & Kleitman, 1957). These startling observations began a whole new era of interest in the laboratory study of sleep, dreaming and, subsequently, sleep disorders. From these new avenues of investigation came an explosion of discoveries and surprises to revision and often outright rejection of established notions in these areas.

This explosion continues today. The number of articles in scientific journals about sleep, dreaming, and sleep disorders in the last few decades easily outnumbers all those that preceded them. New journals devoted to sleep and its related phenomena have recently been born and a number of very fine technical books have been published. However, nothing written within the last decade is suitable for use by undergraduate students as a textbook or course supplement and adequately covers sleep, dreaming, and sleep disorders. This book is intended to fill that void.

I have written this book from several perspectives. First, from the vantage point of a researcher in each of the three areas of sleep, dreaming, and sleep disorders. I have included the results of some of my research in order to show how knowledge about these many facets of sleep has been discovered.

Second, I have written this book out of my experiences with sleep disorders in sleep disorders centers. I have included many actual experiences with sleep disorder patients so that students can better understand the problems that sleep disorders present to their suffers.

Finally, I have written this book from my experience as a college professor who has frequently taught courses on sleep, dreaming, and sleep disorders in the last two decades. This book is written for college students with no prior knowledge of sleep and related phenomena. At the same time, it is not boring for those students that already have some knowledge in these areas. The book begins by examining the natural fascination that most students have for sleep and related topics and builds to its readers to a greater fascination for, as well as increased understanding of, all aspects of sleep. I have avoided using technical jargon as much as possible. At the same time I have tried to avoid overgeneralization and oversimplification. In addition, I have endeavored to involve readers as much as possible by talking about all aspects of their sleep and dreaming, as well as taking them to a sleep laboratory during an all-night recording session and having them present while sleep disorder cases are being reviewed in a sleep disorders clinic.

The organization of the book is logical and straight forward. The prologue is a visit to a sleep lab that is intended to both inform readers and heighten their interest in the topic of sleep. In the rest of the book, the basics of sleep are covered first followed by dreaming and sleep disorders and concluding with an overview of the functions of sleep and dreaming. The first section starts with a chapter on the basics of sleep (Chapter 1) describes the specific criteria for sleep and its substages as measured in the lab, what a typical night of sleep is like, and how it changes with age. This is followed by a chapter on the involvement of the body and the brain in sleep (Chapter 2). Next other characteristics of sleep, sleep loss, and factors that affect sleep or that are affected by sleep are presented (Chapter 3) followed by the exploration of the rhythmical nature of sleep (Chapter 4). This section concludes with a chapter on the sleep in animals (Chapter 5).

The section on dreaming focuses on the process of dreaming rather than dreams themselves although dreams cannot be and are not ignored. Throughout the chapters in this unit, many sample dreams are presented to illustrate points. The unit begins with a chapter that previews the facts (and fictions) of dreams and dreaming (Chapter 6). The next chapter (Chapter 7) summarizes the key aspects of the major theories about dreaming and dream interpretation. The final chapter (Chapter 8) explores three contemporary methods for interpreting dreams including examples and complete instructions for their use.

The following Section focuses on sleep disorders. In Chapter 9 the major types of disorders are each presented in turn usually introduced by illustrative case examples that bring the problems to life for the reader.

The final section is a summary of what sleep and dreams are all about. First, remaining questions and problems about the whole area of sleep, dreaming, and sleep disorders are also presented in Chapter 10. Then on the basis of what has been learned about sleep, dreaming and sleep disorders, the probable functions of sleep are reviewed and discussed (Chapter 11).

I hope that readers will gain increasing fascination and knowledge about sleep while using this book, just as I have from writing it.

Wm. H. Moorcroft, Ph.D.
Decorah, Iowa
March 4, 1993

PS. A special note to instructors who use this text in a course. I continually update the contents of this text and would be willing to share these updates until the successor to this book is available. Write me for details.

Acknowledgments

No one can write a book like this without help. I would like, therefore to acknowledge the invaluable assistance that I received from many, many people and institutions. First, and foremost, I want to say thanks to my wife Christina and my mother-in-law Marcile for all of the strong support, gracious consideration, and enthusiastic encouragement that they have offered me while preparing this book. Thanks, too, to Luther College for allowing me time and use of facilities. Special thanks to the Luther College Library staff (especially Liz Kaschins and Ruth Reitan for help in procuring resources) and the Luther College Computer Center for technical help and support. My thanks also go out to many students who have contributed by helping to write portions of certain chapters (Connie Foxworthy, Elaine Hoversten, and Krista Hennager), editing and indexing (Melinda Emery), being co-researchers (Nancy Nielsen, Sue Stueck, Maria Johnson, Lindsay Jordan, and Krista Hennager), being typists (Heidi Leight), helping prepare graphs (Shriram Chaubal), and making suggestions after using preliminary drafts in class. My gratitude also goes to Lynn Williams and Jeri Laursen who also provided much needed assistance with preparation of the manuscript. Thanks to Mark Mahowald, MD, ACP for reading a chapter and suggesting revisions. A special thanks is due to the many people who allowed me to use their dream interpretations as examples in this book (as promised, they will remain anonymous). Many thanks to Rosalind Cartwright and associates of the Sleep Disorders Service at Rush-Presbyterian-St. Luke's Medical Center in Chicago and to Phil Westbrook and associates of the Sleep Disorders Center at the Mayo Clinic in Rochester, Minnesota for graciously enabling me to spend very fruitful sabbaticals with them. And finally, thanks to any others whom I may have failed to mention by name.

Prologue

A Visit to a Sleep Lab

How do you know if someone is asleep? You can look to see if the person has their eyes closed, looks relaxed and still, is not very responsive to stimuli, is breathing regularly, and so on. But every child has at one time or another done all of these things to fool their parents. The child was pretending to be asleep, although very much awake. At the other extreme, a person in a coma may also be showing all of these signs and thus appears to be asleep. The point is this: you cannot tell very easily if a person is asleep just by observation. You could wake the person up and ask them if they were asleep, but you then depend on that person's subjective experience and, of course, the person is then no longer asleep. It is rather like the joke my father used to tell: "Says one Englishman to another, 'Were you in the boat when the boat tipped over?' 'No, you blithering idiot, I was in the water!'"

Two important things have followed from this inability to be absolutely sure that another person is asleep. First, there was little study of sleep until quite recently because of the difficulty in determining objectively and unobtrusively the presence of sleep in a subject. Thus, much of what is known about sleep is new knowledge, and some of it is surprising since it is contrary to popular beliefs. Second, it is necessary to study sleep in a sleep lab, with the sleeper attached to sensitive instruments, to obtain good, objective data without disturbing the person's sleep. (Although, more recently, miniaturized portable equipment has allowed some sleep research to be conducted outside the lab.) Sleep labs have only been in existence since 1953 when Aserinsky and Kleitman first reported that sleeping people have two different kinds of sleep. Today there are many sleep labs all over the world engaged in exploring the mysteries of sleep every night. Let me first take you on a visit to a sleep lab before we discuss what is known about basic sleep processes.

A Visit to a Sleep Lab

We arrive at the Medical Center (although some sleep labs can also be found in University Research Centers) a little before 10 P. M. and walk down a small, but pleasant, carpeted hallway that has several doors on either side. We continue to one door that is open exposing a brightly lit room.

The "subject" for tonight's study is a paid volunteer who has changed into his pajamas and is sitting next to a small table partially covered by a clean white towel. On this table there are some rolls of medical tape, a few bottles, scissors, a toothpaste-like tube, some gauze, a comb and hair clips, a tape measure, an electrical meter, and other similar things. On the nearby wall hang a dozen or so long wires with disc-like enlargements on one end and metal pins about the size of match sticks on the other end. The subject is male, blond, about 25 years old with a mustache and a nice tan. He looks rather athletic.

Also in the room is a young woman, probably a recent college graduate, in a white lab coat. She is short and small with long black hair and glasses. With a pleasant, warm smile, she turns to us and says, "Hi. I'm Sally, the sleep technician. This is John. He will be our sleeper tonight. John has been here before so he knows what is going to happen. As I get him ready, I will describe what I am doing and why I am doing it."

"First we have to apply several wires to John's head. They are called electrodes, but think of them more as antennae." As she is talking, she takes one from its holder and hands it to us. Up close, the disc end looks about the size and shape of half a pea and is hollow. "Others have plastic ends with just a little silver foil embedded inside and attached to the wire. The one you have is gold plated. They both work the same but the metal ones are easier to put on the hairy scalp, while the plastic ones work well on bare skin."

Meanwhile, she has started to measure John's scalp with the tape measure and marks it with a special, soft red pencil. "The electrodes have to be placed on specific locations on the head several inches above each ear called C3 and C4 and another at the back of the head at O1 or O2. The same measurement technique is used worldwide to apply electrodes. That way we can compare results directly." She carefully marks a spot on each side of the head about one-third of the way down from the center of the top of the head toward each ear. She picks up the comb and several hair clips and parts the hair over the marked area on the right side. Then she picks up a cotton-tipped stick and a bottle of liquid.

"Our bodies are covered with a layer of dead skin plus oil." Turning aside to us with a wry smile on her face, she says in a confidential tone, "That kind of takes the glamour out of looking at a good-looking movie star - all you see is dead skin." Turning back to John, she proceeds to moisten the cotton-tip and to rub the exposed marked area. "This removes the dead skin and oils to enable better electrical reception by the electrode."

She then picks up another cotton-tipped stick and the toothpaste-like tube. After squeezing out a bit of its contents, she puts a small dab on the end of the cotton and proceeds to rub it onto the prepared spot on John's head. "This is electrode gel. It also helps make better electrical contact." With another wry smile she turns to John's face and says, "The green color in your hair will grow out in about nine months."

Laughing, John replies, "You can't fool me. I've been through this before."

Turning to us, Sally explains, "Actually this stuff is very harmless and easily washes out." Meanwhile she has taken the electrode from us and squeezes enough gel into its hollowness to just fill it. Then she carefully places it on the prepared spot on John's scalp and holds it in place with her left forefinger. Working quickly, she takes the top off a glass petri dish and picks up a moistened piece of square gauze about the size of two big postage stamps. "It's soaked with a biological glue." Sally places the gauze on top of the electrode, being careful not to disturb it. Again holding all of this in place with her left hand, she uses her right hand to pick up a metal pencil-sized object attached to a small rubber lab hose. While using the dull tip of the object to hold the electrode and gauze in place, she presses a foot switch and a stream of air hisses through the hose and out of the object toward the glue-soaked gauze. Deftly, she pats her fingers on the gauze around the electrode as it dries. Fifteen seconds later she turns off the air stream and sets the apparatus down. "The electrode will stay in place, air-tight all night now. " She gave a gentle but firm tug on the attached wire causing John to reflexively tilt his head in its direction. The electrode with its now stiff gauze covering stayed firmly in place. "However I can easily remove it in the morning by dissolving the glue."

"What does the electrode do?" you ask.

While repeating the procedure on the other two marked spots on John's head, she tells us, "It allows us to record his brain waves (on what is technically called the EEG or electroencephalogram). As you will see, the brain waves change quite a bit during sleep."

Having finished applying the three scalp electrodes, Sally selects one of the plastic disc electrodes and then peels a dime-sized piece of cellophane tape off a paper roll. It looks like a flat, transparent doughnut with a blue tab on one side. "It's sticky on both sides," she explains as she applies it carefully to the plastic disc and just as carefully lays the prepared electrode and its attached wire on the table. With another moistened cotton-tipped applicator, she cleans the skin near the outer corner of the left eye, then mashes gel on the spot with another applicator. After peeling off a protective layer from the tape on the electrode, she presses it onto the prepared spot. She then takes a piece of hypo-allergenic surgical tape and places it over the electrode and surrounding skin. Giving a little jerk on the wire, she says, "That one will also stay in place all night," as John's head reflexively jerks in her direction.

"She thinks I'm a puppet on a string," he playfully complains.

As she similarly applies another plastic electrode at the outer corner of the other eye, she explains, "These will enable us to measure his eye movements. The eyes are like little batteries with the positive pole in front. When the eyes move, the positive front moves closer or farther from the nearby electrode thus changing the electrical influence on the electrode. In this way we get what you might call `eye movement waves' (actually the EOG or electrooculogram). Like brain waves, the EOG helps us to determine when John is asleep and what kind of sleep he is in."

She then glues two additional electrodes on John's chin as she explains. "These let us record neck muscle tension. When muscles contract, electrical changes occur in them. The more contracted or tense a muscle, the more electrical activity. This enables us to assess how relaxed the muscles of the neck are. You see, as long as we are awake, our neck muscles are more or less contracted in order to hold our heads up. This is true even when we are resting our heads on a pillow. This neck muscle tension or EMG (for electromyogram) gives us another indicator of the presence of sleep and the stage of sleep." Turning to me she asks, "How can you tell when students fall asleep during your lectures, Dr. Moorcroft?"

I reply, "Well, of course they never do." After a few seconds of silence accompanied by stares of disbelief, I continue. "O.K., so once in a while a student may doze off. How do I know? Well, let me see. Ah, they don't answer my questions or take notes and their heads are dropped."

"That's it! Their heads drop because during sleep the neck muscles relax. As we shall see, in one kind of sleep the muscles are almost totally relaxed."

"You mean there is more than one kind of sleep?"

"Yes. We all cycle in and out of different kinds of sleep each night!"

"Is he ready now?" you ask.

"Not quite." Sally replies, as she reaches for three more plastic electrodes. "These will be ground and reference electrodes." As she prepares and attaches one to the middle of the forehead, she continues, "This one prevents other electrical `noise' from interfering with our recordings. Have you ever had a portable radio get louder and clearer as you reach out to adjust the knobs?"

"Yes," you reply.

"What is happening is that you are acting as an antenna for the radio. You see, your body is constantly receiving all sorts of electrical signals - from radio, TV., and all sorts of electrical appliances and motors. Much of this is stronger than brain waves and the rest of what we measure. By applying this electrode, we can get rid of this electrical garbage."

She then proceeds to put the final two electrodes on the bony knob near the bottom of the back of the ear.

"What do those do?" you ask.

"These are called reference electrodes. Anything we record needs two electrodes. Activity on one is actually compared to activity on the other. Sometimes both electrodes are from active areas such as two sections of the brain, and the resulting record is the difference in activity between the two. A lot of other times, it is better if the comparison electrode has no electrical input of its own so that the record shows all of the activity from the active electrode. One of these reference electrodes that I'm applying now is used as a comparison to both eye electrodes and scalp electrodes and sometimes to one chin electrode."

"Wait a minute. What about the other scalp electrode and reference electrode?"

"It is a back-up. We usually don't use all of the scalp electrodes at one time either. The one at the back of the head is useful for determining sleep onset but not of much use otherwise so sometimes we only use it in the beginning of the night or don't even bother to use it at all. We also only use one of the two electrodes over the ears. If something prevents us from recording from one of these we can easily switch to the other one without disturbing John. Otherwise, we might have to wake him up to attach another electrode."

"Can I go to sleep now?" asks John, barely stifling a yawn.

"I have to check the electrodes electrically first," replies Sally. She inserts the other ends of the electrode wires into the receptacles of the what .ooks like an elcetrical testing meter two at a time and looks at the dial each time. When she finishes checking the electrodes, she tapes some of the loose wires to his face directing them all to the back of his head, shaping them into a ponytail with some more tape.

"All set."

"Great. (Yawn) I'm tired."

After John uses the bathroom, Sally leads him to another room with us following. The room resembles a small but cozy motel room with a bed, night stand with a lamp, a chair, florescent overhead lighting, and carpeting. The bed has a brown blanket neatly tucked in at the sides of the mattress and two pillows above the folded over end of the top sheet. At the head of the bed just over the pillows is a blue metal box attached to the wall. It is about the size of a cigar box but not quite as rectangular. It contains several neat columns of holes surrounded by plastic nuts. Over each hole is a number. On the night stand facing the bed is a speaker with an attached microphone. Wires from both the box and the microphone lead through the wall nearby. In the corner of the room opposite the bed is a very small TV. camera mounted near the ceiling.

After John lies down in bed, Sally plugs the color-coded wires into the appropriate places in the box. The wires are long enough to allow John to easily move around in bed.

"Are you comfortable?" she asks.

"You bet," he replies.

Sally leads us out of the room and closes the door.

"How can he sleep with all those wires on him?"

"Most people have little trouble, especially after the first night. Think how hard it is to stay awake all night, especially in a quiet room and in a comfortable bed."

We walk across the hall to another room labeled Control Room. As Sally opens the door, we see a room about the size of the bedroom except lined with a bewildering array of electrical equipment. Three thingsappear to dominate our view - the many knobs on the equipment, the machines with lined-paper lying across their stainless steel table-like tops, and a TV. monitor above each machine. The paper has folds at regular intervals giving it the appearance of a succession of place mats with each one pulling the next one out of a box. On some machines, this paper is as wide as a paper towel. On other machines it is two or even three times as wide. Resting on the paper are pens evenly spaced from one another. Each pen looks like a broad but quickly tapering finger with a gentle curve of 90 degrees at the end where it makes perpendicular contact with the paper. At the other end of each pen, the broad base attaches to the machine, and the paper feeds up from below just in front of where the pens are attached. There are some letters and numbers written earlier on the paper with a felt-tipped pen; faint parallel blue lines, some running its length, others its width, are printed on the paper. There is also a fine trail of dark blue ink on the paper that earlier came from each pen. These pen lines are straight and parallel, but in several places the pens have left a trail of abrupt, cone-shaped deviations. Some lines jumped more than others and some faded faster, but basically the pattern is the same on all.

"These machines are called polysomnographs," Sally explains. "The jack-box into which we plugged the electrode wires leads to this one right here. I previously made careful adjustments for the five channels we will be using; all the writing and pips on the pen lines are a record of these adjustments. The first and second lines are connected to the electrodes near John's eyes. The top line is from his left eye, the second line from his right. The third line is the muscular activity from the chin electrodes. The fourth and fifth lines are for the brain waves - one from above one ear and the other from the back of the head."

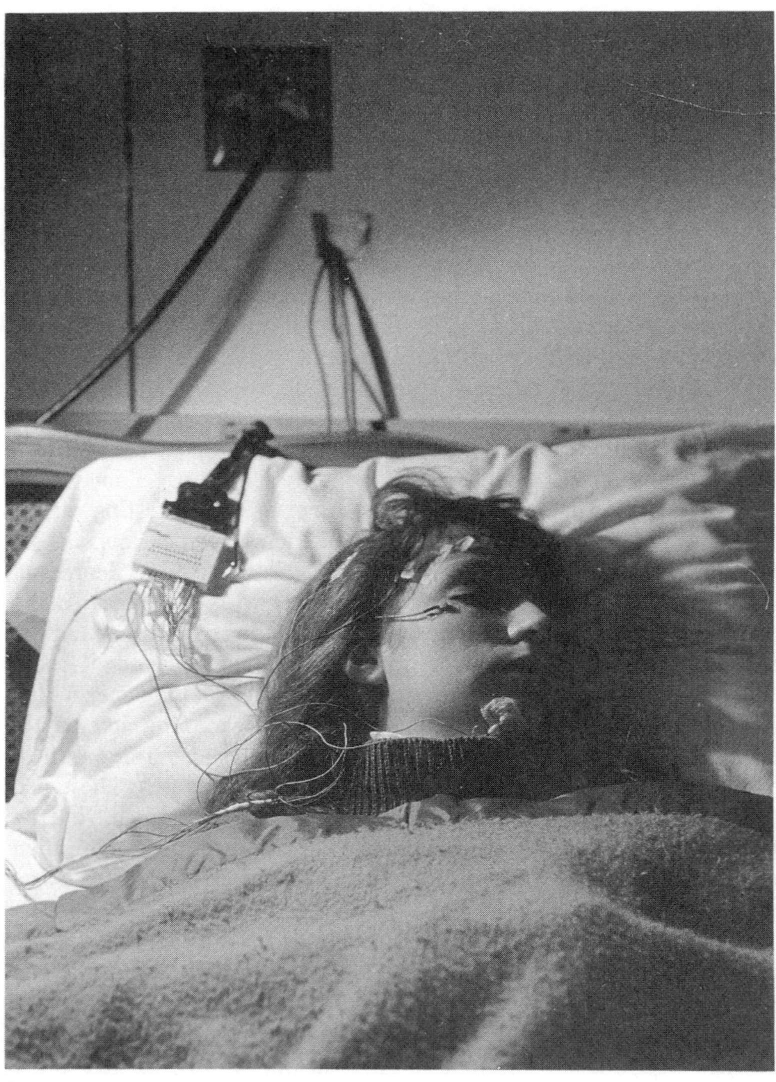

This photograph is a typical view in a sleep lab. It shows a subject's sleep being monitored during an experiment in the author's sleep lab. (Luther College Photo Bureau)

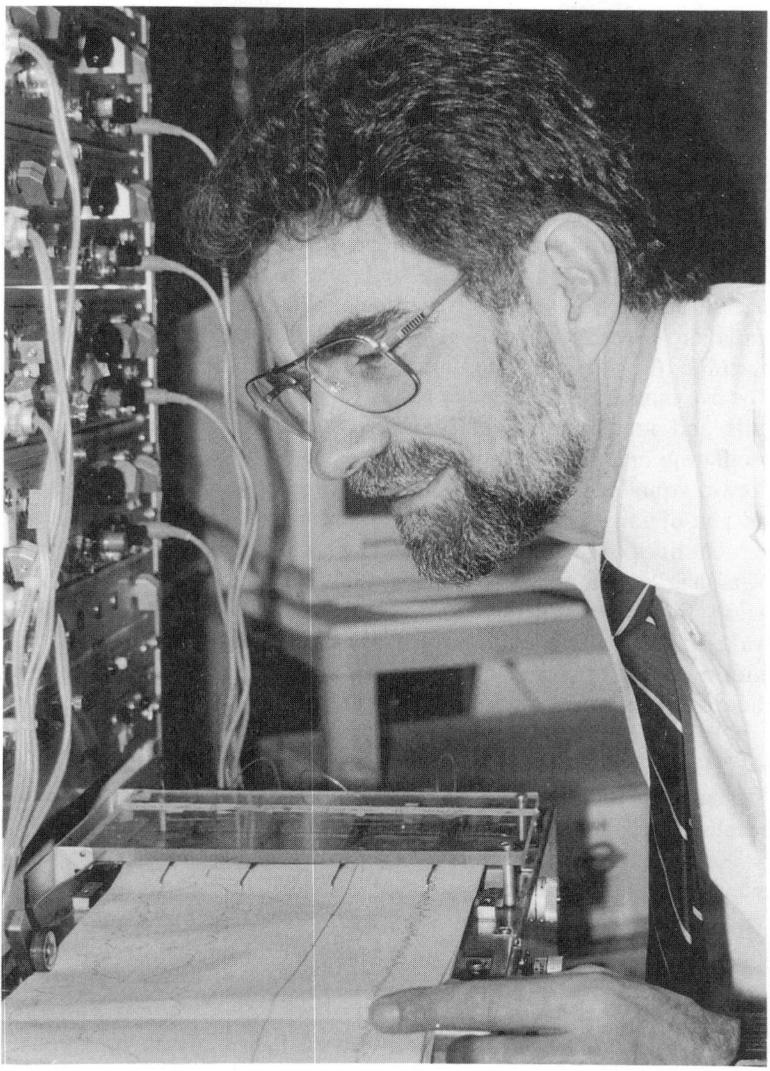

The polysomnograph in this photograph is typical of that found in many sleep labs. In front of the machine is the author examining the sleep record (polysomnogram) of a research subject. (Luther College Photo Bureau)

Sally flips a switch on an intercom next to the polysomnograph. "John, can you hear me?"

"Just barely."She adjusts the volume.

"How about now?""Fine. Real fine."

"O.K. Remember to stay awake while I make adjustments to the machine."

"O.K., but don't take too long or I might be gone."

She then turns a large metal knob on the front lower side of the polysomnograph, and the paper starts moving at about a place mat-size sheet every 30 seconds, the pens leaving their straight dark-blue trails on the paper. As Sally manipulates other switches on the machine, the pens begin to dance, each to its own particular rhythm. The eye movement pens make records that look like mirror images of hills and mountains. The EEGs are small, rapidly but irregularly oscillating lines, such as a very nervous person might make if trying to draw a straight line. The EMG does not look like a line at all; rather the pen literally vibrates leaving a thick band of ink made up of many vertical lines of random heights, somewhat like a magnified side view of a shag carpet. Suddenly, all the pens go out of control, vibrating wildly the full extent of their reach, spitting ink as well as leaving wide, irregular, thick tracings of their activity on the paper. This stops after a second or two as abruptly as it started and the pens return to their previous patterns of movements.

"What was that?" you blurt out.

"He moved. He probably was trying to get more comfortable. We'll occasionally see that all through the night. It actually is useful, because it tells us how restless the sleep is."

Sally continues to look at the record while making some adjustments to the knobs. Finally satisfied, she turns to us and says, "Now, we will see if everything is working as it should." Pulling on the intercom switch she says into the microphone, "John, I'd like you to do a few things for me now."

"O.K."

"First, look up." Pause. "Look down." Pause. "Look up." Pause. "Look down." Pause. "Look right." Pause. "Look left." Pause. "Look right." Pause. "Look left." Each time she gives a command, she makes note of it on the moving paper chart as the eye movement pens seemingly respond to her commands moving toward each other almost touching when John moves his eyes up or to the right and away from each other when the eyes move down or to the left.

"Now blink five times." Again the pens dance in unison, but this time producing what looks like a row of 5 dunce hats. Again, Sally writes her instruction to John on the paper.

"Now grit your teeth." This time, the muscle pen starts to vibrate so much that it hums and spits ink. The thickness of the line it produces triples. "That's fine." Now addressing us she says, "The muscles of the neck contract when a person grits their teeth and the polysomnograph shows this. Next we'll check the EEG and at the same time get a sample of another kind of brain wave."

"John, close your eyes and blank your mind, but don't fall asleep."

"(Yawn) I'll try," came the sleepy voice in return. As Sally marks the chart, the EEG begins to change from its low, fast, random pattern (called beta waves) to a higher, slightly slower, but very rhythmic and regular pattern, looking somewhat like a folded ribbon candy from the side.

"These are alpha waves. They occur when a person's mind is awake but relaxed and not particularly concentrating on anything." When she flips the intercom switch and tells John to open his eyes, the alpha waves change back to the beta waves.

"Alpha waves also occur when drifting into sleep. What you saw before the alpha waves, and are seeing now, are the beta waves of an awake, alert mind."

"Well John, it's time. Call me if you want to get up or need anything, O.K.?"

"O.K."

"Goodnight." She writes the time on the paper, 11:07, as she switches off the room lights with a remote switch near the intercom.

We all watch the chart closely. Not much happens at first other than an occasional body movement. In several minutes, the EMG becomes less thick to about half its original size, more alpha waves appear, and fewer eye movements can be noted. Then the eye channels trace out lines that look like as mirror images of rolling hills and the EEG becomes much more jagged, but the pens do not move as rapidly as in beta nor as rhythmically as in alpha. "These are the signs of the start of sleep - slow rolling eye movements and the replacement of alpha waves with slower, less regular theta waves in the EEG. It's a light sleep called stage 1. He will probably spend very little sleep time in this stage. It's more of a transition between stages."

Soon John's eyes stop moving and the EEG pen gradually moves less rapidly than before, but it is still rather jagged. Then it oscillates for about a second producing a wave that looks like compact alpha. "That's a sleep spindle, a sure sign of stage 2 of sleep." Soon the pen makes a sudden large move up, then down past midline, then back to its previous activity level resulting in a line resembling an upside-down pointed ice cream cone next to a smaller but right-side up cone. "A K-complex, another characteristic of stage 2."

This continues for another 10 minutes - occasional spindles and K-complexes on a background of irregular but slower and slower activity. Then the EEG begins to show occasional large sonorous movements and fewer and fewer spindles and K-complexes. When about 20% of the record was like this, Sally explains, "These are delta waves and they indicate the presence of delta sleep. In many ways, this is the deepest sleep." Soon much of the record contains delta waves and continues this way with little change for about half an hour.

Suddenly startling us, the pens shift into their sudden wild movements indicating a body movement. We confirm this when we look up at the TV monitoring John and see that he is rolling over. When things settle down, the record again resembles stage 2 with moderate, jagged background and spindles and K's.

Exactly 93 minutes after sleep onset, the EMG becomes very quiet, almost a thin, straight line. Suddenly the eye movement channels burst into activity, showing large, jagged, mirror-image mountains for a few seconds, then fall silent. "That is a burst of rapid eye movements. John is now in another kind of sleep called REM (for rapid eye movement). Look closely at the EEG. Notice no spindles or K's are present and the brain waves look like the teeth of a saw blade." Just then there is another burst of eye movement lasting longer than the first. "As you can see, sleep is not a single entity, but is made up of several different states."

The REM period does not last long. After a few minutes another body movement occurs and stage 2 returns for 10 to 15 minutes followed by more delta.

And so it goes throughout the night. John cycles between the stages except there is less and less time spent in delta (in fact, almost none at all in the second half of the night) and more and more time in REM. Most time however is spent in stage 2 - about half of the night. Around every hour and a half, he starts a REM period.

It is interesting to observe what is happening to us as we stay up all night to watch John sleep. It is especially hard to keep awake when nothing exciting is happening, like long periods of stage 2. We have to stand up and keep moving or keep talking otherwise a brief sleep occurs. Several times we catch each other drifting off and in a fun way scold one another. It seems to get cold in the room between 3 and 5 A.M. We check the thermostat and find that the temperature remains unchanged. We later realized that this was also the time when it was hardest to stay awake.

At 6:15 A.M., through blurry eyes, we can see that the pattern on the paper is changing. Several body movements occur and the EMG gets thicker again. The EEG becomes low and fast and random and the eyes start moving, not as rapidly as during REM and more continuously. "He's awake now," Sally informs us. She turns off the chart that had run continuously all night almost exhausting the 6-inch high box of paper. "Good morning," she intercoms to John and turns on the light.

"Ugh - oh, mornin'" (Yawn).

"I'll come in and unplug you now."

"Yeah. O.K."

We follow her in. "How do you feel? Sleep well?"

"Hey, I slept like a log. How about you?"

"Oh, be quiet," she blurts out with a smile.

Now unplugged, John is led back to the room with the equipment table. We follow. He sits in the chair next to the table as Sally soaks some gauze in solvent, then puts a moistened cotton puff over each of the glue-stiffened gauze patches on John's head. In about 30 seconds, she lifts both pieces of gauze and the underlying electrode from the left side of his head, then repeats the procedure on the right side and then the back. With another solvent-wet gauze square, she carefully wipes at the area where each electrode rested, then combs the hair back into place. She removes the other glue-attached electrodes by the ears and chin. Next she next peels off the tape holding the wires close to his face, then, pulling the tab on the double-sticky tape rings, removes each of the rest of the electrodes in turn. Using a tissue, she wipes off the electrode cream that remains on the skin after removing each electrode.

We say good-bye to one another before John heads for the shower and Sally returns to the control room to do some post-sleep polysomnograph checks and then turns off the machine. "See you again tomorrow night," she says as she disappears into the control room. We start to float out of the sleep lab in our sleepless, dazed state toward our own beds in search of our own quota of that sweet commodity that we have been scientifically observing all night.

A Second Night in the Sleep Lab

"I hope you slept well during the day today," I say, "after being up all night."

"Well, I slept but not as well as usual," you reply. "I was kind of restless and woke up a lot, but I'm O.K."

"Sounds typical for daytime sleep. Tonight Sally will awaken John at various times during the night to collect dream reports."

"I can't wait. I hope he has some wild ones."

"You may be surprised," I comment, "at just how dull they are!"

"Hi, Sally. Here we are for another night."

"Oh, hi. I just about have John ready, so it won't be long now." At that moment he came walking out of the preparation room carrying the ponytail of wires leading from the electrodes on his head and face.

"Not a bad way to earn 75 bucks - sleeping," he says to us.

"It's not all sleep tonight," Sally reminds him. "I will be waking you at various times throughout the night and asking you to report whatever is going through your mind at the time. You may be dreaming or thinking or may have nothing at all going on at that time. That's all right. I just want to know what is going on in your mind when I wake you. All reports are equally valuable."

"Oh well, It's still an easy 75. See ya in the morning."

By now he was in bed and the electrodes were plugged into the board. Soon Sally had turned the machine on, made adjustments, and assured herself that everything was working fine and that John was asleep.

"Dreams," Sally says, "can be explored much better in the sleep lab because we can catch them when they are fresh. Tonight we will wake him three times - first during delta, then during stage 2, and finally during REM sleep. Watch for differences in what he reports in each stage. The questions I ask are a bit formal, but they have to be the same every time to be sure we don't miss something.

Soon we see the signs on the moving chart that he is asleep and moving down through the stages. Then at 12:07, ten minutes into the first delta period, Sally turns on a tape recorder and begins. "John . . . John . . . JOHN!"

"Ugh. . ., oh-ah. . ."

"John?"

"Yea." Yawn.

"What was taking place just at the moment you were called?"

"Nothin'. Nothin' was happenin'."

"At that moment would you say that you were awake, drowsy, in light sleep, or in a deep sleep?"

"Deep. It was good sleep."

"Was there any visual imagery? If yes, describe it."

"Well, yea, kinda. A woods, some trees, you know."

"Were there any distortions in the way familiar people or objects were represented?"

"No, not really. It was kinda vague."

"Were you an active participant in what you experienced or just passively observing it?"

"I just saw it."

"Were there any other persons in this experience?"

"No, none; just trees."

"During this experience were you aware that you were here in the laboratory?"

"No."

"During this experience were you aware that you were observing the contents of your own mind, or did you feel that you were observing or participating in events out in the real world?"

"Sort of real world, but fuzzy."

"How vivid an experience was this: very vivid, moderately vivid, or quite vague?"

"Kinda vague."

"How realistic was this experience: very realistic, a mixture of real and unreal, or very unrealistic?"

"A mixture, I'd say."

"How emotional was this experience: very emotional, only mildly emotional, or very unemotional?"

"Not at all emotional. No emotion."

"How pleasant was this experience: very pleasant, neutral, or unpleasant?"

"Neutral."

"Were you dreaming or thinking?"

"I don't know. More dreaming, I guess, but maybe thinking."

"O.K., you can go back to sleep now."

After Sally turns off the tape recorder, you state, "That wasn't really much of a dream, was it?"

"No." she replies, "That's typical though of what you get in delta sleep - something like a fuzzy photograph."

At 3:10 a.m., ten minutes into stage 2, Sally says, "It's time again," as she turns on the tape recorder.

"John."

"Ah, yeah," followed by a strain in his voice indicating that he is stretching.

"What was taking place just at the moment you were called?"

"Nothing. I (yawn) was sleeping till I heard you call."

"Was there any visual imagery? If yes, describe it."

"No, none whatsoever."

"You can go back to sleep now."

Sally turns the tape off as she says to us, "People don't seem to dream constantly. Much of the time they report nothing at all, especially when not in REM."

"What happens in REM?" you ask.

"Just wait."

Five twenty-three a.m., ten minutes into REM.

"John, . . ., John."

"Ugh . . . yea!"

"What was taking place just at the moment you were called?"

"Well, I was in a shed - you know a tin type shed - with many people, some of whom I knew. I was standing on one side of the building around some cars with a couple of middle-aged men and a couple of girls around 20 years of age. Something had happened to one of the cars, an older model, and the girl was upset. At that point my attention was distracted to the other half of the shed where a guy about 20 years of age was showing films of - I guess it was his vacation or something - while others of the same age watched. Right then, the scene shifted to some body of water like a lake or something. I was driving a speed boat while the male who was showing the film was swimming in a scuba suit. It's crazy, but he was going the same speed as the boat. Then you woke me up."

"At that moment would you say that you were awake, drowsy, in light sleep, or in deep sleep?"

"Oh, I was asleep allright; it was sound. I guess I would have to say deep."

"Were there any distortions in the way familiar people or objects were represented?"

"People? No. But, the cars were all funny pastel colors and kinda wavy, shimmering. That's all I can remember."

"During this experience were you aware that you were here in the laboratory?"

"Oh no. It seemed real, like I was there."

"During this experience were you aware that you were observing the contents of your own mind, or did you feel that you were observing or participating in events out in the real world?"

"It seemed real at the time but now that I think about it, things were kind of flat or quiet. You know, not very emotional or something. Like spacey."

"How vivid an experience was this, very vivid, moderately vivid, or quite vague?"

"It was vivid, quite clear."

"How realistic was this experience; very realistic, a mixture of real and unreal, or very unrealistic?"

"It seemed realistic while it was happening, but now not all of it seems like it was real. A mixture I guess."

"How emotional was this experience; very emotional, only mildly emotional, or not emotional?"

"Surprisingly, not very emotional. Things just happened and that was O.K."

"How pleasant was this experience; very unpleasant, neutral, or unpleasant?"

"It was O.K. Kinda neutral, I guess."

"Were you dreaming or thinking?"

"Dreaming. No doubt about it, I was dreaming."

"Goodnight. You can go back to sleep again."

"Night."

Turning to us, Sally says, "That was a fairly typical dream - like a T.V. program with action and a sequence of events but scenes can jump forward, backward, or parallel. I did not have to ask all of the standard questions either since he had already indicated what the answers would be."

We decided to leave early since there were to be no more dream reports collected and we were tired from the night before.

"Thanks Sally and say good-bye to John for me," you say on your way out of the door.

"I will" she replies. "Good-bye."

Turning to me as we walk down the hall, you ask, "Where was all the sex and violence in the dreams?"

"That's just it, there usually isn't any. Most dreams are pretty dull when you get right down to it."

"Do we always dream during REM?" you ask.

"People will give a dream report like this one over 80% of the time when awakened during REM, even if they state before-hand that they never dream."

"Well thanks again," you call out as you turn to head to your car, "I really appreciate your arranging for me to visit the sleep lab."

"Glad to do it," I respond, "and, oh by the way . . ."

"Yes?"

"Pleasant dreams!"

Sleep, Dreaming, & Sleep Disorders

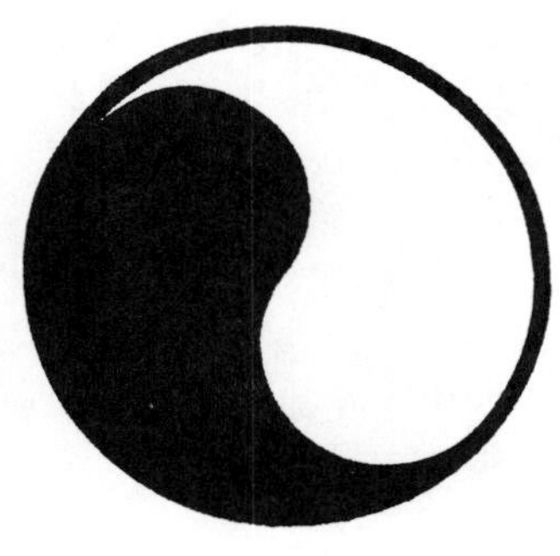

Section 1

Sleep

Chapter 1

Sleep
(as indicated by Electrical Recordings)[1]

Sleep Stage Criteria

One definition states that "sleep is a reversible behavioral state of perceptual disengagement from and unresponsiveness to the environment" (Carskadon & Dement, 1989). Sleep is typically accompanied by lying down, absence of movement, closed eyes, and so on. However, as indicated in the preface, these are inadequate criterion to use for the precise, scientific determination of sleep. For this purpose, most labs use three modes of measurement - EEG, EOG, and EMG - to determine both when a person is sleeping and what kind of sleep is occurring (Kryger, Roth, & Dement, 1989; Rechtschaffen and Kales, 1968). Some labs regularly use another set of EEG leads from the back of the head (over the occipital region of the brain) (Kryger, Roth, & Dement, 1989). Additional measurements such as heart beat, breathing, and leg movements are often employed. Table 1-1 summarizes how the stages of sleep aredetermined from these measurements. Refer to this table during the description that follows.

---

[1] Parts of this chapter are adapted, with permission, from Moorcroft W H (1987). An overview of sleep. In J Gackenbach (Ed.), *Sleep and dreams: A sourcebook* (pp. 3-29). New York: Garland Publishing. Copyrighted by Garland Publishing in 1987.

Table 1-1 Criteria for determining the stages of sleep

		EEG
WAKE		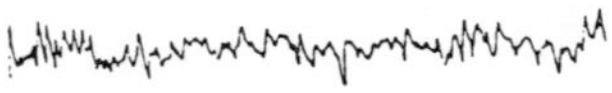 beta waves 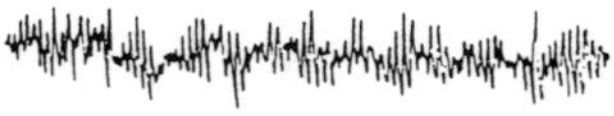 alpha waves
NREM	STAGE 2	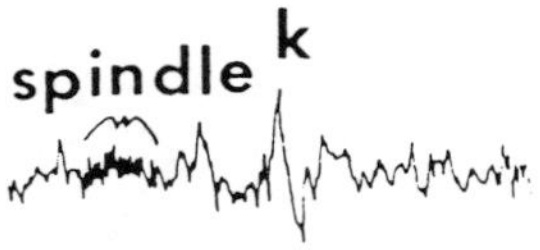 spindle, k theta waves
	DELTA	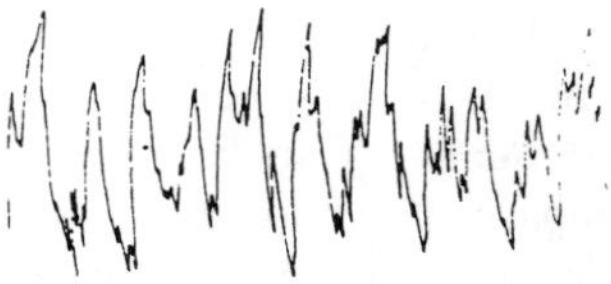 delta waves
REM		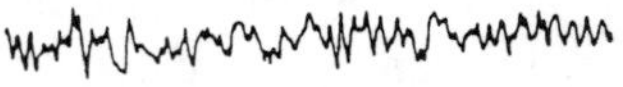 sawtooth waves 50µv 1sec

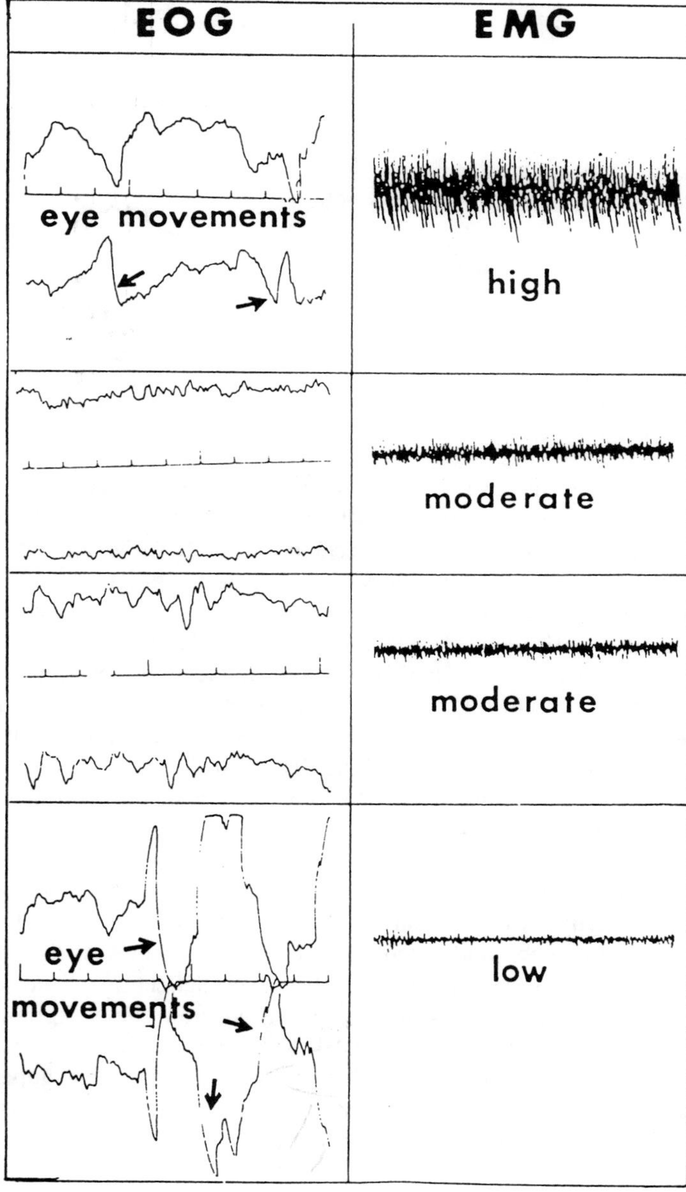

Derived from Williams R L, Karacan I, & Hursch C J (1974). *Electroencephalography (EEG) of human sleep: Clinical applications*. New York: Wiley. Copyrighted © 1974 by John Wiley & Sons, Inc. Used by permission of John Wiley & Sons, Inc

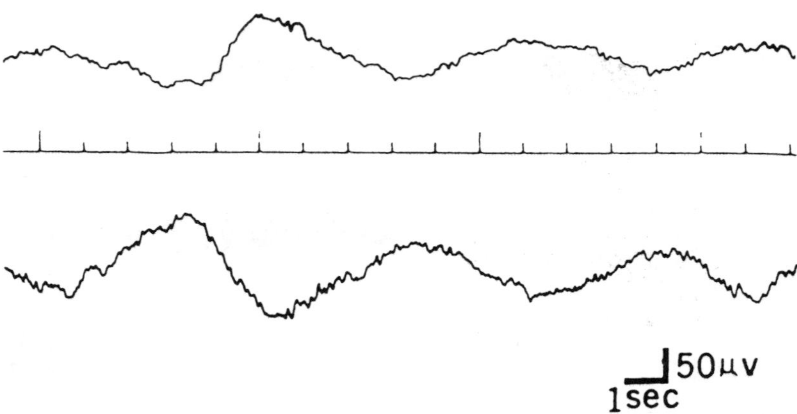

Figure 1-1 Slow eye movements.

The waking state (also often called stage 0 or W) is characterized by high (that is, thick appearing) EMG; eye movements that are rather constant but not as abrupt as those occurring in stage REM; and either low voltage (that is low amplitude on the recording chart), fast, irregular waves called beta waves (over 13 Hz) or moderate voltage, rather regular, fairly slower waves called alpha waves (8 - 12 Hz).

Sleep onset (not shown in Table 1-1) is characterized by slow eye movements (see Figure 1-1) with a duration of at least several seconds, the appearance of a mixture of EEG frequencies of relatively low voltage theta waves (4 - 7 Hz), and the disappearance of alpha waves. These may also be accompanied or preceded by a moderation of the EMG activity (less thick).

In stage 2, eye movements are absent and muscle activity is moderate. The EEG shows theta waves and low voltage, mixed frequency activity (with less than 20% delta waves) accompanied by frequent K-complexes and sleep spindles. A K-complex is a high amplitude sharp negative wave - an upward pen deflection - followed by a smaller, slower positive wave that stands out from the background activity and lasts more than 1/2 second. K-complexes may also occur in other stages of sleep. Although often spontaneous, they may appear in response to sudden stimuli, especially auditory. A sleep spindle is a burst of rhythmic 12 - 14 Hz waves lasting at least 1/2 second.

Delta or slow wave sleep is characterized by high voltage (more than 75 MV), slow (1/4 - 2 Hz) EEG waves called delta waves. At least 20% of the record must show these delta waves to be considered this type of sleep. This stage can be further broken down into stages 3 (20 to 50% delta waves) and 4 (greater than 50% delta waves).

Stages 1 through 4 are collectively known as NREM (pronounced non-REM) sleep. Older reports may use terms such as delta, quiet, slow wave, orthodox, or S in place of NREM (Moorcroft, 1987). (More recently, slow wave sleep (abbreviated SWS) is often used in place of delta sleep and refers only to NREM stages 3 and 4.)

REM sleep is easily distinguished from the other stages. The EEG is low voltage, random, and fast (often "saw-tooth") waves, the EOG frequently shows bursts of sharp waves (reflecting rapid eye movements) alternating with periods of up to three minutes of no eye movements and the EMG is small or absent. This stage of sleep is also known by several other names. It has been called paradoxical sleep (since the EEG resembles the waking EEG yet the person is paradoxically asleep), activated sleep, deep sleep, low voltage-fast sleep, emergent or ascending stage 1 sleep (because the EEG sometimes resembles stage 1 and the sleeper is emerging or ascending from deeper sleep), and D (dreaming) sleep (Moorcroft, 1987).

REM differs from the other stages of sleep in several additional ways. The slow, deep, rhythmic breathing and moderate, regular heart rate that are characteristic of the general physiological tranquillity of NREM sleep give way to sudden changes in heart and breathing rate. Heart and breathing rates show a higher overall average too during REM. Likewise, blood pressure has a higher average level during REM but fluctuates greatly from moment to moment. Males have erections while females show a parallel enlargement of the clitoris and vagina. Finally, and importantly, the muscles used to make body movements are paralyzed to the extent that they are flaccid (Orem & Barnes, 1980). The unchanging characteristics occurring throughout REM, such as low voltage fast EEG, erections of the penis/clitoris, muscle paralysis, and a high arousal threshold are sometimes referred to as **tonic REM**, while the changing characteristics that tend to occur in clusters, such as bursts of eye movements, and other things discussed in Chapter 2 are known as **phasic REM**. Phasic REM bursts of about 2 to 9 seconds occur about every 16 to 120 seconds during REM (Seligman & Yellen, 1987). Chapters 2, 3, and 4 present these aspects of REM sleep more fully.

A clever study by Segalowitz, Ogilvie, Janicki, Simons, & Buetow (1991) shows another distinction between REM and NREM (SWS), namely a difference in the psychological functioning in these two stages. They measured the electrical response of the brain to tones under four different conditions using a new technique called the ERP (Event Related Potential). They compared two awake conditions (paying careful attention to the tones versus concentrating on a reading) and two sleeping conditions (REM versus SWS). Part of the response of the brain to the tones (called the N100 wave) was identical for both wake conditions but was much reduced during both sleep conditions. This is interpreted to mean that the brain is much less attentive to external stimuli when asleep and/or it is generally less aroused. Another slightly later response of the brain to the tones (called the P300 wave) revealed something quite different. The P300 wave during the waking condition when the subjects were paying attention to the tones was similar to these waves when the subjects were in SWS. However, the P300 waves were much reduced during both the wake reading condition and REM which was interpreted as showing that the brain was attending to other things (reading in the wake condition and dreams in the REM sleep condition) and not available to attend to the tones. Thus during REM, unlike NREM, the mental functioning of the brain is more attuned to its own internal perceptual and thinking world, in the form of dreams, than it is to the external world.

Clearly then, sleep is not a single stage. We can easily distinguish differences between REM and NREM. REM can be summarized as a very active brain and internal organs in an immovable body while NREM as a quiet brain and resting internal organs in a movable body (after Carskadon & Dement, 1989). NREM can be further divided into stages 1 and 2, and SWS (also known as stages 3 and 4). As we shall see in subsequent chapters, these distinctions are very important when we assess dreaming and disorders of sleep.

Sleep In The Average Young Adult

In the Prologue, we followed John through a typical night of sleep for a young adult (someone 20 to 39 years of age). Let's review that night and make comments. In doing so we will present some averages.

These may vary considerably from individual to individual but are used here to indicate a general pattern (Carskadon & Dement, 1989; Williams, Karacan, and Hursch, 1974).

When the lights were turned out, John's aroused beta waves became relaxed alpha waves. Some time later, typically 10 minutes, the emergence of slow eye movements signal the approaching onset of stage 1. Stage 1 is identified by a reduction in the number of alpha waves as they are replaced more and more by a mixture of low voltage, mixed frequency waves - especially theta waves. Had we awakened him at that time, he probably would have reported feelings of floating. At other times he may have experienced a myoclonic jerk (a sudden kicking of a leg or thrusting of an arm) which may have awakened him with a start (Dement, 1978). In either case, he probably would have stated that he was not really asleep but rather "almost asleep." John would have reported that (Carskadon & Dement, 1989) his thinking was no longer reality-oriented, he was less self conscious, and he may have reported a "short dream" (Faraday, 1972).

During stage 1, John's reactions to outside stimuli were diminished. Many experiments support this idea including several in which subjects pressed a switch taped to their hands each time they heard a tone played over earphones or (in another experiment) saw a flash from a light placed in front of their eyes. Such responses became slower, more infrequent, or disappeared completely whenever the subject entered stage 1 sleep (Carskadon & Dement, 1989).

Stage 1 can best be thought of as a transition between wakefulness and sleep that lasts 1 to 7 minutes. If it lasts longer it probably will be interspersed with short periods of wakefulness. Stage 1 is certainly is not a deep sleep since the person can be easily aroused.

Sleep onset is actually a rather sudden all-or-none event (Ogilvie, Simons, Kuderian, MacDonald, & Rustenburg, 1991) that we have difficulty accurately perceiving (Carskadon & Dement, 1989; Bonnet, 1990) because we alternate in and out of it several times before it becomes firmly established (Ogilvie, et al, 1991). This is like turning the lights off then on again repeatedly several times before finally leaving them off.

The emergence of K-complexes and/or sleep spindles signals the start of stage 2 sleep. If awakened now, John would more likely have said that he was truly asleep. It would have been harder to awaken him from this stage than it was from stage 1 but still not too difficult. Stage 2 at this point usually lasts 10 to 25 minutes.

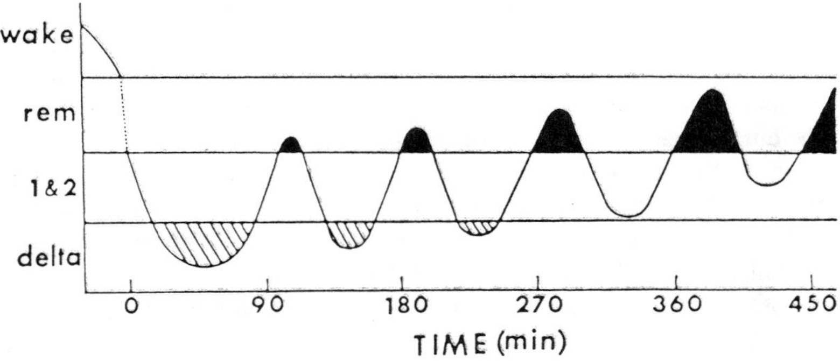

Figure 1-2. A hypothetical night of sleep in an average young adult.

The increasing presence of large delta waves indicates the onset of SWS. Waking John would have been the most difficult at this time; hence, SWS is often considered the deepest stage of sleep. The average length of the first period of SWS ranges from 20 to 40 minutes.

Following the reemergence of a brief period of stage 2 sleep (4 to 10 minutes), which is often preceded and/or ended by a series of body movements, the signs of REM sleep occur. Its onset is 80 to 120 minutes after the beginning of stage 1. This period of REM is typically short (about 1 to 5 minutes). It is usually not as difficult to arouse a sleeper from REM as from SWS but this can vary considerably in this stage. As we saw when John was awakened during REM on his second night, dreaming typically occurs in this stage.

And so the cycle continues throughout the night as shown in Figure 1-2. The length of the first NREM-REM cycle is about 70 to 100 minutes; subsequent cycles are 90 to 120 minutes in length resulting in 4 to 5 REM periods per night. The duration of REM tends to increase with successive cycles (as does the frequency of the rapid eye movements), eventually lasting 1/2 hour or more, while that of SWS decreases. In fact, SWS is seldom seen during the second half of the night. Most of the rest of sleep is stage 2 with very little stage 1 occurring. This entire pattern is punctuated with an average of 55 movements per night, typically occurring at the point of a stage change and numerous brief awakenings of which the sleeper may not be aware. Typically only 1 or 2 of these are long enough to be scored

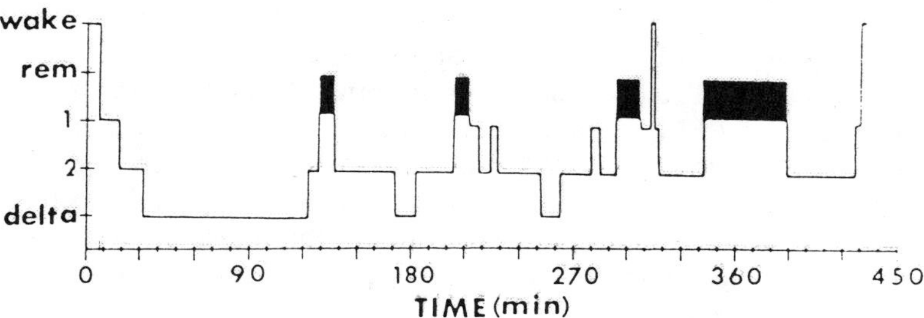

Figure 1-3. An actual night of sleep of a young female.

as wake. (An arousal is scored as wakefulness if it exceeds 30 seconds in duration).

Figure 1-2 is not from an actual subject but represents an ideal night of sleep based on many nights of sleep from many subjects. Actual nights for individual subjects do vary from this. Figure 1-3 shows a single night of sleep for an individual and shows the more standard way of representing such a night.

The average young adult spends about 7 1/2 hours in bed per night. A little over 7 hours of this time is spent asleep (although average total sleep in a nychthemeron[2] approaches 8 hours if naps are taken into account). It takes the average young adult about 10 minutes to fall asleep and they will awaken (for 30 seconds or longer) twice during the night. Total wakefulness between falling asleep and final wake up accounts for 1 1/2 % of the sleep period (about 6 to 7 minutes). REM accounts for about another 25% of this time (or a little less than 2 hours), stage 2 for about 50% (about 3 1/4 hours), and delta about 15% (a little more than 1 hour). Although these figures are averages and normal individuals may differ considerably, it is necessary to be familiar with them because they constitute the standard against which other conditions of sleep are measured.

Now that we have reviewed how sleep is measured in the laboratory, we must make two important statements before going on.

---

[2]We need to introduce a new term here. Not everyone sleeps at night (see chapter 3) nor is sleep always neatly confined to a single period every 24 hours (see chapter 5). It is awkward to have to say "every 24 hours" or "a night and a day" thus we will use the term nychthemeron. A nychthemeron is a full period of one night plus one day (Anch et al, 1988).

First, the stages of sleep are not as discreet as this description implies. In fact, one stage often more or less gradually merges into the next. The frequency of delta waves gradually increases during stage 2 sleep prior to stage 3. The EMG may decrease prior to the first burst of eye movements of REM. K complexes and sleep spindles may continue from stage 2 into stage 3. When a person is falling asleep, signs of stage 1 may alternate with signs of wake for several minutes before stage 1 becomes dominate. At other times, the transition from one stage to another is more abrupt. Abrupt transitions are frequently demarked by body movements.

Second, these lab criteria are used to MEASURE sleep but they do not necessarily DEFINE sleep. When asked to define sleep very few people would mention brain waves and eye movements. Rather, such definitions would include many of the following:

reduced awareness of the environment;
reduced interaction with the environment;
reduced activity;
absence (or near absence) of voluntary movement;
absence (or near absence) of consciousness (Anch, Browman, Mitler, & Walsh, 1988)

(see chapter 5 for a further discussion of this issue when defining sleep in animals). This is what most people think sleep is and what they feel constitutes a definition of sleep. The problem is that these are not easy things to measure and quantify. Most of the time these things that "define" sleep occur simultaneously with changes in brain waves, eye movements, and neck muscle activity. These changes are more easily measured and quantified, so we use them in our sleep labs as polysomnographic indicators of the occurrence of sleep.

However, as described in other parts of this book, in some cases the polysomnographic indicators of sleep are not in agreement with behavioral observations based on the definition of sleep. Thus, we need to take caution so that we do not start to consider sleep as occurring only if the correct EEG, EOG, & EMG signs are present and to rigidly assert that sleep is occurring when these signs are present (Herman, Laljiani, Polokof, Armitage, Roffwarg, & Hirshkowitz, 1992).

There is a more general issue involved here also. We think of sleep as a single entity - a unity. It is becoming more and more apparent (as many other sections of this text will show) that sleep is a collection of many aspects. No one aspect alone is sufficient for sleep to occur (or to characterize sleep) and sleep may be said to be occurring even in the absence of several of its aspects. Put another way, "sleep should be considered a syndrome." In medicine, a syndrome is "a set of symptoms occurring together" (Dortland, 1977). Likewise, sleep is a set of conditions; no single condition is adequate to define sleep nor is sleep any one inclusive set of criteria.

Sleep During Other Ages

This is the average, typical sleep of the young adult. Not all sleep is like this. Some normal young adults, for example, may differ greatly in length and percentage (but not sequence of stages) from these norms depending of things like the amount of time dedicated to work, gender, status, parenting, and satisfaction with health (Harvey & Moldofsky, 1991) and biological sleep need (Hauri & Linde, 1990). And even casual experience with babies indicates a pattern greatly different from this. The elderly typically show differences too (Harvey and Moldofsky, 1991).

Table 1-2 summarizes the patterns of sleep typical for various ages. Before we follow through these age related changes we must note the missing information for the newborn. This lack of information does not reflect a lack of study on the sleep of infants. Quite the contrary; they have been much studied (Hoppenbrouwers, 1987). Rather, their sleep patterns are so different that one researcher once queried, "Do infants really sleep?" Let's see what prompts this question.

Sleep in Infants

When the sleep of infants is measured, the same basic EEG, EOG, and EMG measurements are taken (although the brain waves produced by the immature infant brain are very different from those discussed so far) plus measurements for respiration via additional sensors applied to the chest. In addition, every 30 seconds an observer must mark on the moving chart the condition of the baby - either quiet or active and either eyes open or closed and whether it is crying, making body

Table 1-2 Average Patterns of Sleep for Various Ages

Variable	Age					
	Newborn	Pre-school	Grade School	High School	Young Adult	Retired
Time in Bed (hrs., mins.)		10h 18m	9h 54m	8h 12m	7h 21m	7h 38m
Total Time Asleep (hrs., mins.)	(17)	9h 53m	9h 30m	7h 48m	7h 4m	6h 46m
Time to Get to Sleep (mins.)		14	15	16.5	9	13
Number of Awakenings (30s or more)		1.5	1.1	2.3	2	5 (♀ less)
Percent of Time Awake		1.3	1.0	1.3	1.2	8.5
Percent REM	(50)	31	28	24	26	22.5
Percent Stage 2		45 (♀ less)	48	48	51	56
Percent Delta		20.5	21	23	16	5
REM Cycle (mins.)	(60)	90 (♀ less)	111	112	105	100
Sleep Efficiency		.96	.96	.95	.96	.88
Number of Stages		34	33	39	36	41

Derived from Williams R L, Karacan I, & Hursch C J (1974). *Electroencephalography (EEG) of human sleep: Clinical applications.* New York: Wiley.

movements, yawning, making facial expressions, etc. These measurements and observations allow the discrimination of two stages of wake (wake and drowsy) and three stages of sleep (active, quiet, and indeterminate). (The criteria for infant sleep reported here are from Anders, Emde, and Parmelee, 1971. Other sets of criteria are quite similar [see Hoppenbrouwers, 1987]).

Since the criteria and, indeed, the stages are so different for infants, the question about the validity of sleep in infants is a good one. If we say sleep is what we see in young adults, then the question can be answered "no" since infants do not meet adult criteria. Others respond by pointing out that quiet sleep (QS) and indeterminate sleep (IS) transform into NREM as the infant matures. Likewise, active sleep (AS) gradually becomes REM sleep. Thus since the sleep of infants merges gradually and smoothly into adult sleep, we can say infants do sleep although their sleeping is immature. This is not unlike the maturation of language in children in that the coos and babbling of infants is unlike adult speech but is the important, immature precursor of it.

Now we can return to Table 1-2. The figures for the infants that are present in the chart are in parenthesis because they are either gross approximations or are based on the criteria for infant sleep. The rest are absent simply because nothing in infant sleep clearly resembles those categories of adult sleep (Moorcroft, 1987).

At thirty-six weeks post conception the sleep of the fetus begins to become more recognizable (Hoppenbrouwers, 1987; Coons, 1987). (Ultrasonic visualization of fetuses in the uterus has been an important technique for being able to observe sleep behavior in the fetus while still in the uterus. The data obtained in this way has been compared to polysomnograms from premature infants.) The various components of sleep begin to occur together at this age and the sleep is more sustained. There are high levels of AS and IS but not much QS.

During the first few months of life[3] there is much maturation of sleep but with a great deal of variation between individuals. Most sleep is AS (45% of the nychthemeron is occupied by this stage) with considerable QS also occurring (20%) and significant amounts of indeterminate sleep (higher in premature infants). These various

---

[3]This and other ages are averages that assume normal gestation length. Premature infants maintain the same schedule based on gestational age (based on time of conception) not birth age. Individuals may, however, vary quite a bit from these averages.

stages are more or less evenly distributed throughout the nychthemeron, but an approximate a 60 minute cycle can be discerned. Sleep onset AS is frequent (often following a feeding) but begins to decline at one month of age and becomes almost nonexistent by two months of age. Sleep begins to consolidate (become less randomly scattered throughout the 24 hour day) and there are fewer brief interruptions of sleep caused by movements, awakenings, brief stage changes. Yet the sleep seems to follow the infants' four hour feeding cycles rather than its own sleep rhythm. Soon (at about 6 weeks) sleep begins to occur more frequently at night with the longest sleep period being about 3 1/2 hours (1/4 of the total sleep in the nychthemeron). As the infant ages, AS declines (because of a decrease in the number of episodes) as QS increases (due to an increase in both the number and duration of episodes).

Three months of age is a major turning point. At this age, the sleep of children can be compared with that of adult sleep (Coons, 1987). As can be seen in Table 1-2, the time in bed declines with advancing age in children as does total time asleep. Concurrently, in the first five years or so of life, the number and timing of sleep periods changes (see Figure 1-4). In the 24 hour day the newborn has multiple periods of sleep separated by shorter (at first) periods of wakefulness. By 1 year of age much of the sleep has "consolidated" into the evening and night (much to the relief of parents) but a daily nap period or two remains and usually is of NREM sleep. Ninety five percent of 2 year olds and 50% of 5 year olds nap regularly (Rosen, 1990). By four years of age, the waking time is longer partially because the nap is later and shorter. Usually by age six the regular nap disappears and all sleep occurs at night. (See Chapter 3 for the surprising prevalence of naps in other cultures and even among adults in our culture.)

Sleep in Preschoolers and Gradeschoolers

Returning to Table 1-2, we can see that the time it takes to get to sleep remains relatively stable until young adulthood, as does, percent of time awake after going to sleep. Number of awakenings during sleep dips from 1 1/2 in the preschooler to about 1 in the gradeschooler and rising to two in the high schooler. Sleep is very deep during these ages. It is very difficult to awaken children from sleep and almost impossible to do so during the first cycle of SWS.The percent of REM starts high, going from 75% in premature infants to

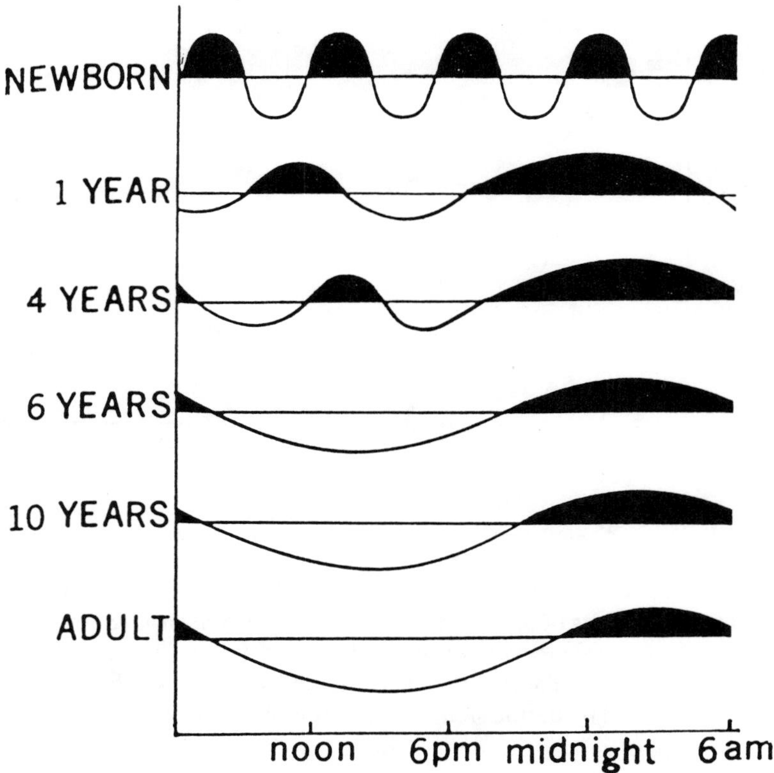

Figure 1-4. The number and timing of sleep periods in 24 hours at different ages (after Kleitman, 1972

to 50% in term infants, and settling down to around 25% in adolescents. Stage two stays steady at around 50% throughout maturation and adulthood. Percentage of SWS is likewise stable but does drop somewhat between high school and adulthood. Finally, the REM cycle (time from the start of one REM cycle to the next) increases from 60 minutes in newborns to over 100 minutes in children of grade school age.

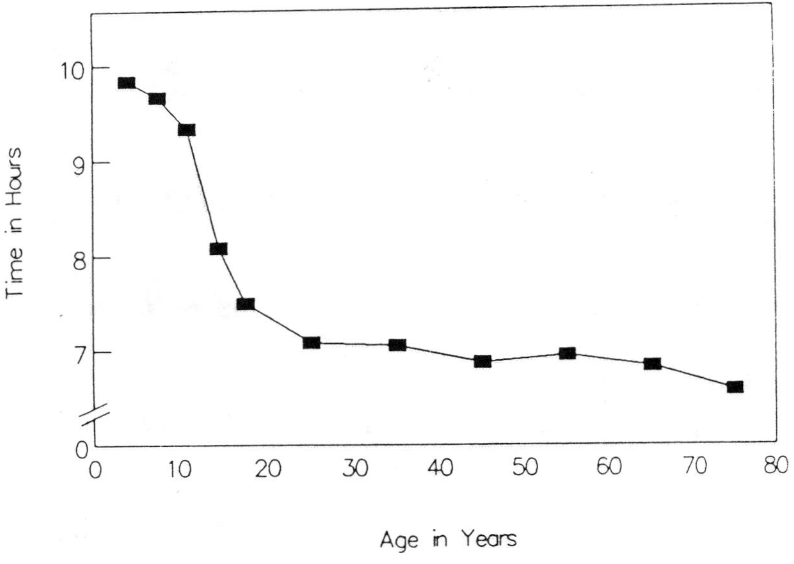

Figure 1-5. Average amount of total sleep time per night from three to seventy-nine years of age. After Williams R L, Karacan I, & Hursch © J (1974). *Electroencephalography (EEG) of human sleep: Clinical applications*. New York: Wiley. Copyrighted © 1974 by John Wiley & Sons, Inc. Used by permission of John Wiley & Sons, Inc.

A somewhat different pattern of sleep changes with age is seen when looking at total amounts, rather than percentages, of time spent n each stage. This is because total sleep time during each nychthemeron decreases with age up to adulthood (Table 1-2 and Figure 1-5). This different pattern is especially true for some of the percentages that change very little with age. For example, while the percentage of the total sleep time occupied by stage 2 increases insignificantly from preschool age to high school age (Table 1-2), the absolute amount of stage 2 decreases from about 275 minutes to near 200 minutes (Figure 1-6). A comparison of Figures 1-7, 1-8, and 1-9 with Table 1-2 reveals that REM and delta also show declines in absolute amounts in the early years of life but little change in percentage of total sleep time. The decline in REM is greatest during

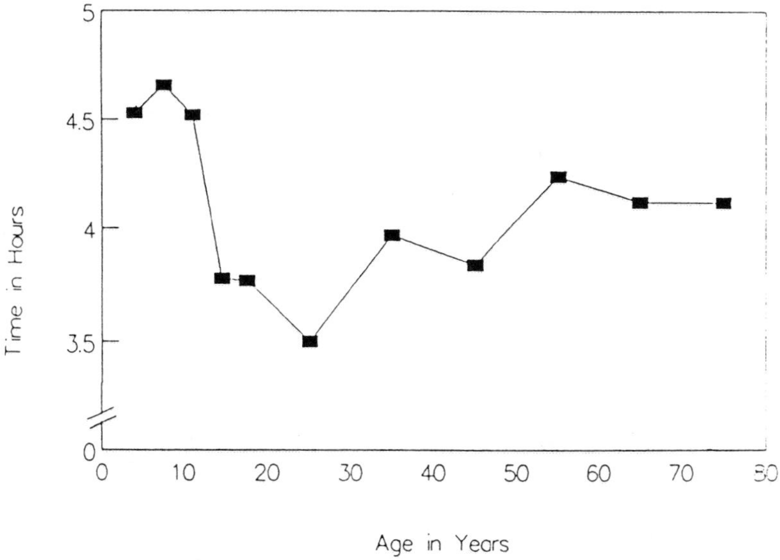

Figure 1-6. Average time per night spent in stage 2 from three to seventy-nine years of age. After Williams R L, Karacan I, & Hursch C J (1974). *Electroencephalography (EEG) of human sleep: Clinical applications*. New York: Wiley. Copyrighted © 1974 by John Wiley & Sons, Inc. Used by permission of John Wiley & Sons, Inc.

these years but continues until late teens. The stage 2 decline occurs almost entirely during preadolescence and gradually increases beginning in the middle of young adulthood. The decline in delta begins during grade school and continues slowly but steadily throughout the rest of life.

The second decade of life has been investigated more intensively recently (Carskadon, 1982). This is a time of dramatic changes in both physiology and behavior in humans; these changes could also cause changes in sleep.

Sleep in Teenagers

There are several important changes in sleep during the second decade of life that have been noted (Carskadon, 1990a; Carskadon,

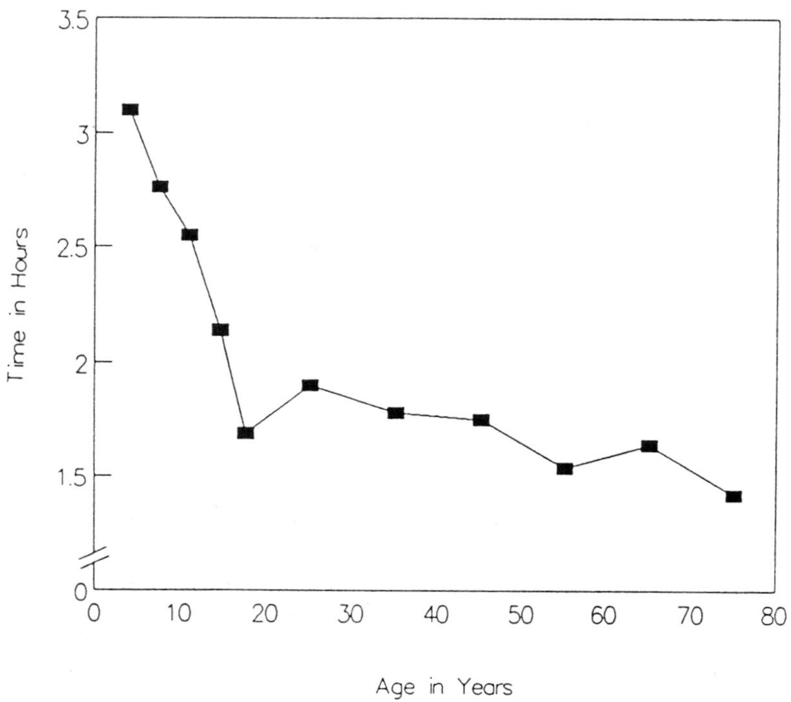

Figure 1-7. Average time per night spent in REM Sleep from three to seventy-nine years of age. After Williams R L, Karacan I, & Hursch C J (1974). *Electroencephalography (EEG) of human sleep: Clinical applications*. New York: Wiley. Copyrighted © 1974 by John Wiley & Sons, Inc. Used by permission of John Wiley & Sons, Inc.

1990b; Carskadon & Davis 1989; Carskadon & Dement, 1987). The changes in total sleep during this period of life, as they appear on a graph, have been described as "a general drift downward with two big drops followed by a drift upward" at the same time that sleep need (contrary to common belief) actually increases.

The first big drop occurs early in the decade (in pre-teens). Preadolescents average over 9 1/2 hours of sleep every night. Before long this drops dramatically, especially on school nights.

Accompanying this, older preadolescents go to bed later on non-school nights but get up much later the next morning. The result is 2 1/2 hours less sleep on school nights and over one hour less on non-school nights compared to younger preadolescents. In addition there is an increase in napping that can be observed at this age but not in sufficient amounts to eliminate the increase in sleepiness during the day (Carskadon & Dement, 1982; Levine, Lumely, Roehrs, Zorick, & Roth, 1988). This dramatic drop in sleep appears to be a result of several factors: the individual rather than the parent becomes responsible for setting the bed time (the role of the parent often shifting to terminating the sleep period now!), cultural and social forces (especially having a job but also increased interest in socializing with friends, watching favorite television programs, and the like), and physiological changes (such as the onset of puberty, brain maturation, and so forth).

Most teenagers are chronically sleep deprived. A group of German adolescents was studied every two years for ten years beginning at 10-14 years of age. Over half to three-fourths expressed a wish for more sleep. However, it was not always the same individuals who expressed

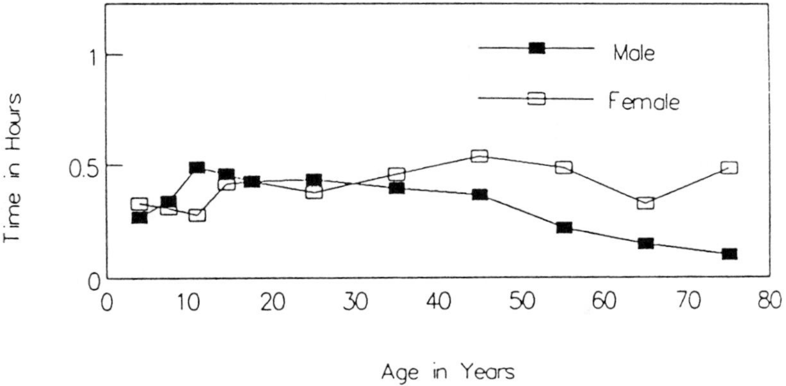

Figure 1-8. Average time per night spent in stage 3 in males and females from three to seventy-nine years of age. After Williams R L, Karacan I, & Hursch C J (1974). *Electroencephalography (EEG) of human sleep: Clinical applications.* New York: Wiley. Copyrighted © 1974 by John Wiley & Sons, Inc. Used by permission of John Wiley & Sons, Inc.

this wish nor were any significant trends noticed (such as getting more sleepy or less sleepy as the study went on). Most of these tired students said they felt tired upon awakening, wanted to stay in bed, and needed 15 minutes to feel alert. A fair number also reported being in a "trough" the rest of the morning. Surprisingly, the tired students did not report spending less time-in-bed than the rested ones during the week or weekends but did during vacations.

In the United States, 70% of senior high school students report that they do not get enough sleep (Carskadon, Seifer, Davis, & Acebo, 1991). They report getting an average of about one hour less per night then desirable. The typical bedtime on weeknights is 23:00 hours and 1:00 hours on weekends (20% go to bed even later) resulting in an average total sleep time on weekdays of seven hours and nine hours

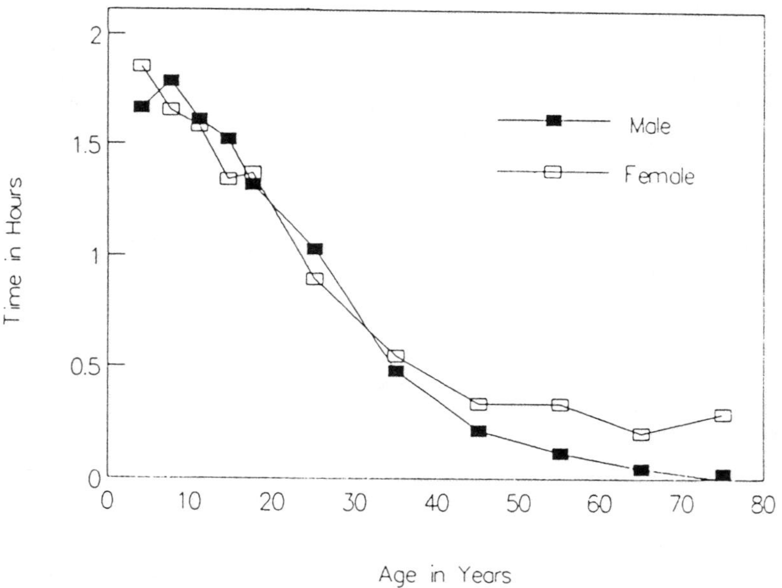

Figure 1-9. Average time per night spent in stage 4 in males and females from three to seventy-nine years of age. After Williams R L, Karacan I, & Hursch C J (1974). *Electroencephalography (EEG) of human sleep: Clinical applications.* New York: Wiley. Copyrighted © 1974 by John Wiley & Sons, Inc. Used by permission of John Wiley & Sons, Inc.

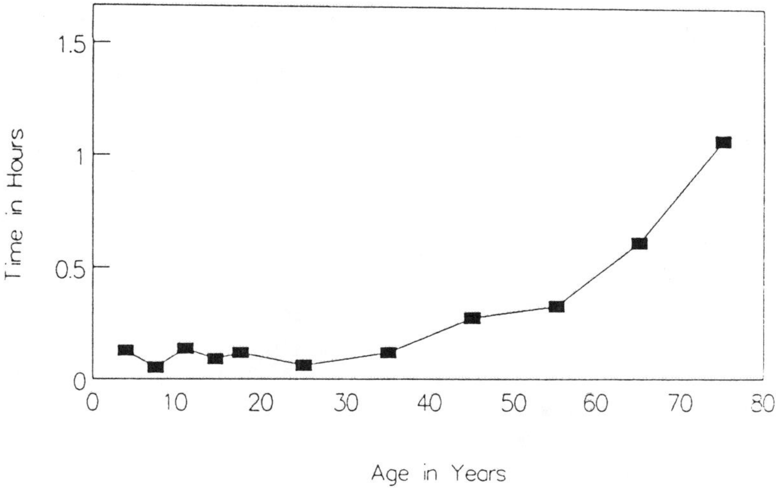

Figure 1-10. Average time per night spent awake after initial sleep onset from three to seventy-nine years of age. After Williams R L, Karacan I, & Hursch C J (1974). *Electroencephalography (EEG) of human sleep: Clinical applications.* New York: Wiley. Copyrighted © 1974 by John Wiley & Sons, Inc. Used by permission of John Wiley & Sons, Inc.

average on weekends (Allen & Mirabile, 1989). There is a direct relationship between having a part-time job and complaints of insufficient sleep and sleepiness.

A second "big drop" occurs upon entrance to college (those who do not go onto college have not yet been studied sufficiently to know what happens to them, although Levine et al (1988) suggest that they too are sleepy from sleep restriction but not to the same extent as college students.) The transition from high school to college results in many changes in a young adult's life including their sleep patterns. A study by Carskadon and Davis (1989) examined sleep in this transition. They found that the total sleep time of these young adults after going to college was 20 to 36 minutes less than before college. There was a greater change in when this sleep was obtained. After entering college, the average bed time changed to 2:30 am, but with a wide variation between and within individuals. Bedtimes for college students are

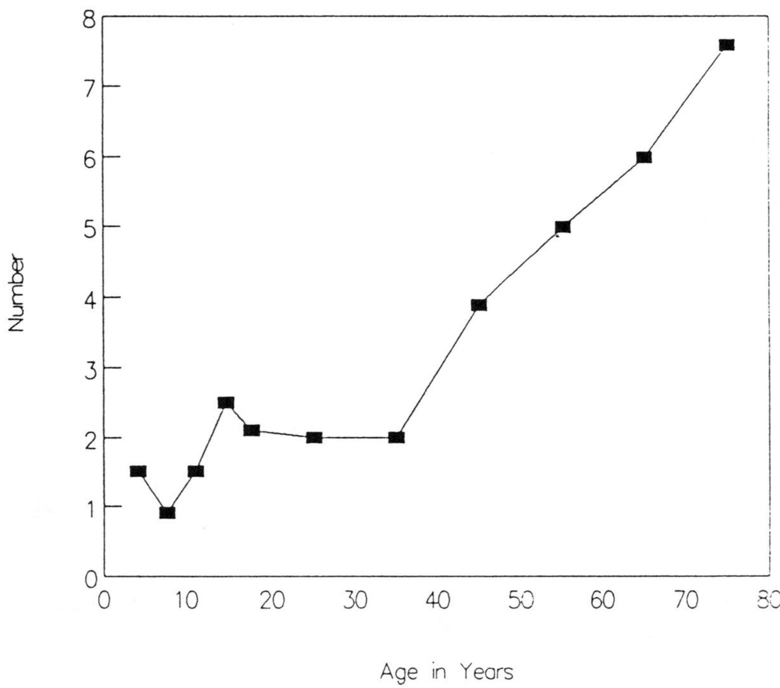

Figure 1-11. Average number of awakenings during the night from three to seventy-nine years of age. After Williams R L, Karacan I, & Hursch C J (1974). *Electroencephalography (EEG) of human sleep: Clinical applications*. New York: Wiley. Copyrighted © 1974 by John Wiley & Sons, Inc. Used by permission of John Wiley & Sons, Inc.

considerably later than for working adults. (This is called a "phase delay" [see chapter 4]. As many as 20% of college students develop a sleep disorder called "Delayed Sleep Phase Syndrome" [see chapter 8] that has a negative impact on grades). The average daytime sleepiness of college students throughout the day is at the level that has been shown to result in impaired performance (Carskadon, 1990a).

Once in college, the sleep patterns of students are very interesting to study because of the flexibility of their work/rest schedules. An example of this flexibility is the incidence of naps (Bigler &

Carskadon, 1990). On the average about 20% of the days contained naps and they were even more frequent on weekdays. The average length was 90 minutes but many were much shorter and many were much longer. Bigler and Carskadon also observed that students woke up earlier and slept less on the weekdays (408 minutes) than on weekends (455 minutes), yet the average bed time did not change significantly between weekdays and weekends. In general, students went to bed earlier and woke up earlier when using an alarm, but alarms were used on weekdays 50% of the time and only 26% of the time on weekends. Another difference between alarm use and non-alarm use were the reasons for going to sleep. On alarm days, students went to sleep in order to get a certain amount of sleep, while on non-alarm days it was more of an "overwhelming" need to sleep. Some of the reasons Bigler and Carskadon's college students gave for falling asleep were: 1) "overwhelmed by sleep" (52%) 2) finished socializing, homework, work (29%) 3) to get a certain number of hours of sleep (15%) 4) "it's bedtime" (4%). The reasons for waking included: 1) alarm (43%) 2) spontaneous (38%) 3) others (19%). The use of an alarm did not always result in waking the subjects since students overslept on almost half the days that they had set their alarm!

But as students progress in their college careers, they drift toward more sleep per night and less self reported daytime sleepiness (Acebo et al, 1991; Osborn & Moorcroft, 1981 unpublished observations). This probably results due to progressively earlier bed times. Eventually, for many students the sleep obtained approximates sleep need by senior year (and the start of the third decade of life). The pattern of more sleep on weekends than weekdays continues to persist though. However, weekday sleep comes closer and closer to sleep need as the college years progress and weekend bedtimes and arising times get earlier and earlier.

Contrary to widespread belief, there is no decrease in the need for sleep during adolescence. In fact the opposite appears to be true - the need for sleep increases during adolescence (Carskadon & Dement, 1987). (This was shown in an experiment in the sleep lab by adolescents who were all required to be in bed for 10 hours (22:00 to 8:00); all adolescents, regardless of age, slept for about nine hours under this condition!) However, the amount of delta sleep decreased by 35% during this decade and stage 2 sleep increased, but REM remained stable. The only gender difference shown during adolescence was more delta sleep in males than females. At the same time the mid afternoon increase in sleepiness (see chapter 4) emerges suggesting a physiological change in sleep need. Feinberg (1989) summarizes evidence suggesting that dramatic brain changes during the second decade of life may be responsible for the dramatic sleep changes seen then also. This "global reorganization" of the brain in the adolescent includes: a dramatic decrease in the density of cortical synapses, considerable changes in cerebral metabolic rate, changes in some indices of electrical functioning, and a loss of plasticity following brain injury. These changes are seen as a normal part of brain maturation and are probably genetically controlled via changes in hormones.

There are several consequences of the high level of sleepiness seen in adolescents (Carskadon, 1990a). As sleepiness gets worse, so do things like driving, academic performance, and substance abuse. In addition, anxiety and depression increase in females (Carskadon et al, 1991). This results in higher levels of school failure and drop out rates and more accidents. This is a significant problem in our society today.

Sleep in the Elderly

To this point we have examined changes in sleep from infancy through adulthood but have not said anything about retirement age. This is because so many changes occur during this time that it requires special emphasis. Wilse Webb (1975) aptly described these changes as a fraying of sleep. Think of a rope whose various strands are tightly woven when new but begin to loosen up at the ends as the rope gets older. This is what happens to many individuals as they reach, and then go beyond, retirement age. However, individuals differ more from one another with respect to sleep during this era than at any other time. Some people experience little change in sleep as they get older, while others notice considerable changes in sleep which are often alarming to the individuals. This widening range of individual differences of sleep in older age must be kept in mind during the following discussion (from Bixler, Kales, Jacoby, Soldatos, & Vela-Bueno, 1984; Carskadon & Dement, 1987; Feinberg, 1989; Horne, 1988; Prinz, 1980; Spiegel, 1981; Vitiello & Prinz, 1990; Webb, 1975).

Contrary to popular opinion, the elderly do **not** need less sleep during each nychthemeron. Although total sleep time at night does decline slightly (Table 1-2 and Figure 1-5), total sleep time during the nychthemeron does not decline if nap time is added to nighttime sleep time. Sleep differences in the elderly can be summarized by noting five types of changes: changes in EEG, sleep stages, sleep cycles, the rhythm of sleep, and sleep quality.

EEG. Delta waves (the major sign of SWS) are not as intense, have a higher wave frequency, and do not occur as often as they did at earlier ages. Spindles are often not well formed, are lower in amplitude, are of slower frequency, and occur less than half as often. There is also a decrease in the average number of eye movements during REM sleep (often called "rem density").

Sleep Stages. SWS (often considered the deepest stage of sleep) is weaker and of shorter duration. There is a decrease in stage 4 sleep both in terms of minutes per night (Figure 1-9) and percent of sleep (Table 1-2). Most of these changes in SWS occur before fifty years of age. This increase in SWS is much less (but nevertheless still significant) if less rigid criteria are used for counting delta waves (Horne, 1988) since their amplitude is often less than the 75uV criterion level. REM shows slight decreases in minutes per night (Figure 1-7) and percent of sleep time (Table 1-2). The amount of wakefulness during the sleep period increases in the elderly (Figure 1-10), because both the number of awakenings (Figure 1-11) and the average length of each awakening increase dramatically. The awareness of awakenings increases also. Returning to sleep after awakening gets more difficult for the elderly as the night goes on and sometimes results in shortened sleep. Stage 1 sleep also increases considerably in the elderly (Figure 1-12). Since stage 1 is more of a transitional state between sleep and wakefulness, its increase contributes to the lessening of the depth of sleep in the elderly. There is an increase in the number of stage shifts which disrupts the continuity of all sleep stages, but especially REM.

Other stages of sleep show little change in the elderly, and the time it takes to get to sleep changes very little. Stage 2 sleep may change slightly in both absolute amounts and percent of sleep time, but this is insignificant compared to other changes.

Cycles. The first NREM-REM cycle is shorter in the elderly possibly due to the reduction of SWS. The duration of the REM portion of sleep does not increase with successive cycles as it does in younger ages. That is, there is a shift of REM to earlier portions of the sleep period. Less sleep continuity occurs because of the greater

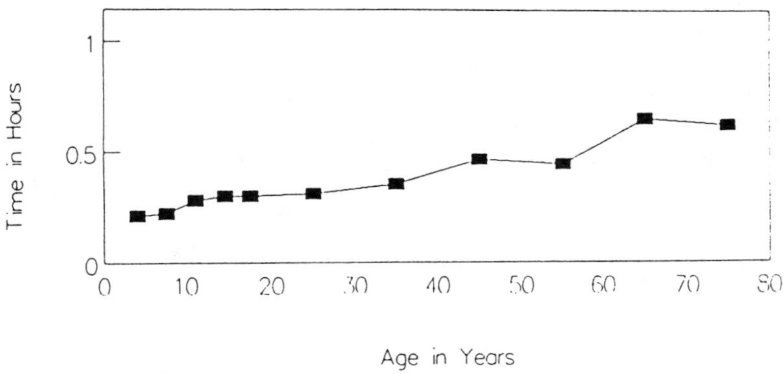

Figure 1-12. Average time per night spent in stage 1 from three to seventy-nine years of age. After Williams R L, Karacan I, & Hursch C J (1974). *Electroencephalography (EEG) of human sleep: Clinical applications.* New York: Wiley. Copyrighted © 1974 by John Wiley & Sons, Inc. Used by permission of John Wiley & Sons, Inc.

number of stage shifts and the increased number and duration of awakenings as well as an increase in brief (about 15 seconds) arousals which tend to fragment sleep, and an increase in the number of stage shifts. Also contributing to the fraying of sleep may be the decrease in arousal threshold (at least to noise). Furthermore, an elderly person can awaken abruptly without the grogginess usually seen in the young.

Rhythm. The elderly tend to fall asleep earlier and awaken earlier. The average elderly person does get less sleep at night but more sleep during the day. The re-emergence of the nap seems to occur in the elderly (Webb, 1975). The significance of this is debatable, however. Later (in Chapter 3) we will explore napping in general, but suffice it to say that napping may be more common and more normal at all ages than is generally believed. The relative infrequency of naps in the young and middle aged may be due more to social endeavors and work schedules than anything else. Their re-emergence in retirees may be a result of the absence of the rigid schedule demands of the workplace which prevent the possibility of napping. On the other hand, napping, especially excessive napping, may be both the cause as well as the result of the "fraying" of sleep in the elderly (Prinz & Raskin, 1978) because at any age, sleep tends to reduce the efficiency of subsequent

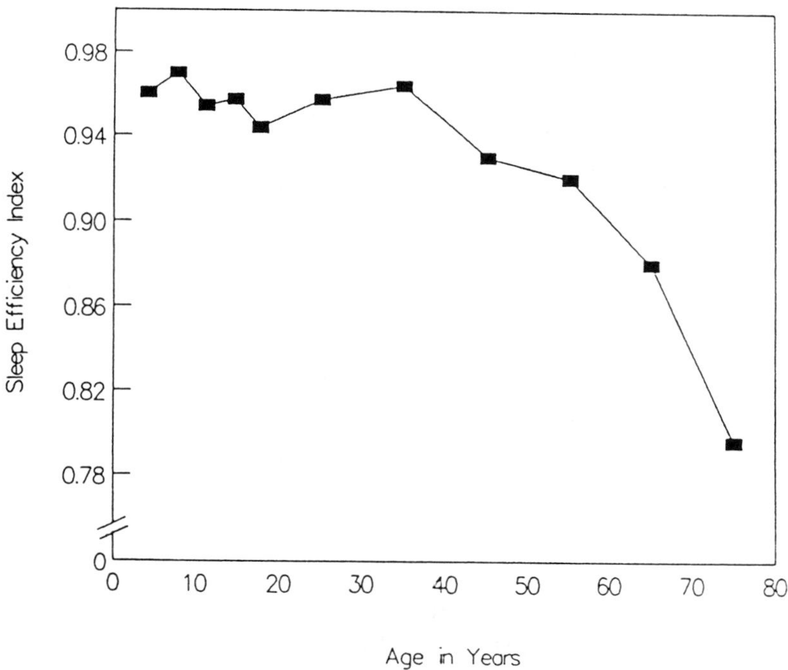

Figure 1-13. Average proportion of time in bed spent asleep (sleep efficiency) from three to seventy-nine years of age. After Williams R L, Karacan I, & Hursch C J (1974). *Electroencephalography (EEG) of human sleep: Clinical applications.* New York: Wiley. Copyrighted © 1974 by John Wiley & Sons, Inc. Used by permission of John Wiley & Sons, Inc.

sleep unless substantial wake time accumulates prior to the second sleep period. However, this issue is not fully resolved. There appear to be wide differences among individuals that make a definitive analysis of the function, cause, and consequences of napping in the elderly difficult.

Quality. A measure called sleep efficiency (derived by dividing total sleep time by time in bed) dramatically summarizes many of these changes (Figure 1-13). A general decline in this index begins at about 30 years of age when it is .96, with the decline accelerating after

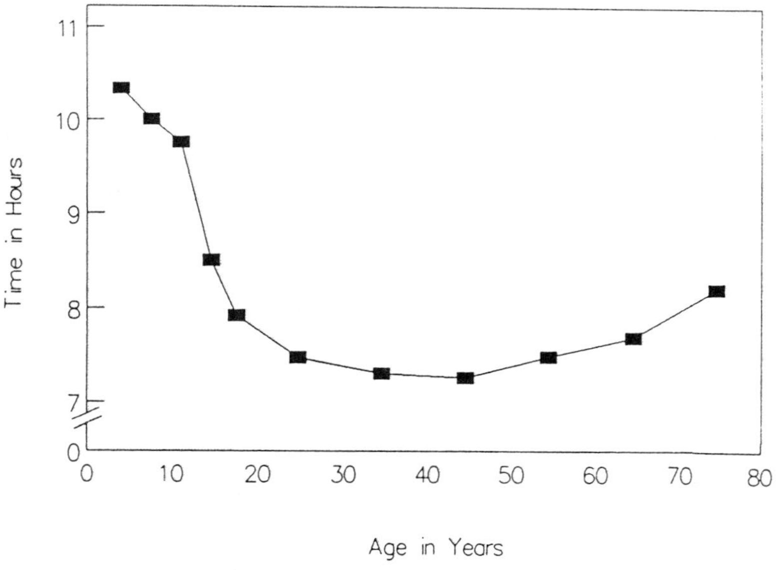

Figure 1-14. Average amount of time in bed from three to seventy-nine years of age. After Williams R L, Karacan I, & Hursch C J (1974). *Electroencephalography (EEG) of human sleep: Clinical applications.* New York: Wiley. Copyrighted © 1974 by John Wiley & Sons, Inc. Used by permission of John Wiley & Sons, Inc.

50 years of age to less than .80 in the eighth decade of life. Much of this decline in sleep efficiency is due to the increased number and duration of awakenings. The increased wake time also explains the increase in the time in bed during the retirement years (Table 1-2 and Figure 1-14).

The end result of all of these changes is a greater dissatisfaction with sleep among the elderly than is seen at any other age.

There appear to be two causes for these changes in sleep in the elderly. First, many of these changes are a normal part of the aging process. In many ways we would not expect to see retirees do what they did when younger. This should include sleep. Second, sleep disorders (see Chapter 9) tend to become more prevalent with age and many of these disrupt normal sleep.

Conclusion

Looking back over all of the information in this chapter, what can we conclude? First, it should now be obvious that sleep is more than a **passive** reduction of bodily processes (Dement, 1978). Prior to 30 years ago most sleep experts would have said that sleep is a passive phenomenon and, even today, most people would agree with this statement. Indeed, it seems that way since we do everything possible to reduce our body activity and internal activation when we attempt to go to sleep. We usually seek a quiet, dark place in which to sleep. We place our bodies in a reclining, muscle relaxing position. We try to arrange as few disturbances as possible. We close our eyes and let our minds "go blank." And if we fail at any of these things, we tend to find sleep to be elusive and difficult. In short, we reduce body effort and any stimulation as if attempting to settle down to an easy "idle".

But in the laboratory we have already seen that sleep is anything but passive. The most compelling illustration of this is the recurrent REM episodes with active mind content and aroused body functions. In fact, during REM our bodies need to **actively** inhibit our muscles which produce movement in order to prevent us from acting out our dreams (see chapter 2)! While it is true that NREM appears to more closely conform to the notions of passive sleep, the study of brain functions (see Chapter 2) suggest that this is not entirely true. During sleep, some parts of the brain are **more**, not less, active than during wakefulness because they are **actively** producing sleep. Thus, during sleep the brain does not reduce its activity to a low level; rather, some areas become more activated. Literally, during sleep the night shift of the brain actively takes control from the day shift.

This knowledge is important. It changes our whole attitude toward sleep. Sleep is not as simple as it seems. We begin to think of it differently and ask different kinds of questions when we become aware that sleep is more than the absence of wake. It also changes our approaches on how to correct sleep problems. For example, the widely used sleeping pills are merely chemicals that reduce all of the brain's activity. It should not surprise us then to learn that sleeping pills do **not** produce normal sleep. Currently, the search is for a sleeping medication that will **activate** those areas of the brain that produce sleep.

Second, the information in this chapter is consistent with the idea that there are important functions that occur during sleep. The organization of structure and the energy required to produce sleep and its regular alternation of REM and NREM would hardly occur if there was not some great purpose to it all. Also, the great changes in the sleep of the young, in kinds of sleep, their amounts, and in patterns of sleep suggest an underlying functional purpose. This is followed by relatively stable or only very gradual changes in adulthood, but the golden years again show many changes with sleep beginning to fray and greater individual differences in the amounts and patterning of sleep. It is also during these years that great changes in the body and mind are often noticeable suggesting that some of these bodily and mental changes might be related to the changes in sleep occurring at the same time. We will pursue the idea that there are important functions to sleep throughout this book but especially in chapter 10.

Differences between males and females have not been mentioned in this chapter because there are very few until late adulthood. As retirement age approaches, sleep begins to fray in males before females. By post-retirement ages, changes in the sleep of females may occur as much as 10 years later than similar changes in the sleep of males.

In this chapter we have reviewed the basic characteristics of sleep and how they change with age. But sleep is rich with many other aspects beyond the basics. We will explore these aspects in the rest of this book.

Chapter 2

The Body and Brain in Sleep[1]

To the observer, sleep appears to be a passive state - simply a reduction of activity and reactivity during which an organism all but "turns off." Our ability to record the electrical changes within the brain and measure physiological processes in the rest of the body during sleep shows that this is far from true, there is in fact much activity taking place. Often this activity is quite different from what it is during wakefulness. We shall look at the differences in bodily physiology first, then look at how the brain produces sleep.

The Body During Sleep

In recent years it has become apparent that sleep is a different state not only mentally, but also physiologically. Quantitative, and sometimes qualitative, differences have been noted between sleep and wake in many body systems. Changes in the cardiovascular system,

---

1 Adapted with permission from Moorcroft, W.H. and Clothier, J. (1987). The Body and Brain in Sleep. In J Gackenbach (Ed.) *A Sourcebook of Sleep and Dreams* (pp. 30-61). New York: Garland Press. Copyrighted by Garland Press in 1987.

alimentary system, the motor system, and, most notably, respiration have been documented during sleep in recent years.

Breathing

Of all the physiological differences in sleep compared to wakefulness that have been discovered in the last decade, the changes in respiratory control are most dramatic. The complex and overlapping neural and biochemical mechanisms that regulate respiration in awake humans and other mammals were assumed to function equivalently during sleep (see Guyton, 1976 for example). Recent evidence refutes this notion (Anch et al., 1988; Grunstein and Sullivan, 1990; Kryger, Roth, & Dement, 1989; Moorcroft & Clothier, 1987; Mendelson, 1987; Orem, 1985; Parmeggiani, 1991).

Not only are there differences in the level of the functioning of these respiratory systems, there are even changes in how they function. Movements of the rib cage for breathing are reduced during sleep making the contractions of the diaphragm more important. Yet because of the physics of laying down; the stomach applies weight against the diaphragm and makes it more difficult for the diaphragm to do its job. However, there are many other changes that affect respiration when asleep.

During wake breathing is controlled by two interacting systems. The first is an automatic, metabolic system whose control is centered in the brainstem (see later in this chapter for a description of parts of the brain). It subconsciously adjusts breathing rate and depth in order to regulate the levels of CO_2 and O_2, and the acid/base ratio in the blood. The second system is the voluntary, behavioral system. Its control center is based in the forebrain and it regulates breathing for use in speech, singing, sighing, and so on. It is capable of ignoring or overriding the automatic, metabolic system and produces an irregular pattern of breathing.

During NREM breathing becomes deeper and more regular but there is also a decrease in breathing rate resulting in less air being exchanged overall. This occurs because during NREM sleep the automatic, metabolic system has exclusive control over breathing and your body uses less oxygen and produces less carbon dioxide. Also, during sleep the automatic metabolic system is less responsive to carbon dioxide levels and oxygen levels in the blood. Two things result from these changes in breathing control that occur during sleep. First, there may be a brief cessation or reduction of breathing when falling asleep as the sleeper waxes and wanes between sleep and wakefulness and their differing control mechanisms. Second, once sleep is fully obtained, there is an increase of carbon dioxide and a decrease of oxygen in the blood that persists during NREM.

But that is not all that changes. During all phases of sleep, several changes in the air passages have been observed. It takes twice as much effort to breath during sleep because of greater resistance to air flow in the airways and changes in the efficiency of the muscles used for breathing. Some of the muscles that help keep the upper-airway open when breathing tend to become more relaxed during sleep, especially during REM. Without this muscular action, inhaling is like sucking air out of a balloon - the narrow passages tend to collapse. Also there is a regular cycle of change in resistance between the two sides of the nose. If something blocks the "good" side, such as congestion from allergies or a cold, then resistance increases dramatically. Coupled with these factors is the loss of the complex interactions among the muscles which can change the route of air flow from nose to mouth (Tangel, Mezzanotte, Wheatly, & White, 1992).

Other respiratory regulating mechanisms apparently cease functioning during sleep. For example, during wakefulness there is an immediate, automatic, adaptive increase in breathing effort when inhaling is made more difficult (such as breathing through a restrictive face mask). This reflexive adjustment is totally absent during NREM sleep. Only after several inadequate breaths under such conditions, resulting in the considerable elevation of carbon dioxide and reduction of oxygen in the blood, is breathing effort adjusted. Finally, the coughing reflex to irritants in the airway produces not a cough during sleep, but a cessation of breathing. If the irritation is severe enough, a sleeping person will arouse, clear the airway, then resume breathing and, hopefully, return to sleep.

Additional breathing changes occur during REM sleep that are even more dramatic then those of NREM. The amount of air exchanged is even lower in REM than NREM because although breathing is more rapid in REM, it is also more irregular with brief episodes of shallow breathing or absence of breathing. In addition, breathing during REM depends much more on action of the diaphragm and much less on rib cage action. The arousal response to irritants in the throat is slower during REM. Beyond this there appear to be dramatic differences between tonic and phasic REM in respiratory control. During tonic REM the automatic, metabolic system is in control of breathing but it is even less sensitive than during NREM. During phasic REM the voluntary, behavioral system seems to take over control of breathing. The result is highly irregular, rapid but shallow bursts of breathing with dramatic pauses. The overall result is less air exchange during REM causing further increased levels of carbon dioxide and decreased levels of oxygen in the blood. All of these changes during REM sleep are most dramatic in the infant.

Body Temperature

Temperature regulation also shows some dramatic changes during sleep (Horne, 1988; Kryger, Roth, & Dement, 1989; Moorcroft & Clothier, 1987; Parmeggiani, 1991). Body temperature tends to gradually decline until near the end of sleep, but may vary a bit with the REM-NREM cycle.

During NREM, and especially during the SWS portion, the body still regulates its temperature but at a lower level (about 0.4°C lower [Wehr, 1990]). Both heat production and heat conservation mechanisms are slightly less effective during NREM sleep. The blood vessels on the surface of the body dilate which results in more heat loss and causes the shivering response to lessen. If the room temperature is warm, then more exaggerated and persistent sweating and blood vessel dilation may accompany the onset of sleep. It is as if the thermostat regulating body temperature is turned to a lower setting during sleep.

During REM the situation is dramatically different, for there appears to be an almost total loss of thermoregulation. For example, during REM there is no shivering, greatly reduced sweating unless the temperature gets very high, and no vasodialation or panting in response to dramatic changes in ambient temperature. Although overall heat production during REM is similar to that seen during stage 2, it does not vary in response to body temperature changes. These differences in thermoregulation in human REM sleep occur because the temperature regulation mechanisms located in the brain are not functioning during REM. It is as if the thermostat was disconnected yet the furnace is still working. Actually, rather than a furnace it is more like having a wood burning stove as the source of heat; it produces heat at a constant rate with little regulation. This is the type of temperature regulation found in the fetus. The fetus is in a relatively constant environment of high heat and 100% humidity, so it does not need a sophisticated temperature regulatory system - only something to become activated in extreme emergencies. In other words, thermoregulation during REM sleep is more primitive.

During sleep your body temperature usually drops during NREM. When in REM it may increase if you are in a warm room or decrease if you are in a cold room. (In contrast, the temperature of the brain increases during REM due in part to heightened neuronal activity) If the ambient temperature is low enough, the body temperature may drop too much during REM resulting in warming during the subsequent NREM. These changes in temperature regulation do not account entirely for the circadian fluctuation in body temperatures (see Chapter 4), for such daily changes still occur under conditions of continuous bed rest or sleep deprivation. However, the difference between daily high to daily low temperature was attenuated by such conditions 25% and 45% respectfully.

Heart Rate and Blood Pressure

There are also changes that occur in the cardiovascular system during sleep (Moorcroft & Clothier, 1987). Blood pressure, heart rate, and output from the heart are at their daily lows throughout the sleep cycle but most especially during SWS with decreases of 25% or more. During this stage of sleep there is also less variability in both heart rate and blood pressure; in contrast, there is considerable variation in these factors during REM. Blood pressure may show as much as a 40 mm Hg. increase during phasic REM. Recently, a somewhat similar phenomenon has been observed in NREM; heart rate briefly increases and constriction of the blood vessels of the fingers accompany K-complexes. Other differences occur in the internal rhythms of the heart during sleep as measured by the ECG (electrocardiogram).

The changes in blood flow in the brain during sleep are especially noteworthy. During NREM some parts of the brain show increased blood flow of 25 to 50 percent or even more. Simultaneously, many other areas may show simultaneous reductions of between 20 to 25 other areas may show simultaneous reductions of between 20 to 25 percent (especially in the brainstem). For example, blood flow to the cortex decreases 10-15% in stages 1 and 2 and drops 30% in SWS. During REM the overall flow of blood to the brain increases by 50 to 175 percent and further brief increases may occur in addition to this during rapid eye movements and other phasic occurrences.

Why do these blood flow changes occur in the brain? One theory is that many of these changes are in response to local changes in metabolism and brain cell activity during sleep, but recent research has failed to confirm this. In fact, during NREM glucose use in the brain drops about 1/3 from waking values (Chase & Roth, 1990). Another theory is that many of the changes in body and brain blood flow occur to maintain adequate oxygen to the brain during sleep in the face of lowered blood oxygen levels (see above). Finally, during NREM the blood flow to the brain increases in proportion to the amount of carbon dioxide in the blood just as it does during wakefulness. Such a relationship does not occur during REM, however, since the blood flow is much greater than changes in carbon dioxide levels in the blood would account for.

Hormones

Changes in the hormones of the body during sleep (Mendelson, 1987; Moorcroft & Clothier, 1987) fall into three patterns. Sleep is strongly related to the levels of some hormones, especially those that tend to build and restore the body (such as growth hormone - and many sex hormones) and those that are produced by the anterior pituitary gland. Levels of these hormones tend to follow changes in the sleep period relatively easily and are susceptible to sleep deprivation. A prime example is growth hormone.

The onset of sleep is associated with the major release of growth hormone in humans (but not all mammals) during the nycthemeron. Other bursts of this hormone occur when sleep resumes after brief awakenings, multiple periods of sleeping and waking, or significant shifts in the time of sleep. Growth hormone output is significantly reduced by sleep deprivation and sleep following sleep deprivation contains extra secretion of growth hormone. (A question often arises here; can lack of adequate sleep stunt growth? The answer seems to be yes. Sleep disrupted children have lower levels of growth hormone and stunted growth. Also, dwarfs resulting from a lack of growth hormone have less powerful delta waves during SWS.)

But this relationship between sleep and growth hormone levels shows developmental and other variations. After three months of age, almost all of the release of growth hormone by the pituitary gland occurs during sleep. During puberty, some is also secreted while awake. In adulthood, most is secreted during early sleep (probably the first SWS period). With aging, less and then eventually none, is secreted during sleep, probably related to the decline of SWS in the elderly. And finally, it is interesting to note that administration of growth hormone prior to sleep inhibits SWS and increases REM suggesting (1) some kind of feedback regulation between the amount of growth hormone and the stage of sleep from which it is predominantly secreted and (2) a relationship between growth hormone secreted early in sleep and the amount of subsequent REM. Recent research suggests that the relationship of growth hormone with sleep is more dominant in males than in females (Kupfer & Reynolds, 1989).

Another group of hormones are only weakly related to sleep in the sense that they reluctantly follow changes in the sleep period, often taking several days to do so. They are probably more directly related to the circadian rhythm of the body (see Chapter 4) than to sleep itself. They include the hormones that tend to activate body structures and use body resources (such as thyroxin and cortisol). Melatonin is another example. Melatonin from the pineal gland shows a circadian rhythm with high levels at night. This rhythm only reluctantly follows changes in sleep time and it may never completely shift away from a night time propensity since melatonin production is inhibited by light. Melatonin is higher in children than adults. Since melatonin has been shown to cause sleepiness in humans, the higher levels of sleep in children may be in part due to their higher levels of this hormone.

In summary, several hormones show concentration peaks tied to sleep onset or offset and a regular sleep-wake cycle seems to be important in maintaining normal hormone cycles (growth hormone, prolactin, also to some extent luteinizing hormone, testosterone, and follicle stimulating hormone). For other hormones, though, sleep appears to be less important in their regulation (thyroid stimulating hormone, cortisol, melatonin), and there are still other hormones that bare no relationship to sleep at all.

Other Effects

The physiology of your other organ-systems has also been found to be different in sleep (Moorcroft & Clothier, 1987). One example is the excretory system. During sleep less urine is produced than when awake which may be due to the reduced blood flow through the kidney during sleep. Other mechanisms function to keep this reduced volume of urine from becoming too concentrated.

One of the more curious physiological differences that occurs during sleep is a reduction in digestive acid secretion in most people; this is contrasted with an increase of 20 to 30 times normal levels in patients suffering from duodenal ulcers. Swallowing greatly decreases during sleep resulting in less effective clearance of fluids from the throat region but salivation ceases in sleep.

One obvious aspect of going to sleep is a reduction of bodily movement. Yet muscle tone and simple reflexes are at about the same level in NREM as in wakefulness. In REM many reflexes and general muscle tone are reduced and there is almost total absence of bodily movement. All of this is due to the inhibition (hyperpolarization) by the brain of the motor neurons of the brainstem and the alpha motor neurons (the cells of the nervous system that stimulate muscles causing them to contract). Yet in spite of this inhibition, muscle twitches and jerks occur due to a variety of spontaneous action potentials and other brief excitations of the alpha motor neurons.

Parts of the genital regions are also affected by sleep. During REM there is an erection of the penis in males and the clitoris in females as well as lubrication of the vagina. In adolescents, these same events sometimes may also occur during NREM.

In NREM the overall low, steady levels of physiological activity appear to be the result of a activation of the parasympathetic nervous system and suppression of the sympathetic nervous system[2]. But, there are exceptions. First, the galvanic skin response (GSR) which is

---

[2] The sympathetic nervous system, together with the parasympathetic nervous system, make up the autonomic nervous system. This system controls the glands and internal organs. In general the two portions have opposing functions with the sympathetic arousing the body, mobilizing its energy in stressful situations. The parasympathetic portion, on the other hand, calms the body, conserving its energy.

controlled by the sympathetic nervous system begins to rise in stage two and peaks in SWS but is remarkably low and steady in REM. At the same time, the GSR is much greater on one side of the body than the other during sleep. Also GSR "storms" during SWS are related to pre-sleep stress and personality (Anch et al., 1988). Second, in some sleepers, K-complexes of stage 2 are accompanied by brief increases in heart rate, constriction of the blood vessels in the fingers, and sudden changes in the GSR. Third, the sympathetic system comes into action if, and when, necessary for homeostatic regulation.

During REM sleep the sympathetic nervous system is further depressed, but the balance between it and the parasympathetic nervous system is less stable (Parmeggiani, 1991; Siegel, 1990). This accounts for the large changes in heart rate, breathing rate, blood pressure, and so on that occur during REM. Typically, the sudden changes in these sympathetically controlled responses occur at the same time as bursts of the rapid eye movements that characterize phasic REM.

More recent discoveries have added to the list of the effects of sleep on the body. An increase in the ability of the blood to clot is associated with morning awakening and may partially account for the high incidence of sudden cardiac death in the morning (Willich, Tobler, & Muller, 1987). Some immune functions increase during sleep, especially during SWS (Moldofsky, Lue, Eisen, Keystone, & Gorczynski, 1986).

Bodily Effects On Sleep

It is also becoming apparent that certain physiological processes may affect sleep (Moorcroft & Clothier, 1987). For example, people who have higher daytime body temperatures sleep longer than the average, and there is a high correlation between basal metabolic rate and sleep length (Walker & Berger, 1980). Warm ambient temperatures tend to induce sleep probably because the body loses more heat during sleep and thus is able to use sleep as a means of cooling itself. Extremely cold or, to a lesser extent, extremely warm room temperatures (Parmeggiani, 1987), however, will increase awake time during sleep and alter the structure of sleep with REM being most vulnerable to a too warm or too cold room (Szymusiak & Satinoff, 1985). Some hormones affect sleep/wake (Borbély & Tobler, 1989; Horne, 1988;Krueger, Obál, Opp. Cady, Johannsen, Toth, & Majde, 1990). People with hypothyroidism show a decrease in SWS and stage 2 sleep and those with hyperthyroidism have more SWS. Vasopressin and hormones associated with the adrenal cortex promote wake. Growth hormone, vasoactive intestinal peptide, and somatostatin increase REM. Prolactin promotes sleep. Sensations from the internal body cavity (such as a full stomach) have been shown to induce sleep. Although lethargy is commonly reported by women before and during menstruation, laboratory sleep studies show no clear and consistent changes in sleep during the menstrual cycle (Mauri, 1990). Menopause produces changes in sleep noted by women themselves and in polysomnographic studies (Mauri, 1990). Stress during the waking hours before sleep reduces stage 4, increases awakenings, and disturbs REM (Anch et al. 1988; Koulack, 1991).

Changes in weather may affect sleep although little research has been done on its effects (Whitton, Kramer, & Eastwood, 1982). Weather, including temperature, humidity, barometric pressure, wind, ions, electric fields, electromagnetic fields, geomagnetic storms, lunar phase, infrasound, and solar disturbances has been shown to have effects on behavior (Persinger, 1980) and some aspects of weather (for example changes in barometric pressure [Borbély, 1986; Hauri, 1982]) may also have an effect on sleep. People who are undergoing dramatic gains of weight have long and generally uninterrupted sleep while those dramatically losing weight experience shortened and fragmented sleep (Danguir, 1988). Poor sleep may follow going to bed on an empty stomach and good sleep with a full stomach, but this may depend on your typical eating habits and what is eaten (Adam, 1980) since indigestion disrupts sleep. A snack prior to bed may disrupt sleep if you do not typically eat late in the evening. Hunger decreases total sleep time (Danguir & Nicoloides, 1985) and malnourished infants have less SWS and more REM (Brown & Price, 1988), but acute starvation increases SWS (Fagioli,Baroncini, Ricour, & Salzarulo, 1989). Thirst increases body movements and decreases REM (Koulack, 1991). Even dietary composition has been reported to change sleep (Hauri & Linde, 1990); for example, a diet with low carbohydrates and high fat intake produces an increase in REM, but eating carbohydrates prior to bedtime increases body temperature and

SWS time (Bunnell, Phillips, & Berger, 1991). It has been recently hypothesized that sleep varies with the overall metabolic rate of the body. Many other medical conditions, as well as physiologically toxic substances too numerous to detail here, are also known to affect sleep - usually detrimentally.

Exercise also affects sleep, but its effects depend on such factors as time of the nycthemeron and the fitness of the person, as well as type, duration, and intensity of the exercise (Anch et al., 1988; Broman, 1980), and the effect is only on the first NREM-REM cycle with no effect on TST (Anch et al., 1988). For example, in non-athletic individuals, intense aerobic exercise (swimming, running, bike riding, etc.) prior to bedtime arouses an individual and results in a longer sleep latency and a decrease in both REM and SWS (Montgomery, Trinder, Paxton, and Fraser, 1987). On the other hand, static exercise (weight lifting, push-ups, etc.) in the evening shortens sleep latency due to fatigue and causes SWS to occur earlier in the night. Overdoing any exercise can cause muscle pain which could disrupt sleep. The effects on sleep of exercise done earlier in the day are minimal. In trained athletes and other "fit" people, regular exercise has been observed to increase the overall amount of SWS. Regular aerobic exercise for anyone is thought to improve sleep (Trinder, Montgomery and Paxton, 1987). Horne (1987) has given convincing evidence that the increase in SWS produced by exercise or fitness is an indirect effect of an increase in body temperature produced by the exercise. This occurs only if there is a high rate of energy expenditure for at least 1/2 hour under conditions that cause the body to not easily lose heat (i.e. hot and humid air) (Horne, 1988). Extreme exercise can affect sleep for several days. Shapiro, Bortz, Mitchell, Bartel, & Jooste (1981) compared sleep in marathon runners before and after an 8 to 10 hour race. For the four nights after the race, sleep length increased as did the amount of SWS. REM decreased for the first two nights. Sleep latency was lower only on the first night, but wake-after-sleep-onset was also higher on that night (probably because of pain).

Pregnancy

The changes that occur in sleep during pregnancy dramatically demonstrate how changes in the body can affect sleep, and have been a special research interest of mine.

Interest in sleep and pregnancy started (for me at least) in 1979 when Don Jensen and I discovered that we lived about an hour apart from one another. Don and I had graduated together from college some 13 years earlier where we were in the same fraternity, had double dated together, and so on. But we had lost touch with one another as he went off to medical school and I to graduate school. Don was now an OB-GYN and I was intensively developing my interests in sleep disorders. Sitting in front of his fireplace that fall, we were reviewing our lives since we last saw one another. Don turned to me and asked, "What do you know about the sleep of pregnant women?"

"Nothing," I replied. "Why do you ask?"

"Well, a lot of my pregnant patients complain about changes in their sleep and dreams."

"Interesting. I'll see what I can find out about that."

With the help of computerized searching, I gathered together all of the existing reports of sleep and dreaming during pregnancy, about three dozen all told, and began to piece together a picture.

Almost at once I began to see problems with the research. Much of it focuses only on the third trimester of pregnancy. Some of the rest was retrospective, asking pregnant women to look back over their pregnancies and describe the changes in their sleep. Until recently, almost all of the sleep research (but not dream research) was done primarily for purposes other than to study sleep in pregnancy; pregnancy just happened to be a convenient way to study what was of primary interest. These interests included the effects of hormones on sleep (since there are many hormonal changes during pregnancy), contributions of late pregnancy sleep changes toward producing post-partum depression, and the parallels of the sleep-wake cycle of the fetus and mother (looking for a blood born sleep factor in the mother that would influence the sleep of the fetus). Much of the dream research was more directly aimed at dream changes during pregnancy but was not always carefully done.

Because of these flaws in prior research, I began in 1980 to do careful, systematic research of the changes in sleep and dreams that occur during pregnancy, paying special attention to the time of conception and the time of birth. The experiments were done both in the laboratory and through the use of subjective self-report forms which the women filled out at home. This work was done with the collaboration of Don Jensen, M.D., Sue Stueck, and Nancy Nielsen.

The following represents a composite of both the literature search (American Sleep Disorders Association, 1990; Anders & Roffwarg, 1968; Billiard & Passouant, 1973; Branchey & Petre-Quadens, 1968; Hertz, Fast, Feinsilver, Albertario, & Schulman, 1992; Hoppenbrouwers, Ugartechea, Combs, Hodgman, Harper, & Sterman, 1978; Karacan, 1968; Karacan, Heine, Agnew, Williams, Webb, & Ross, 1968; Karacan & Williams, 1970 a,b; Karacan, Williams, Hursch, McCaulley, & Heine, 1969; Petre-Quadens, DeBarsey, Devos, & Sfaello, 1967; Petre-Quadens & DeLee, 1974; Petre-Quadens, Hardy, & DeLee, 1969; Pivik, Azumi, & Dement, 1969; Schweiger, 1972; Sterman, 1967; Williams, Karacan, & Hursch, 1974) and my research.

Changes in sleep of any kind were recalled to have occurred during the first trimester by 13% of women, second trimester by 19%, third trimester by 68%, and all 3 trimesters by 11%. Polysomnographic studies of pregnant women generally show many changes in sleep as the pregnancy progresses. The most noticeable change is an increase in sleepiness and sleep (longer night sleep and increased napping) early in pregnancy. By the middle of pregnancy sleep has returned to typical-for-age levels but falls below these levels later in pregnancy. REM sleep may either increase or decrease during the middle of pregnancy but usually always is increased later in pregnancy. (Interestingly, both total sleep time and REM sleep levels may (but not always) return to typical-for-age during the last month of pregnancy). Meanwhile, during the middle of pregnancy, the level of SWS begins to drop, often (but not always) disappearing completely during later pregnancy. The levels of stages 1 and 2 sleep increase as SWS decreases. The number of awakenings begin to increase in mid-pregnancy, eventually reaching over four per night by the end of pregnancy; the awakenings are also of longer duration. As a result, sleep efficiency decreases. Sleep latency becomes longer toward the end of pregnancy, but REM latency shortens during this time.

Looking at these data another way, we can say that when a woman first becomes pregnant she will experience an increase in sleepiness and probably sleep more. As the pregnancy enters its second trimester, this excess sleepiness disappears, but she begins to wake up more during the night. Other less obvious changes in sleep are simultaneously beginning to occur in the second trimester in REM (increase or decrease), SWS (decrease) and stages 1 and 2 (increase). During the third trimester sleep is quite changed. Total sleep time is below typical-for-age levels, SWS is low or sometimes non-existent, it is harder for the woman to get to sleep, and she wakes up more and for longer periods of time. Yet REM occurs sooner and lasts longer, and there is more stage 1 and 2 than ever before. During the final month of pregnancy total sleep time and, sometimes, the amount of REM return to typical-for-age levels and the amount of SWS improves.

What happens following birth to the sleep of the mother? The picture is muddled by factors such as breast feeding versus not breast feeding, use and type of anesthetics during delivery, and so on. It will take more research to sort out the answer to this question. However, in one recent study (Hertz et al., 1991) women whose sleep was measured in the laboratory during late pregnancy were again studied 3-5 months later. They showed improvement in waking during sleep and sleep efficiency, but were still low in REM.

What is it about pregnancy that changes sleep in these ways? Changes in body size undoubtedly have an effect, but so do the metabolic and hormonal changes that accompany pregnancy. Disruptions to physical comfort, especially lower back pain, indigestion, leg cramps, uterine contractions, and pressure on the bladder become more and more disruptive to sleep as the pregnancy progresses.

(The changes in dreams during pregnancy are summarized in chapter 5.)

Alcohol and Caffeine

The effects of alcohol and caffeine on sleep and wakefulness are especially worthy of discussion. Both are widely known to have effects on sleep and wake, but recent research has expanded our understanding of their effects (Anch et al., 1988; Mendelson, 1989; Plath, Roehrs, Zwyghuizen-Doorenbos, Sidlesteel, Wittig, & Roth, 1989; Roehrs, Zwyghuizen-Doorenbos, Zwyghuizen, Timms, Fortier, & Roth, 1989; Walsh, Humm, Muehlbach, Sugerman, & Schweitzer, 1989; Walsh, Muehlbach, Humm, Stokes, Dickins, & Schweitzer, 1989; Zarcone, 1990; Zwyghurizen-Doorenbos, Roehrs, Russo, Buzenski, Wittig, Lomphere, & Roth, 1989).

Alcohol has a potent affect on sleep. A couple of drinks shortens the time to get to sleep, which has often prompted people to use it as a sleep medicine. But actually, any amount of alcohol disturbs sleep. It increases the latency to REM, decreases the percent of REM sleep, and decreases the density of eye movements during REM. Depending on the amount of alcohol consumed this may last only half the night (with compensatory rebound in the second half) or the entire night. There is also an increase in the number of awakenings during sleep and maybe more SWS. Total sleep time is unaffected. It has been reported that it may take four days for sleep to return to normal after an episode of drunkenness. After only a few days of continued moderate use of alcohol REM gradually returns to normal levels or to slightly above normal. When alcohol use is subsequently discontinued there is greatly higher levels of REM for a few days (called REM rebound). Alcoholics have more arousals from sleep, more stage changes, and more REM. During abstinence, alcoholics will experience disturbed sleep for several months and less SWS with more stage changes for as long as two years.

More recently attention has focused on the effects of alcohol on wakefulness (Knox, Roehrs, Claiborne, Stepanski, & Roth, 1991; Roth, 1990; Zarcone, 1990). Severity of sleepiness is directly related to the degree of sleep deprivation and the amount of alcohol consumed. That is, as prior sleepiness increases, it takes less alcohol to make a person sleepy. But this effect also depends on the time of day (circadian rhythm effect) - drinking during the late afternoon increases sleepiness more than drinking during the early evening. Consumption of an excessive amount of alcohol tends to make people sleepy regardless of time of day or prior sleep deprivation, and severely sleep deprived people do not become sleepier following alcohol intake.

Surprisingly, the sleepiness induced by alcohol has been shown to outlast the blood (breath) levels of the alcohol. It is as if the alcohol stimulates a sleep drive that continues until something alerts the person (such as obtaining some sleep or a circadian wake zone [see Chapter 4] is entered). The practical consequences of such effects have been demonstrated in experiments using simulated driving in the laboratory (Beare, Roehrs, Battle, Waller, Zorick, & Roth, 1992). In one experiment half of the subjects were allowed a full night of sleep but the other half only half a night of sleep. Half of each group were given alcohol and the other half drank something that seemed to contain alcohol but did not. In simulated driving tests several hours later, only the half-a-night-of-sleep-plus-alcohol group had more difficulty keeping the car on the road and several had "crashes" even though their blood alcohol levels approached zero at the time of testing.

Caffeine also affects sleep/wake (Gaillared, 1990). Caffeine impairs sleep and promotes wakefulness. It tends to lengthen sleep onset time, increase amount of wakefulness after sleep onset, and increase numbers of awakenings. It also decreases the amount of SWS and decreases REM latency. But as many people realize, there are marked individual differences in its effects. I have to be careful not to consume caffeine in the evening, or I will have trouble getting to sleep. (Some people are so sensitive to its effects that coffee in the morning makes sleep at night difficult.) My wife, Christina, can drink several cups of coffee right before bed and then get to sleep quickly and easily because "the warmth makes her sleepy."

Caffeine helps keep people alert and awake. This is not a new and surprising statement, but actually little research has been done to confirm this until recently (Muehlbach, Schweitzer, Stuchey, & Walsh, 1991; Platt et al., 1989; Walsh, Muehlbach, Humm, Dickins, Sugerman, & Schweitzer, 1990). This research does confirm the beneficial effectiveness of caffeine in making people more alert and less physiologically sleepy during a night of sleep deprivation and following a night of partial sleep. Specifically, two to four cups of coffee is equivalent to 3.5 hours of mid-afternoon nap prior to a night without sleep. However, four things need to be noted. (1) Caffeine does not replace sleep or entirely eliminate sleepiness. For example, as a night without sleep wears on, subjects who drank coffee with caffeine became more and more sleepy just as did those who had no caffeine in their coffee, but there was always a magnitude of difference between the two groups (i.e. lines on the graph of sleepiness of the two groups paralleled each other and increased at the same rate but were always a fixed distance apart). (2) Unlike alcohol, caffeine does not seem to interact with the degree of sleepiness. It seems to add a constant amount of alertness to your current level of alertness much like adding a gallon of gas to a car's gas tank will raise the level of gas a fixed amount regardless if there is 1/4 or 3/4 of a tank initially. (3) However, like the effects of alcohol on sleepiness, the arousal effects of caffeine on wakefulness outlast its presence in the blood as if it triggers an alertness drive, but continued presence of caffeine is not necessary to sustain it. (4) Although objective measurements show that caffeine reduces the physiological drive for sleep and improves the accuracy and speed of performance during a night of sleep deprivation, subjects own subjective feelings of sleepiness were very much less affected. They reported increasing tiredness as the night went on that was indistinguishable from the tiredness reported by subjects who drank coffee without caffeine.

(The negative effects of other drugs on sleep, including nicotine and recreational drugs, can be found in chapter 9.)

Elements of the Brain Important for Sleep

Certainly a thorough understanding of sleep requires a review of what is known of the brain mechanisms in sleep. While this can be enormously complex (so much so that students are often fearful of even approaching the subject), we will emphasize a less complicated, yet substantial understanding of how the brain participates in sleep. Just as you do not have to be an electrical engineer to understand the essentials of how a computer works or a physiologist to understand the basic ideas of digestion, you don't have to be a brain scientist to become acquainted with how the brain is involved with sleep. With this in mind, let us seek understanding of how the brain participates in sleep.

During the last fifty years there has been intense interdisciplinary scientific study of the physiology of sleep (Jones, 1989). Early investigators used the research tools available to them (brain damage, brain stimulation, and recording brain waves) which led them to a focus on certain parts of the brain as having a role in sleep/wake. As the technology of the tools improved (e.g., recording of the electrical activity of single neurons, drugs capable of selectively influencing certain types of cells, and stains for specific kinds of cell components), so did the detail of the knowledge of the involvement of the brain in sleep. Over the last 25 years there has been a shift in focus to specific neurotransmitters involved in sleep and the cells that produce and receive them. As these efforts led to more knowledge about the neural basis of sleep, our image of the nature of sleep has changed. Most dramatically, it changed from seeing sleep as a single, passive entity to seeing it as a multifaceted, active state.

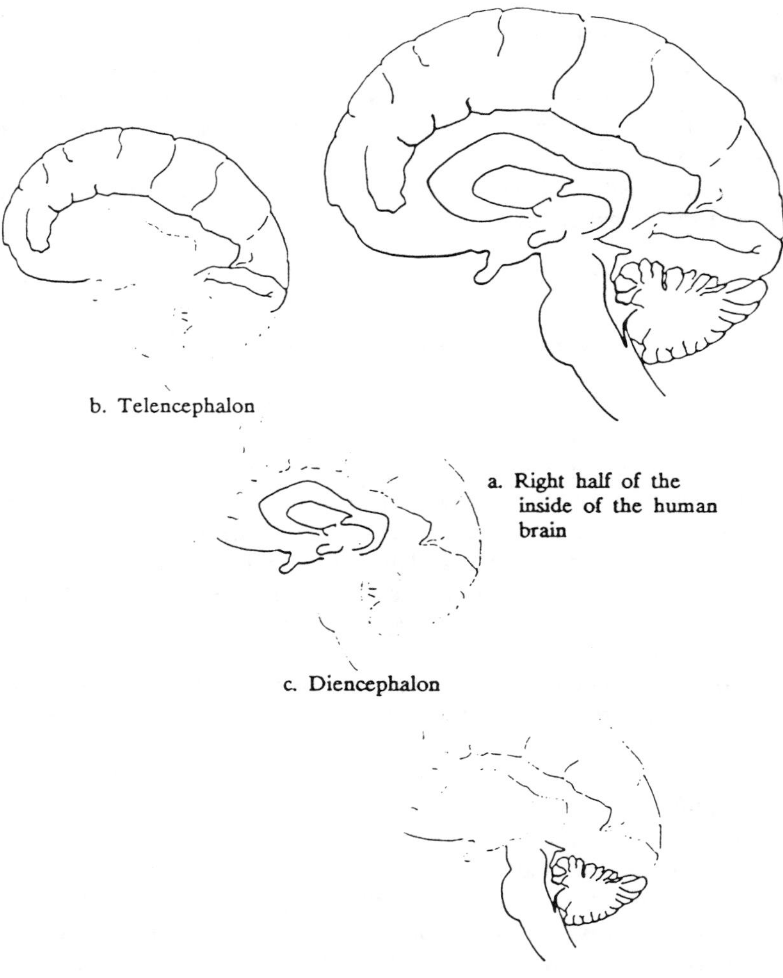

Figure 2-1. The three layers of the brain.

The initiation and maintenance of sleep requires the coordinated activity of brain structures that often differ from those responsible for wakefulness. While no single physiological or chemical model can as of yet totally illustrate the mechanisms controlling sleep, research has provided much knowledge of the role of brain structures in the sleep-wake cycle. But before we proceed to review this research, we first must review the basic structure and chemistry of the brain placing an emphasis on those elements especially important in the control of sleep.

Brain structures. There are many ways to describe the levels of the hierarchy of the brain. The following, however, is most convenient for discussing the brain's involvement in sleep.

Think of the brain as being put together like an onion that has three layers, each of which can be peeled away revealing the layerbelow. The top layers are capable of producing more variations in functions than lower layers. Further, the top layer generally controls and modifies the activity of the layers below. This arrangement of both structure and function is called a hierarchy and is not unlike the structure of a corporation or army. On the lowest layer are the workers or soldiers who rather routinely do the work by following the rules and commands of their supervisors. Next is middle management or officers who monitor the activity of the workers or soldiers and make corrections and adjustments where necessary to meet the goals and requirements set by those superior to them. Finally, at the top is executive management or commanding officers. They are in charge of formulating the goals and making major modifications in how the goals are met or even changing the goal if necessary. Additionally, the lower levels have the responsibility of informing higher levels of how things are going, especially if they are not going well. All of these have parallels in the brain.

Figure 2-1 shows the three layers of the brain: the outermost TELENCEPHALON, a middle layer called the DIENCEPHALON, and the central BRAINSTEM (midbrain and hindbrain). The telencephalon is superior anatomically and functionally. The most striking and obvious structure in the telencephalon is the CEREBRAL CORTEX (refer to Figure 2-2 to find the location of this and any other brain areas mentioned is this section) which covers most of the outside surface of the brain. It plays an important role in sleep/wakefulness as well as in most other behaviors. Lying below the cortex, towards the front of the brain, is the BASAL FOREBRAIN AREA, another part of the telencephalon important in sleep. The hippocampus is a ram's horn shaped structure lying towards the back of the brain above the thalamus and below the cortex. (It is not shown in any of the figures.)

The diencephalon is the layer below the telencephalon. Important structures here include the midline group of the THALAMUS and portions of the HYPOTHALAMUS (lying just below the thalamus), including its anterior (front) PREOPTIC AREA, SUPRACHIASMATIC NUCLEUS, and POSTERIOR HYPOTHALAMUS. Anterior portions of the hypothalamus are a part of the BASAL FOREBRAIN AREA. The thalamus is an important communication link between the cortex and lower brain structures. The hypothalamus also controls functions that are necessary to life such as eating, drinking, body

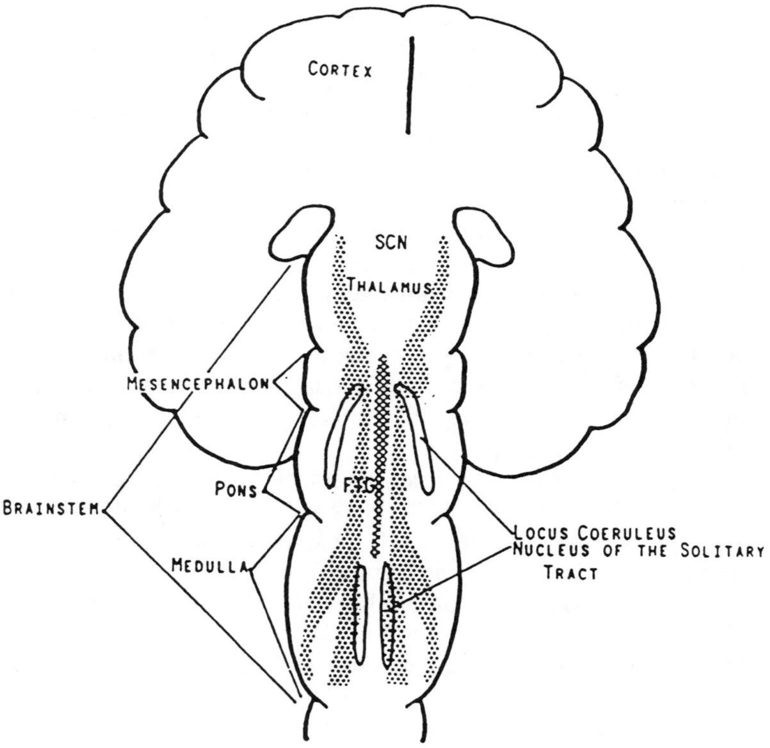

Figure 2-2. The parts of the human brain involved in sleep and waking. The view on the left is from the front looking somewhat down

temperature regulation, and hormone production.

The brainstem projects back (down in humans) from the diencephalon. In addition to containing major lines of communication between the brain and body it also has areas of importance in the control of very basic body functions such as heartbeat and breathing. A number of its divisions are also important in sleep/wakefulness including the RETICULAR FORMATION which runs through the core of the brain stem, the PONS which is the central section of the brainstem, the RAPHÉ which is a group of cells in the midline in the

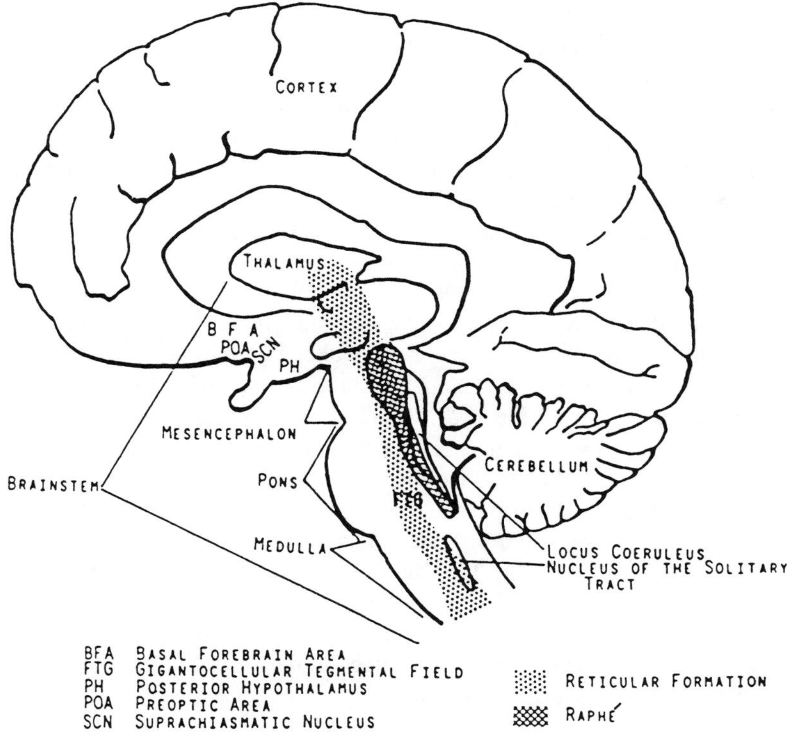

at the back half of the brain. The figure on the right is from the left looking at the inside of the right half of the brain.

center of the brainstem, the NUCLEUS OF THE SOLITARY TRACT located in the lower brainstem, the AREA POSTREMA which occupies a small site at the top of the lower brainstem, and the LOCUS COERULEUS in the front middle of the brainstem.

Brain chemistry. While information is conveyed electrically **within** brain cells, communication **between** these cells is chemical. That is, cells release chemicals called neurotransmitters that have a brief but important effect on adjacent cells. That effect is electrical (electrochemical) and the entire process conveys information from one cell to the next. Although there are many kinds of transmitter chemicals, a single cell is limited in the number it can manufacture. The transmitter chemicals are made from other chemicals called precursors. After the receiver cell is affected by the chemical, other substances may render it ineffective by breaking the chemical apart into what are called metabolites. Among the important neurotransmitters of the brain are acetylcholine, serotonin, norepinephrine, dopamine, histamine, glutamate, and GABA. Drugs (such as sleeping pills) that affect behavior are but substances that act on the transmitter chemicals, their precursors, or the release/reception process in such a way that the message carrying function is disrupted, enhanced, modified, or mimicked.

When discussing the sleep/wake mechanisms in the brain there is a need to distinguish between sleep/wake facilitating mechanisms, sleep/wake inducing mechanisms, and sleep/wake maintenance mechanisms (after Karacan & Moore, 1985). Sleep/wake facilitating mechanisms are neither necessary nor sufficient to produce sleep but can cause drowsiness and facilitate sleep onset and/or increase the duration of sleep if sleep inducing factors (chemical or neural) are active. Sleep/wake inducing mechanisms are a part of the executive mechanisms of sleep in the brain or have a powerful effect on executive mechanisms that result in a change of state. Sleep/wake maintenance mechanisms act to continue the existence of a particular state. In some cases two or all three of these mechanisms may be served by the same brain circuit.

Wakefulness

The areas of the brain important for the state of wakefulness include the portions of the reticular formation that are located in the

PONS and midbrain (often known collectively as the Ascending Reticular Activating System or ARAS), the posterior hypothalamus, the basal forebrain, and, in some sense, the cortex (Jones, 1989).

Of these, the ARAS is arguably the most influential. The ARAS is located in the core of the brainstem (see Figure 2-2 for this and other brain areas mentioned here) and extends upward into the forebrain via two circuits. The first travels from the cortex through a part of the thalamus (the most medial parts called the midline thalamus) and on to diffuse areas of the cortex. This is known as the "dorsal system" (Jones, 1990), and is important for physiological indicators of wakefulness in the cortex (such as beta waves).

The second circuit leads from the ARAS to and through areas below the thalamus including the posterior hypothalamus on to the basal forebrain and nearby areas, which in turn project widely to the cortex and hippocampus. Known as the "ventral system", this circuit is important for the behavioral aspects of wakefulness and alertness. The higher parts of the circuit are able to cause arousal even without ARAS inputs. For example, research on laboratory animals shows that stimulation of the posterior hypothalamus causes a sleeping animal to awaken. This suggests that while the ARAS influences wake, it is not essential for it. All of these areas just mentioned are more electrically active during wakefulness compared to sleep. Stimulation of the ARAS caused EEG desynchronization (low voltage, fast waves such as beta waves) and behavioral arousal, while its destruction results in a slow, synchronous EEG (such as SWS waves) and a coma state. It receives direct information from almost all of the senses of the body. It also receives a great deal of input from the cortex. Although it is incapable of interpreting the sensory information beyond the level of "something different or important is going on out there", it can inform the cerebral cortex that it needs to be alert in order to assess what is happening.

Certain neurotransmitters are known to be important in specific portions of these wakefulness circuits. Norepinephrine is used by the ARAS to influence the cortex via the dorsal system and dopamine is used in the ventral system. Acetylcholine is used by parts of the ARAS to influence the diencephalon and basal forebrain and by the basal forebrain to influence the cortex and hippocampus. Histamine is used by the posterior hypothalamus to influence the cortex (and is thought to account for the drowsiness effects of anti-histamines). Glutamate is influential in the cortex and many areas below it, including the midline thalamus, for wakefulness, and serotonin is also thought to be important in wakefulness (Jones, 1990). Also found in many of these same areas are various neuropeptides which may enhance and prolong the effects of the neurotransmitters in their arousal functions. Many blood born factors (such as epinephrine, histamine, and peptides) enter the cerebral spinal fluid (CRF) and influence many of these brain areas to heighten alertness.

C. H. Vanderwolf (1990) maintains that activation of the cells in the cortex and hippocampus characteristic of wakefulness is caused by acetylcholine and serotonin influencing pathways from subcortical structures. These in turn may be regulated by norepinephrine, dopamine, and histamine pathways. This is in opposition to the ARAS notion of cortical activation.

Sleep

Sleep onset can be viewed as a two stage process (Karacan & Moore, 1985; Sterman, Szymusiak, & McGinty, 1990): inhibition of the arousal system and facilitation of the sleep induction system. First a generalized reduction of activity in the cortex occurs as shown by a slowing of the frequency of the EEG waves. This is followed by intermittent higher frequency activity (sleep spindles - see Chapter 1). Both of these involve changes in the thalamus (Anonymous, 1991). The slowing of brain waves is important for the behavioral (both cognitive and motor) suppression by the cortex that is so necessary for sleep onset and maintenance. The spindles may be a manifestation of the near-isolation by the thalamus of the cortex from the normal sources of potentially excitatory sensory input (Steriade, 1990). Sleep spindles are a result of the activity of pacemaker cells of the reticular cells in the thalamus (McCarley & Massaquoi, 1992; Steriade, 1990). Spindles seem to be intermediate between the low voltage, fact activity of wake (and REM) and the slow (delta waves) of SWS. Delta waves are the result of cortical cells being paced by cells of the thalamus (aided by local cortical cells) in the absence of activating influences from areas of the brain that produce wake and REM (see above and below). Sleep is facilitated by a decrease in most sensory input normally relayed by the thalamus to the cortex, but is aided by an increase in certain other sensory input (such as warmth and a full stomach) on areas of the brain that cause sleep (Jones, 1989). These processes set the stage for the sleep induction system to take control.

NREM induction appears to be controlled by multiple parallel systems spread throughout the brain but especially by portions of the basal forebrain area, hypothalamus, thalamus, and nucleus of the solitary tract in the brainstem (Siegel, 1990). (The role of the raphé, once considered to be a key area for the initiation of sleep, is now unclear.) Although in the minority, there are cells in these areas that are more active during sleep than during wake (Jones 1989). There is evidence that these cells are interconnected with one another (Jones, 1989).

Cells in the basal forebrain area seem to have a key role in the initiation and maintenance of NREM sleep. The basal forebrain area has many connections to brainstem, limbic, and cortical areas by which it can perform its sleep functions (McGinty & Szymusiak, 1989). The sleep initiating neurons of the basal forebrain are located close to neurons involved in temperature regulation (especially heat loss) which may provide the neural mechanism that links sleep with temperature regulation (Jones, 1990; McGinty & Szymusiak, 1990a in Mancia & Marini). (Recall that the basal forebrain was also mentioned as important for wakefulness. The same area can have seemingly opposite functions because different populations of cells within it have different functions utilizing different neurotransmitters [Jones, 1990]. Some, but not all, cells in the basal forebrain area are maximally active during NREM [Siegel, 1990].)

In the brainstem area, the nucleus of the solitary tract may also have a role in the facilitation of sleep. Its role may be in attenuating the arousal effect of the ascending reticular activating system resulting in drowsiness. This area receives input from the vagus nerve, whose stimulation results in sleep-like brain waves. Since the vagus nerve transmits a variety of information to the nucleus of the solitary tract from the stomach and intestines, a large meal may result in stimulation of this brain area and in turn drowsiness.

There are several neurotransmitters thought important for NREM (Jones, 1989). Adenosine is used especially by hypothalamic neurons for this purpose. It is blocked by caffeine, hence the ability of coffee and other caffeine containing beverages to ward off sleep. GABA is used greatly in the hypothalamus and basal forebrain area. Cells that produce both spindles and delta waves rely on this neurotransmitter.

The effects of GABA are enhanced by one type of sleeping pill. Spindles and delta waves are blocked during other states by acetylcholine from pontine cells. Neuropeptides, including the endorphins, are found in many of these "sleep" areas. Other substances thought involved with NREM include somatostatin, prostaglandin, serotonin, insulin, sleep peptides (such as DSIP), and hormones. More recently, GABA-containing neurons that inhibit the ARAS arousal function have been found interspersed within the ARAS itself (Jones, 1990).

REM Sleep

There is little doubt that the pons contains the cells that are necessary, if not sufficient, for the occurrence of REM (Siegel, 1990). The brain above or below the pons can be removed, yet REM persists. Only when the integrity of the pons is violated does REM cease to occur.

REM ON. A population of cells in the pons is responsible for initiating and maintaining a REM episode (Hobson, Lydic, & Baghogan, 1986; McGinty et al., 1989; Siegel, 1989, 1990; McCarley & Massaquoi, 1992). These cells tend to be important for one or more of the components of REM, yet no single group of them is the chief executive that initiates REM. They do not lie close to one another, but they are linked to one another. They function more like a committee whose members communicate with one another by phone. Although these cells are necessary for REM, they are in contact with, rely on, and are influenced by, other parts of the brain both above and below for the complete and normal manifestation of REM. A major component of these influential cells exists in the reticular formation in the medulla. The neurotransmitter acetylcholine is much used by these cells to communicate with one another.

REM OFF. Another diffusely scattered yet interconnected set of cells (another committee) are antagonistic to the function of the REM ON cells (Hobson et al., 1986; McGinty et al., 1988; Sakai, 1986; Siegel, 1989; 1990). When active, they turn REM off and keep it off, but in the process they gradually turn themselves off to permit REM to occur. Some REM OFF cells are scattered among REM ON cells in the pons, with other major concentrations in the locus coeruleus, dorsal raphé, and other parts of the pons. The REM OFF cells rely on serotonin and norepinephrine for their communication. REM OFF cells are very active during waking and NREM to prevent the occurrence of REM or its components. However, they are silent during REM.

Other cells in the dorsal raphé (using serotonin) are thought to be especially important for the timing and coordination of the events of REM by disinhibiting various REM ON neurons (Hobson et al., 1986; McGinty et al., 1988; Sakai, 1986; Siegel, 1989;1990). This same area also seems to play a role in terminating a REM episode since they increase firing just before the end of REM. They are also important for "gating" PGO spikes (see below). Other evidence suggests that the posterior hypothalamus, using the neurotransmitter histamine, may also be a part of the REM control system (Lapierre, Montplaisir, Lamarre, & Bedard, 1990; McCarley, 1990). (The locus coeruleus and pontine gigantocellular tegmental field (FTG), once considered the REM ON system, are themselves no longer considered important for REM [Sakai, 1986]).

In the 1970s J. Alan Hobson and Robert W. McCarley developed a model to explain the alternation of NREM with REM during sleep (McCarley & Hobson, 1975). They hypothesized a lawful relationship in the way that REM OFF and REM ON areas influenced one another. Although in succeeding years the description of the lawful relationship changed, as did the knowledge of the exact identity and location of REM OFF and REM ON components (McCarley & Massaquoi, 1986), this Reciprocal-Interaction Model (most recently named the Limit Cycle Reciprocal Interaction Model or LCRIM [McCarley & Massaqueri, 1992]) has been very important and influential. The current version is shown in Figure 2-3. The characteristics of the REM OFF and REM ON cells were described above. The relationship between these two pools of cells is such that the REM ON cells excite the REM OFF cells as well as being self excitatory. The REM OFF cells inhibit the REM ON cells using serotonin, as well as tending to inhibit themselves. The regular alternation and duration of REM and NREM depend on the rate of strength build up of the various inhibitory and excitatory loops.

The sequence of events shown in Figure 2-3 can be described (McCarley, 1990; McCarley & Massaquoi, 1986; 1992) as a gradual reduction in activity of the REM OFF cells reducing the inhibition of the REM ON cells eventually permitting them to become increasingly

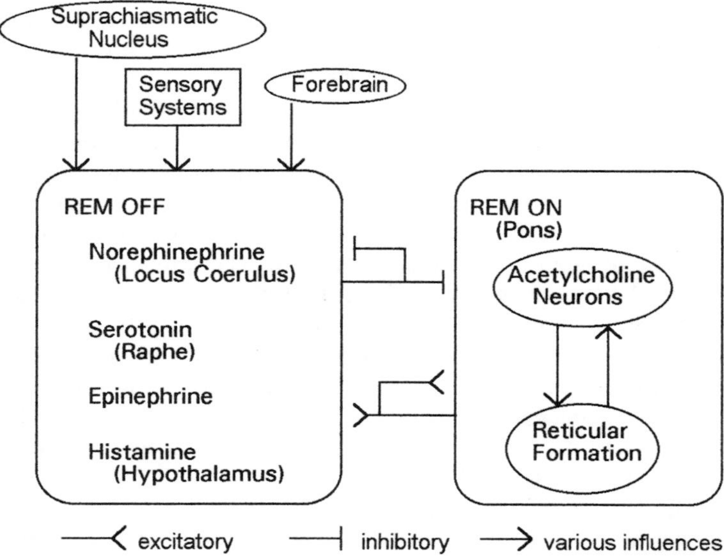

Figure 2-3. The revised version of the Hobson-McCarley Model. After Hobson, 1988 and McCarley & Massaquoi, 1992.

active and start a REM episode. When REM ON cells are active, they strongly excite themselves but also gradually strengthen excitation of the REM OFF cells. Eventually, the excitation of the REM OFF cells reaches a threshold and they suddenly become active and strongly inhibit the REM ON cells at which point the REM episode ceases. But the REM OFF cells also begin to inhibit themselves. As this self inhibition gradually becomes stronger the REM OFF cells begin to lose their ability to inhibit the REM ON cells permitting another REM episode to begin. (See Figure 2-4 for a graphic representation of the outcome of these relationships which is analogous to the population cycles of rabbits and wolves). These relationships are more fully described in mathematical terms as a "limit cycle" (see McCarley & Massaquoi, 1986; 1992a). The REM OFF cells remain active during wakefulness to prevent the components of REM from occurring during wake. The turning on and off of this entire reciprocally interacting system is under the control of circadian mechanisms (McCarley & Massaquoi, 1986), mainly the suprachiasmatic nucleus (described below), and also under the control of other influences (McCarley & Massaquoi, 1992) including: (1) body temperature, (2) inputs from many sensory systems allowing both internal and external sensory influences that are known to interrupt REM, and (3) inputs from forebrain areas (especially the frontal lobe) involved in emotion and cognition which are known to influence REM.

This model describes how REM as a whole is generated and terminated. Other evidence can be used to describe how the various components, both tonic and phasic, of REM are generated. They are the result of activity in subsystems that are directly controlled by both excitatory REM ON and inhibitory REM OFF neurons (Sakai, 1985; Jones, 1985).

The EEG of REM is characterized by desynchronized activity (irregular, low voltage brain waves). This is driven by cells in the reticular formation (mainly midbrain, but also anterior pons and medulla) via midline thalamic nuclei (the same mechanism that produces awake arousal EEG) aided by a second pathway involving the posterior hypothalamus which then projects to the cortex (Hobson et al., 1986; McGinty et al., 1989; Sakai 1985, 1986; Siegel 1989, 1990). At least a part of this system is importantly receptive to, and releases, the neurotransmitter acetylcholine.

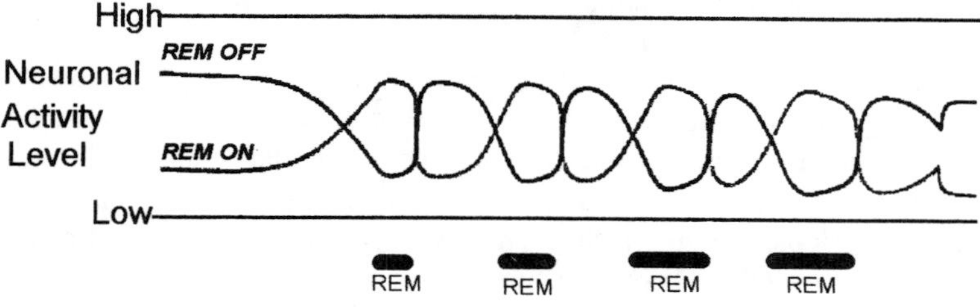

Figure 2-4. A graphic representation of the outcome of the Hobson-McCarley model showing the alternation between NREM and REM. Adapted with permission of the author from Hobson J A (1983). Sleep: order and disorder. *Behavioral Biology in Medicine, 1*, 1-36.

One of the strongest and most dramatic components of REM is the virtual paralysis of the muscles of movement. At one time it was thought that the locus coeruleus was the source of this paralysis, but more recent evidence places the command neurons in areas near the locus coeruleus (Drucker-Colin & Prospero-Garcia, 1990; Hobson et al., 1986; McGinty et al., 1986; Siegel, 1992). These cells excite a group of cells in the reticular formation of the medulla (using acetylcholine and glutamate) that, in turn, excite spinal cord inhibitory interneurons. The spinal cord inhibitory interneurons cause a hyperpolarization of the alpha motor neurons (using glycine) which effectively stops any motor commands from reaching the muscles. A parallel system may originate in another portion of the pons. Although paralyzed in this way, muscle twitches do occur during REM especially in animals and babies. This occurs when motor neurons in the brain are phasically excited enough to briefly overcome the tonic inhibition. This often occurs in conjunction with a burst of rapid eye movements. Another explanation involves the fact that glutamate can have different effects on different cells - resulting in motor inhibition generally, but occasional motor excitation in others.

Experiments with cats show that small damage near the locus coeruleus eliminates the muscle inhibition associated with REM (Sastre & Jouvet, 1979). Such damage causes an animal to "behave" during REM sleep as if acting out its dreams! Especially prominent was predatory attack, but rage, flight, grooming and exploration have also been observed. Figure 2-5 shows photographs taken during REM sleep of a cat with damage to a portion of the brain near the locus coeruleus; it appears to be acting out a dream.

The third hallmark of REM is the rapid eye movements, for which this stage of sleep was named. Phasic firing of neurons in the reticular formation of the pons, and cells in the vestibular nucleus, in turn excite the oculomotor neurons, which control the muscles that move the eyes (Hobson et al., 1986). These muscles are not inhibited as are other muscles of the body, because the neural circuits that control eye movements are devoid of the inhibitory interneurons that are found in the control circuits of other muscles (Feinberg, 1987).

Related to rapid eye movements, but less obvious, is activity called PGO waves that occur in parts of the brain (Drucker-Colin & Prospero-Garcia, 1990; Hobson et al., 1986; Horne, 1988; McGinty, Drucker-Colin, Morrison, & Parmeggiani, 1985; McCarley, 1991;

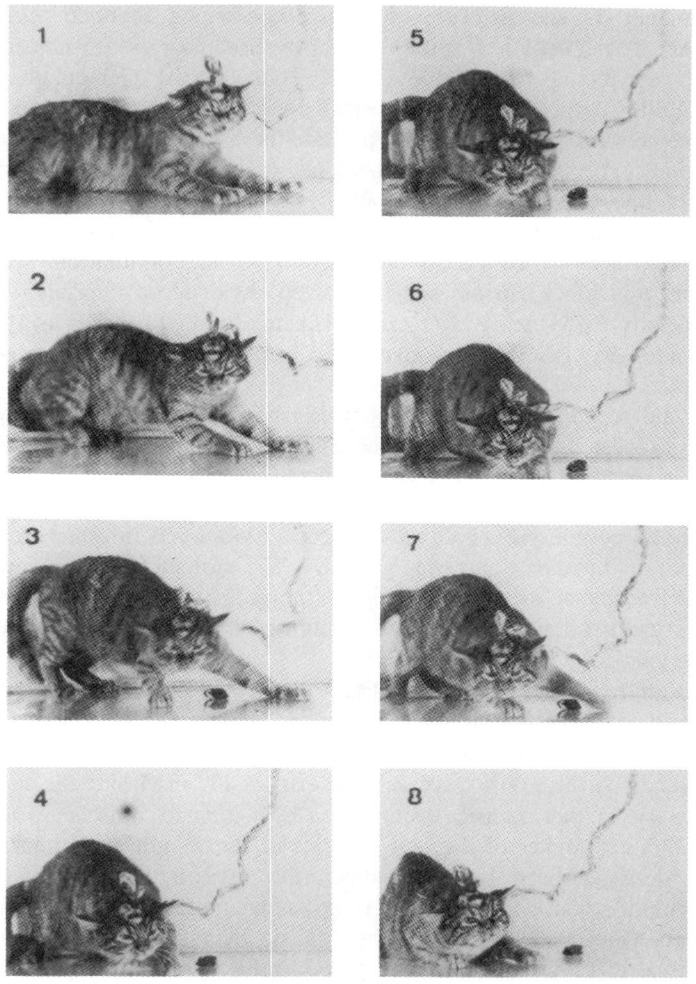

Figure 2-5. A series of photographs is shown of a cat whose brain near the caudal locus coeruleus has been removed. The cat is in REM sleep and appears to be acting out a dream. (From Jouvet M [1980]. Paradoxical sleep and the nature-nurture controversy. *Progress in brain research*, *53*, 331-346. With permission.)

Mamelak & Hobson, 1989; Siegel, 1989; 1990; Steriade & Pare, 1990). These negative, spikey appearing brain waves are named for their sequential appearance in the Pons, lateral Geniculate, and Occipital cortex. They occur just before a burst of rapid eye movements. They typically also precede the onset of REM by 30 to 90 seconds. They are more prominent on the side of the brain towards which the eyes move. PGO waves may convey information to the forebrain about the direction of intended eye movements. They are spontaneous in REM but can be driven by sensory stimulation (such as sound and touch) in any stage of sleep. After sleep deprivation, or especially REM deprivation, the frequency of PGO waves increases dramatically. PGO waves have never been satisfactorily recorded in humans.

The so called burst cells (because of their pattern of firing in bursts) located in the region of the border of the pons and midbrain are the generators of PGO waves. These cells project to the lateral geniculate nucleus in the diencephalon, which in turn projects to the occipital cortex, but activity has also been observed in other areas of the brain including the hippocampus. The system seems to rely on acetylcholine as its neurotransmitter, but is disinhibited by REM OFF cells using norepinephrine and facilitated by REM ON cells using acetylcholine.

Rapid eye movements and PGO waves are major components of the phasic events of REM. So named because of their occasional, irregular occurrence in distinction to the constant (called tonic) presence of the brain waves characteristics of REM and the muscle paralysis. Other phasic events of REM include muscle twitches, MEMAS (twitches of the tiny muscles of the middle ear), and PIPS (electrical activity recorded about the eyeball). There is some speculation that PGO waves are the pacemakers for many phasic REM events (Siegel, 1989; 1990), but phasic events may occur in the absence of PGO waves (Seligman & Yellin, 1987) and PGO waves have been observed apart from rapid eye movements when certain parts of the brain are damaged (Siegel, 1990). The phasic events of REM may be "modified versions of the startle reflex" (Glenn, 1985) or orienting responses (see chapter 11) that occur in both wake and sleep (Morrison & Reiner, 1985).

Our discussion of the brain mechanisms involved in the production of REM was longer than for other sleep states. Not only did this occur because more is known about REM, but also because REM may be more complex. It also just may be a convenient assemblage of components (McCarley & Massaquoi, 1992) that need to be recruited in a specific order rather than a unified state (Hobson et al., 1986). Not only is this shown by the fact that various and separable brain systems are involved, but also because several of the many components of REM can be dissociated from it using various experimental techniques in the lab (Morrison & Reiner, 1985; Siegel, 1989). For example, REM without muscle paralysis can be produced by brain damage near the locus coeruleus (as discussed previously) and muscle paralysis without REM can be produced by extra acetylcholine in these same brain areas.

Circadian Rhythms

A number of experimenters have looked for the brain area or areas that are a part of the circadian system controlling sleep and wakefulness (Moorcroft & Clothier, 1987). Studies have shown the suprachiasmatic nucleus of the hypothalamus (SCN) to have circadian rhythms in its metabolic activity, in the firing rate of isolated groups of its cells, and even in the firing rate of some of its isolated single cells. Damage to the SCN abolishes the circadian rhythm of sleep without changing the proportions of NREM and REM. The SCN appears to be an important link for entraining the circadian cycle of wake/sleep to the light/dark cycles of the external environment because it receives direct connections from the retina (separate from the primary visual pathway) which report on amount of light (Czeizler & Allen, 1988) and indirect connections via the lateral geniculate nucleus. Without these visual inputs, the circadian rhythm of sleep still occurs but is not entrained (Karacan & Moore, 1985). The SCN sends output to many of the brainstem areas that affect the timing of sleep, especially the REM OFF areas, and to areas of the hypothalamus that control hormone release (Hobson et al., 1986). The pineal gland is especially affected by the SCN in its production of the hormone melatonin (Mendelson, 1987; Mirmiran & Box, 1990). (Interestingly, melatonin tends to inhibit the SCN [Mirmiran & Box, 1990].) Destruction of these outputs from the SCN abolishes circadian rhythm of sleep (Karacan & Moore, 1985).

Neurotransmitters and Sleep

Some information about the involvement of neurotransmitters in sleep has been presented in our discussion of the areas of the brain involved in sleep. Other research has been concerned with what neurotransmitters are involved more generally in sleep and wakefulness, even if the specific loci of their involvement is less clear. Neurotransmitters are not the only chemicals in the brain that seem to influence sleep. Such chemicals are known as endogenous (meaning normally found within the body) sleep substances and include hormones, as well as other substances, known to have many effects throughout the body. Our discussion shall focus on substances for which there is reasonably strong experimental support and general agreement (Drucker-Colin & Prospero-Garcia, 1990).

Acetylcholine. Acetylcholine is a neurotransmitter found in many parts of the nervous system including many areas of the brain involved with sleep (Benington & Heller, 1991; Shiromani, Gillin & Hendriksen, 1987). Cells of the basal forebrain area use it to communicate with other portions of the forebrain, diencephalon, and somewhat to the brain stem, with at least some of these circuits being involved with sleep and wakefulness. The dorsal lateral pons, as well as other areas, uses acetylcholine to initiate and maintain REM and the components of REM including brain waves, PGO waves, and muscle paralysis. It is also important in alertness (wake) especially the brain waves characteristic of this state.

Serotonin. The understanding of the role of serotonin has evolved over the years (Monti, Piñeyro, Orellana, Boussard, Jantos, Labraga, Olivera, & Alvariño, 1990). In the 1970's it was thought responsible for the onset of SWS and the "priming" of REM, because damage to the raphé (the main source of serotonin in the brain) and drugs that deplete the brain of serotonin both resulted in less sleep. However, other evidence showed that the cells that use serotonin as their neurotransmitter were much less active in NREM and virtually silent during REM. Thus in the 1980's Jouvet (1984; 1989) revised his theory on the involvement of serotonin in sleep to state that serotonin cell activity during wakefulness initiates the production of other substances subsequently necessary for sleep. Specifically, serotonin from the raphé acts on the basal forebrain, which in turn is important for the production of SWS. Serotonin during wakefulness is also important for inhibiting PGO waves and preventing other aspects of REM from occurring at the wrong time (Shiromani et al., 1987).

Now in the 1990's serotonin is seen as acting on one type of receptor to increase wake and on another to decrease sleep (Monti et al., 1990) and to play a role in modulating the timing of REM onset attempts (less serotonin lengthens the time between REM transitions) (Benington & Heller, 1991).

Norepinephrine. The view of the role of norepinephrine in sleep has been controversial, but it is no longer seen as the agent of sleep (Gaillard, 1990). One population of norepinephrine cells (especially the locus coeruleus) is seen as the agent of wakefulness and as involved in the "gating mechanism" for REM (that is reduction in norepinephrine cell activity is necessary before REM can occur). Another population of NE cells (scattered near the locus coeruleus) is active during REM. Norepinephrine is also seen as being necessary for the production of the low voltage, fast brain waves of both wake and REM although there is some evidence that is inconsistent with this view (Karacan & Moore, 1985).

Other. Other neurotransmitters have been implicated with sleep. The involvement of **GABA** in the production of SWS was noted above. Many sedative and hypnotic drugs have their sleep inducing effects due to their action on GABA synapses (Jones, 1990). **Dopamine** may be important for the behavioral arousal (but not brain waves) characteristic of wake (Gaillard, 1990). **Histamine** may also be important for arousal (Gaillard, 1990) which is why antihistamines often make people feel drowsy. **Adenosine** on the other hand is sleep inducing (Radulovacki, Virus, Djuricic-Nedelson, Baglajewski, Meyer, & Green, 1985; Gaillard, 1990). Caffeine antagonizes adenosine, which may account for its stimulating effects. GHB (Gamma-hydroxybutyrate) increases SWS and improves the efficiency of REM while decreasing stage 1 (Lopierre et al., 1990). Glutamate is influential in the cortex and many areas below it including the midline thalamus, for wakefulness and the inhibition of the muscles of movement during REM.

Sleep Factors

The belief that sleep is the result of the accumulation of a substance in the body during waking is very ancient (Krueger, et al.,

1990a; 1990b). The ancient idea that something builds up in the brain during wake is based on the common observation that going without sleep results in profound sleepiness that can be almost overpowering, which subsequent sleep reverses (Krueger et al., 1990a). Such substances have been called by several generic names including hypnotoxins (i.e. sleep poisons), sleep substances, and endogenous sleep promoting substances. Sometimes these beliefs have been called "bottle theories" as if the body is a bottle that gets filled when awake and drained when asleep. We will use the term Sleep Factors (SFs) in this review. A SF is a substance found in the body that can influence the likelihood (positively or negatively) of sleep/wake. In addition, the concentration, metabolism, and/or receptivity of a SF depend on prior sleep/wake (Krueger et al., 1990a; 1990b).

Very early in the twentieth century, Ishimore and Pierson independently published results from their labs which they believed showed SFs to be present in the cerebral spinal fluid (Borbély & Tobler, 1989; Inoue, 1989; Krueger et al., 1990a; 1990b). During the next fifty years there was some replication of this research but otherwise little attention was paid to SFs, probably because scientific focus was on the electrical and anatomical (cells and synapses) basis of sleep. Also, there were several studies of human Siamese twins (and laboratory created animal analogues) that shared a common blood supply yet showed independent sleep cycles (Borbély & Tobler, 1989) (but see Lahmeyer, 1988 for more recent contradictory evidence). Only in the last twenty years has there been renewed intense interest and effort concerned with finding SFs. As a result, a number of SFs have been identified and several more proposed (Borbély & Tobler, 1989; Inoue, 1989; Krueger et al., 1990a; 1990b). But the very fact that so many have been elucidated (more than 30 so far) has eliminated the notion that there is a single dominant SF.

DSIP

In 1977, Monnier and associates isolated a substance that chemists call a nonapeptide from the cerebral blood of rabbits kept asleep by electrical stimulation of the thalamus (Monnier, Dudler, Cachter, Maier, Tobler, & Schoenenberger (1977). When this substance was injected into the cerebral ventricles of normal rabbits, the general locomotive activity of these animals was reduced. An enhanced EEG delta wave activity typical of NREM sleep was also noted. The substance was named delta sleep inducing peptide (DSIP).

DSIP is the most extensively studied SF (Borbély & Tobler, 1989) with the number of research reports studying DSIP approaching 200. Facilitating the research effort is the fact that DSIP can be synthesized in the lab (Borbély, 1986). DSIP has been found to induce sleep in rabbits, rats, mice, cats, and humans, but some research has failed to replicate these results (Borbély, 1986; Borbély & Tobler, 1989). These negative findings may be due to circadian or seasonal influences on the effectiveness of DSIP (Yehuda & Carasso, 1988) or which analogue of DSIP is used (Kimura-Takeuchi, Kovalzon, & Inoué, 1990).

The sleep induced by DSIP has a rapid onset (within one hour) and persists for several hours. The median thalamus, nucleus of the solitary tract, and parts of the reticular formation seem to be particularly sensitive to it. Beneficial results have been reported when using DSIP to treat insomniacs, but these studies have not included adequate controls and negative evidence has also been reported, thus more research needs to be done before it can be considered for use as a sleeping pill (Borbély & Torber, 1989).

Factor S, Muramyl Peptides, Interlukin-1, Prostaglandins

Another possible sleep promoting substance (S) was isolated in 1967 by J. P. Pappenheimer and associates (Pappenheimer, Miller, & Goodrich, 1967). This substance (called a peptide) was collected from the cerebrospinal fluid of goats, rabbits and cattle. When injected into the ventricles of rats, cats, or rabbits, several hours of sleep followed. It appeared to increase the duration of NREM sleep and decrease locomotive activity (Drucker-Colin, 1981; Kelly, 1981). Recently, research on factor S has led to an interesting and enlightening trail of research (Anch et al, 1988; APSS, 1989; Borbély, 1986; Borbély & Tobler, 1989; Hayaishi, 1988; 1989; Horne, 1988; Krueger, Toth, Cody, Johannsen & Obal, 1988; Krueger, Obal, Johansson, Cady, Foth, & Kruege, 1989; Krueger et al, 1990b)

Later it was discovered that the sleep-active component of Factor S was a substance called a Muramyl peptide (MP). Injections of MPs in animals produce sleep that resembles the recovery sleep following sleep deprivation (see chapter 2) including an increase of SWS, and a greater amplitude of delta waves. This induced sleep seems natural since the animals were in normal sleep postures and could be easily awakened. They sometimes spontaneously awakened and then would behave normally, such as eat or groom, but soon return to sleep. Although many MPs also produce fever, MPs still produce sleep in the absence of fever. MPs are found in all animals and can be extracted from human urine. One MP can be synthesized in the lab which makes it much more available for research.

Here the story takes a curious turn. People of all times and places have experienced sleepiness when ill, and sleep and bed rest have long been recognized as recuperative. Thus it seemed reasonable that the body reacts to illness by becoming sleepy which facilitates bed rest which promotes to the return to health. But the mechanisms for this chain of effects remained a mystery until recently.

Although MPs are found in the body as mentioned above, the body cannot manufacture them. They have been likened to vitamins - necessary for normal body functioning but they must be acquired from outside the body. So the search was on to find their source. The result was the discovery that MPs come from bacteria. The bodies defense against bacteria is to have a type of white blood cell attack, consume, and destroy these potentially harmful invaders. When the cell walls of bacteria are destroyed, one of its key components - MPs - are released intact into the blood stream. Our mucous membranes, especially those of the intestines, are a constant scene of this battle and thus a continuous source of MPs for the body. But in the face of bacterial infection the battle rages on new fronts. The result is a massive increase of MPs in the body that begins early during the infectious assault. This increase of MPs in turn increases sleepiness and NREM sleep. Hence, a link between illness and sleepiness has been discovered.

MPs are transported to the brain by the blood where they are known to influence activity in the raphé and hypothalamus and other areas as well. There is however a 1 to 3 hour latency between the increase of MPs in the brain and sleep onset. Such a latency suggests that the MPs themselves may not directly cause sleep but do so by their activity on other SFs. Thus another scientific search commenced for an additional link in the chain of effects.

Interleukin-1 is the name of a family of cytokines that were already known to be very importantly involved in the body's immune system.

IL-1 is found in almost every part of the body, including the brain, where it is produced by glial cells. IL-1 was found to also produce natural sleep similar to that produced by MPs but with a much shorter latency (well within one hour). IL-1 is at its nycthemeral peak at the start of NREM in humans and is even higher following sleep deprivation. MPs in their general role as stimulants of the immune system can alter the production of cytokines including IL-1. Hence MPs can increase sleepiness indirectly by increasing the level of IL-1 in the body. (IL-1 has also been reported to be produced directly by white blood cells when destroying bacteria).

But we are not done with this chain yet. IL-1 has an effect on the production of prostaglandins (PGs) (Hayaishi, 1989; 1991). PGs play an important role in inflammation and fever generation. They can be found all over the body and can be manufactured by glial cells in the brain. Cells with receptors for PGs are found mainly in the forebrain.

One type of PG called D_2 has been found to be connected with sleep production. It has an especially high concentration in the mammalian brain, particularly in the basal forebrain area. When injected into the preoptic nucleus, a few hours of normal sleep results almost at once, whereas reducing the normal level of PGD_2 in the brain causes a reduction in sleep.

(Interestingly, another PG called E_2 produces opposite effects and thus is considered a sleep inhibitory or a wake maintenance substance. It seems to be more effective in the posterior hypothalamus. PGE_2 and PGD_2 are stereoisomers - that is they are chemically identical except for the placement of one element on opposite sides of the molecule. It is not unusual for the body to have similar elements simultaneously active that oppose one another. Better control can be achieved in this way since the outcome depends on the relative levels of each rather than absolute levels of one or the other.)

Now the description of the chain is complete. When illness-causing bacteria invade the body, white blood cells counter-attack, killing many bacteria resulting in a massive increase of MPs. The MPs influence the production of IL-1, which in turn influences the production of PGD_2 which induces sleep. However, we are still not done, for illness (resulting in increased sleepiness) can be caused by agents other than bacteria. Although not as well researched, there is evidence that viral related agents can affect sleepiness by altering cytokine production. Fungal and protozoa infections can also increase sleepiness perhaps by also influencing cytokines. For example, Smith (1992) reports results from the Canadian Common Cold Unit (a research facility) that, while both influenza and common cold viruses increased sleep duration (but not sleep quality or night awakenings) on days when symptoms were obvious, different effects were noted during the incubation period (flu decreasing sleep, colds increasing sleep).

Still the question remains unanswered: Is the extra sleep induced by illness helpful in recovery? Recent research is suggesting that it is (Smith, 1992; Toth & Krueger, 1992). Rabbits with a greater increase in sleep when challenged by bacterial infections had a more favorable recovery. This correlation, although not conclusive, is consistent with the possibility that sleep has a direct healing effect of sleep. It has also been noted that sleep deprivation increases the susceptibility to viral challenge (Palmblad, Petrini, Wasserman, & Åkerstedt, 1979; Toth & Krueger, 1990).

DSIP, MPs, IL-1, PGD_2 are only a few of the many recognized or suspected SFs. They are the most researched. These SFs appear to be continuously present in the brain and are important in sleep/wake. While each may, more or less, have a specific effect on sleep/wake, their actions are liable to be modified by many factors (i.e. circadian rhythms, presence of other sleep substances, current state of sleep/wake, age, sleep deprivation, and more). Overall, some SFs have been shown to intensify NREM without increasing REM. However, SFs that specifically increase REM have not yet been convincingly demonstrated. None of these SFs affect only sleep. but rather are related to many other functions in the body such as temperature regulation, metabolism, and even learning and memory. See Borbély and Tobler, 1989 and Inoue, 1989 for more complete reviews of all of the SFs found or suspected to date.

Krueger and associates at the University of Tennessee (see for example Krueger et al. 1990b and Krueger, Toth, Johannsen, & Opp, 1990) have developed a model involving complex, although poorly understood, interactions involving the production, metabolism and biological activity among these and other substances that include multiple feedback loops. They call it the Sleep Activation System. This model emphasizes that it is not the specific substances that influence sleep/wake but their interactions with each other and their effects on the brain at multiple levels. The model also recognizes that behavioral, psychological, and environmental factors influence sleep/wake often by influencing SFs. Most sleep factors have (or are assumed to have) circadian variations their levels and effects.

According to this model, the multiplicity of SFs and their interactive and parallel pathways of activity provide an inherent stability to the sleep/wake system. Normal sleep/wake may be the sum of variations of multiple SFs acting on brain mechanisms. Minor challenges to the system such as a small variation of a single SF are buffered resulting in minimal effects on sleep/wake. But a large variation of a SF (especially one of considerable importance), or simultaneous variation of several SFs may interact with other components (such as sleep deprivation or circadian cycle phase) to start a cascade of events that challenges normal sleep/wake. Overall, the integration of these multiple influences on multiple networks of neurons results in states of sleep/wake, just as similar integrations work in all other physiological systems of the body.

CONCLUSION: The BRAIN and SLEEP

A new view is emerging among sleep researchers of how the brain is involved in sleep (Borbély, 1986; Karmanova, 1982; McGinty et al 1985; Mendelson, 1987; Parmeggiani et al., 1985). Rather than trying to relate specific, localized areas of the brain and specific neurotransmitters to the stages of sleep, current thinking views sleep as the result of several influences. First, it involves the synchronization of the activity of diffuse sites in the brain. Second, a variety of physiological influences may modulate the activity of these cells, especially the places previously identified as sleep centers. Third, the levels of neurotransmitters may not be as important as where in the circuits of the brain they are used, what receptor types are affected by the transmitters, and the levels of other transmitters present at the same time. Fourth, many sleep factors also influence the sleep/wake circuits in the brain. The result, is that sleep is now viewed as an aggregation of elements regulated and controlled by several redundant systems. Normal sleep is the simultaneous or sequential recruitment of these components, with perhaps some components playing more dominant, but not indispensable, roles in this process.

Likewise, the wake systems of the brain are diffuse yet interconnected. They can be affected by most other brain sites and psychoactive substances. Whether we are awake or asleep is not simply the cessation of one state and the onset of the other, but rather depends on the overall pattern of brain activity.

Opp and Krueger (1991) summarize this thinking with what they call "a simile for sleep/wake: the language of sleep/wake." Each neuron, brain area, or substance involved in sleep/wake is like a word. Some (but not all) individual words communicate messages by themselves. Most messages are, however, more like sentences, where the combination, sequence, and context of the words convey the information.

Chapter 3

Sleep as Homeostatic[1]

Now that we have seen how sleep is measured in the laboratory, what is typical sleep, how it changes with age, and its relationship to the body and brain, let's explore some other sleep phenomena. In this chapter we will consider sleep as homeostatic. Homeostasis is the "tendency to maintain some variable, such as temperature, within a fixed range" (Kalat, 1992, p. 413). Breathing is a good example; its rate and depth are varied in order to keep the levels of oxygen and carbon dioxide regulated in the body. When these vary, breathing is automatically adjusted in an attempt to bring these levels nearer to optimal.

Certain motives such as hunger and thirst have also been described as homeostatic (Kalat, 1992). When we are in need of nuitrition or water, we feel driven to find and consume food or water. Sleep also seems to fit the definition of homeeostasis, since without its regular occurrence in adequate amounts, we do not feel at our best and our body urges us to make-up deficits. We also suffer if we have not achieved adequate sleep and are driven to obtain more.

[1]Parts of this chapter appeared earlier in Moorcroft W H (1987). An overview of sleep. In J. Gackenbach (Ed.), *Sleep and Dreams; A Sourcebook* (pp. 3-29). New York: Garland Publishing. Copyrighted by Garland Publishing in 1987. Used with permission.

Sleep Needs

How much sleep does a person need? Why do some people need more sleep and others less? We will explore the answers to these and similar frequently asked questions now.

"Sleep as much as necessary so you do not feel tired the next day," is the answer to the first question. This is probably not the kind of answer you expected, but it is the best answer. While 7 1/2 hours per night is the average amount of sleep required for young adults, there are wide individual differences (Kryger, Roth, & Dement, 1989; Williams, Karacan, & Hursch, 1974). Some people do well with 6 hours or less per night, while others cannot live comfortably with less than 10 or 11 hours of sleep (Webb, 1975). Only you can determine how much sleep you require, since only you know when you feel good the next day. Neither differences in will power, latitude, climate, time of day chosen for sleeping, nor demands of society are responsible for the differences among people in the amount of sleep they need. Rather, these differences in sleep need appear to be individual biological differences. Some people are tall, others short; some people need more sleep, others less. Each and every one of us does not need 8 hours of sleep per night to be healthy.

You may have heard or read of a person who does not sleep. Newspaper reports of such persons seem to occur every few years and prompt the question, "Do we really need sleep?" Only one of these reports indicated any kind of brain wave monitoring (Coleman, 1986), and even then it was clear that the record was evaluated using the standard criteria for sleep (see chapter 1). In most other cases, when monitored with a polysomnogram on a 24-hour basis, such "non-sleeping" individuals do sleep. They may not go to bed to do so, the sleep may be spread throughout the 24 hour day and they may not even be aware of sleeping, but they do sleep.

In another example, Horne (1988) relates the story of a lady who claimed she never slept, although she went to bed each night. She knew this because she heard a nearby church clock strike each hour while she laid in bed. However, when her sleep was monitored, she was observed to regularly awaken a few minutes before each hour, and promptly return to sleep after the clock struck the hour.

Some people may have ulterior motives for their claim of not sleeping, such as the man who had received a large amount of money in compensation for an automobile accident that left him sleepless for over 10 years. In the sleep lab, he did go almost four days without sleeping, but then succumbed to the pressure and slept for several hours accompanied by snoring (Borbély, 1986). Until recently, the documented record for the least amount of sleep needed is about 3 hours every 24 hours (Anch et al, 1988). Over one half of this sleep time was spent in delta sleep and another quarter in REM. More recently, a 70 year old woman was documented to sleep only 1 hour every 24 hours, half of which was delta. She simply did not feel tired or show any signs of sleep deprivation (Borbély, 1986).

These are extreme cases. In a poll of 800,000 American adults, one out of every thousand reported sleeping less than 4 hours per night, and another four out of every thousand reported sleeping between 4 and 5 hours. The vast majority of people need a substantial amount of sleep each night (see Figure 2-1).

Very few people sleep too much. Sleep tends to be self regulating - when you have had enough, you tend to wake up more easily and more often. Also, most people tend to shorten sleep in order to gain more wake time rather than vice versa. Too much sleep, for those few who do get it, can be as bad as too little sleep (Kleitman, 1972). After oversleeping, most people report feeling lethargic and slow moving, with their head in a fog. These unpleasant sensations may last the rest of the wake period or slowly diminish with time and exercise. (See also Chapter 9.)

There are some people that need a considerable amount of sleep. In many cases there are medical causes for this excessive sleep (see chapter 8). However, just as there are some naturally very short sleepers, there are some naturally very long sleepers (See Figure 2-1). About 16 people per thousand report needing more than 10 hours of sleep per night just to feel refreshed and alert (Borbély, 1986).

Individuals tend to show consistent percentages of the various stages from one night to the next, although their polysomnograms may look different (Anch et al., 1988). Sleep may be considered a fairly stable trait within individuals, with some people characterized as "sleepy" and others as "alert" (Lavie & Segal, 1989), although others interpret these data as showing that sleepy individuals are not obtaining the quota of sleep they need (Rosenthal, Krstevska, Roehrs, Kontich, Fortier, & Roth, 1992). The "sleepy" people fall asleep more easily, sleep more efficiently, get more sleep each night, are able to

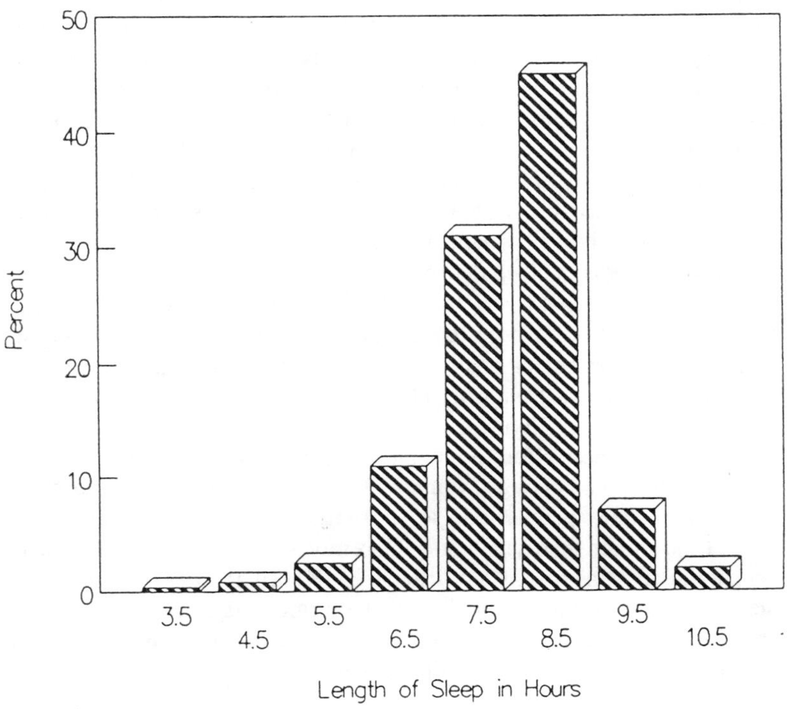

Figure 2-1. Sleep duration in one million adults. (After Kripke, D F, Simons R N, Garfinkel L, & Hammond (1979). Short and long sleep and sleeping pills: Is increased mortality associated? *Archives of General Psychiatry*, 36, 103-116.

nap more easily, but often find it harder to stay awake. "Alert" individuals show the opposites of these traits.

Sleep needs and sleep/wake cycles appear to be essentially inherited (Anch et al., 1988; Partinen, Kaprio, Koskenvuo, Putkonen & Langinvainio, 1983). Identical twins (whether reared together or apart) are more similar in their sleep length, REM characteristics, and number of stage shifts than fraternal twins or unrelated to children of the same age (Benoit 1985, p. 438; Partinen, Kaprio, Koskenvuo, Putkonen & Langinvainio, 1983; Anch et al., 1988). Heritability of sleep has been shown in humans and animals for total sleep time as well as the amount of REM and NREM (Anch et al., 1988). Yet, sleep needs are not so rigidly determined by genetics as to be unchangeable. For example, stress can vary sleep length a little (less SWS and/or REM accompanied by more and more awakenings ([Anch et al., 1988]), and depression can either shorten or lengthen sleep (Reynolds & Shipley, 1985).

Children's sleep needs require special mention. Generally, as seen in Chapter 1, children sleep more than adults. But they too show individual differences, and their sleep needs change with age. Sleep patterns do not become stable until about 20 years of age (or later if the person is still in school). The best advice for parents is to, first, get their child up at the same time every morning and, second, insist that they go to bed when they show signs of being tired at night. This should be modified appropriately if the child shows signs of tiredness or of having over-slept during the awake hours. Older children will invariably protest that it is not fair that they have to go to bed a) earlier than Johnny or Joan down the street, b) before their brothers or sisters, or c) before "everybody else in the whole world". A good reply to this is, "True, it's not fair, but different people need different amounts of sleep and you need to go to bed right now!"

Length of Sleep and Wakefulness

Although individual sleep need has a strong genetic component the actual amount of sleep obtained is easily and frequently varied by volitional and environmental factors (Carskadon & Dement, 1989). What are the effects of variations in the length of wakefulness on subsequent sleep? The major effect is simple (Webb, 1975). Generally, the longer we are awake, the more quickly we fall asleep. People who decide to "sleep in" one morning often report difficulty getting to sleep the following night. A similar result can happen if they take a long nap during the afternoon or evening (Webb, 1975).

But doesn't staying awake longer cause us to subsequently sleep longer? The effects of duration of wakefulness on subsequent sleep length are less well known, due to a lack of research and more complicated interactions with other factors (Webb, 1975). We can only sleep for so long before we start to wake up. It is as if sleep is self-terminating. Our circadian rhythms (discussed in the next chapter) make it easier and more efficient to sleep during a certain part of every

24 hours. When we attempt to sleep too long, our sleep starts to encroach upon our natural awake time and tends to make continued sleep more difficult. Finally, environmental influences, such as daylight, traffic noises, and the activity of other people, tend to make prolonged sleep more difficult. Nevertheless, we can probably safely say that prolonged wakefulness does tend to lengthen subsequent sleep, and, conversely, shortened wakefulness tends to shorten the sleep that follows. We cannot be more specific, however, about whether a lot of wakefulness results in only a little more sleep or a lot more. Nobody knows for sure.

What are the effects of changing the length of the sleep period? Since SWS is present only in the first few hours of sleep, the sleep period must be drastically shortened before SWS can be affected. On the other hand, the amounts of stages 1, 2, and REM vary directly with sleep length (Webb, 1975). Think of a clock with several springs. One spring is for SWS and another for REM. When you sleep, the SWS spring is wound first. Only when it is tight can the REM spring be completely wound. Thus, shortening sleep will greatly reduce the winding of the REM spring before the SWS spring begins to be affected. Stages 1 and 2 are fillers between the winding periods, so they are reduced in proportion to the amount of sleep lost. During wakefulness, the springs slowly unwind. If they have not been wound enough the night before, we may feel the effects. However, a little extra rewinding the next night or two seems to correct previous insufficient winding. (See the section on sleep deprivation and recovery in this chapter for more related information.)

Changes in the amount of sleep one night affect sleep on the subsequent night (Gillberg, 1992, personal communication; Levine, Lumley, Roehrs, Zorick, & Roth, 1988). When sleep is shorter for a night, it is more efficient the subsequent night, but alertness during the intervening wake period is compromised. Conversely, extended sleep one night causes greater alertness during the next period of waking, but less efficient sleep on the subsequent night, without having an effect on the total amount of sleep.

Long Versus Short Sleepers

Most of us are close to the average for our age in the amount of sleep needed per night. The rest fall into three groups: short sleepers, long sleepers, and variable length sleepers. People from each of these groups have been studied in an attempt to find out if they differ in any other way besides sleep needs. They do (Cartwright, 1978; Hartmann, 1973).

Short sleepers, for research purposes, are people who need an average of less than 5 1/2 hours of sleep per night. Insomniacs and voluntary self-deprivers of sleep were excluded from study. Only those people who felt good and performed well with that amount of sleep were studied. Likewise, long sleepers were people who must have over 8 hours sleep (with 9 hours spent in bed) each night to feel good and function at their best. Variable length sleepers were people who required short nights of sleep for long periods of time (months) but long nights of sleep during other long periods. The results of studying these kinds of sleepers are presented as averages from each group. No one individual showed all, or even many, of the characteristics to be described. Furthermore, the subjects were post-college age at the time they were studied. (The relationships reported below between sleep length and personality have been questioned [Stuss & Broughton, 1978; Hicks & Pellegrini, 1977] and similar research [Webb, 1975] done on college students did not produce the same results. However, most college students have not stabilized their sleep patterns and, thus, observations on them are difficult to generalize.)

Let us consider the sleep of the short and long sleepers first (Hartmann, 1973; Horne, 1983c). When their sleep was analyzed in a sleep lab, all subjects in both groups showed the same basic REM/NREM sleep cycles, and in about the same distribution throughout the night. In these respects, both groups resembled each other, as well as normal length sleepers. However, the amount of REM sleep the subjects in each group obtained was different. Short sleepers accumulated a less than average amount of REM sleep, while long sleepers obtained an above average amount of REM. The long sleepers had twice as much REM as short sleepers. Long sleepers also had more stage 2 sleep than average, but short sleepers less. Long sleepers had three times as much wake plus stage 1 and short sleepers very little, suggesting that the quality of sleep in the short sleepers is higher. Furthermore, long sleepers showed more rapid eye movements per minute (called rem density). They also had slightly less SWS (Borbély, 1986), more time awake in bed, longer time to get to sleep, and did not feel as refreshed in the morning.

More recent research has shown that long and short sleepers differ during recovery from sleep deprivation, although no differences were noted during the deprivation itself (Horne, 1988). Following 36 hours without sleep, average and short sleepers increased their sleep time by 25% and 33% respectfully, but long sleepers only increased by 5%. All of the subjects increased their time in SWS by 40%, but REM sleep increased very little in long and short sleepers (3%) ,but increased greatly in average length sleepers (33%). Horne interpreted these results as showing that short sleepers are down to their minimum sleep need per night, whereas long sleepers are obtaining a lot of extra sleep beyond minimum (see chapter 9 discussion of core and optional sleep) and can make up lost SWS without adding sleep length.

Returning to Hartmann's results, short sleepers reported themselves to be efficient and energetic, were satisfied with themselves and their lives, and liked to keep busy and work hard. They were more physically active when awake. They viewed sleep as a chore. Long sleepers were less easy to categorize as a group, except that they viewed sleep as a luxury and found it was very desirable and necessary to get the "right amount."

On psychological tests, short sleepers revealed themselves to be ambitious, decisive, and extroverted. Furthermore, they were somewhat conformist and tended to deny, rather then worry about, problems. Other than denying problems, they showed little psychological pathology. In contrast, long sleepers were mildly to moderately "neurotic". Some were anxious, inhibited, and depressed. Others were not very self assured. They tended to be worriers. There were some suggestions of high creativity among members of this group.

Short sleepers were socially adept persons. Long sleepers were nonconformists, social critics, and politically active. They also complained about aches and pains. When awakened during their dreams, long sleepers felt quiet and passive early in the night, but more active and energetic later. Short sleepers were the same throughout the night during dream wake-ups. Thus, it appears that the long sleepers were experiencing psychological change within sleep which the short sleepers were not experiencing. In contrast to Horne's findings, Hartmann found that long sleepers also showed more negative effects when deprived of REM accompanied by greater later recovery of lost REM. (See the discussion of "REM pressure" later in this chapter.)

Although interesting, it is not possible to distinguish causes from effects these findings. Do the sleep characteristics determine the personality characteristics or do the personality characteristics determine the sleep characteristics? Or are both perhaps caused by something else, or are they totally unrelated? The study variable length sleepers (Hartmann, 1973) provides some answers.

When variable length sleepers need only short nights of sleep, their personality and behavioral characteristics resembled those of short sleepers. Conversely, when they needed long nights of sleep, they closely resembled long sleepers in personality and behavior. Furthermore, their sleep needs increased during times of stress, depression, job changes, increased mental work, increased physical work, increased emotions, and general inward focusing. Their sleep needs decreased if all was going well, work was stable and pleasant, and so on. In other words, except for few a of these individuals who denied reality by "keeping busy," sleep needs increased in variable length sleepers when they were stressed, worried, or changed their lifestyle. Importantly, the changes in the physical or emotional events of waking life seem to precede, and thus cause a change in, sleep needs.

Similar kinds of changes can be seen in the sleep of average length sleepers, although to a lesser degree (Hartmann, 1973). For example, there is a modest but real increase in REM during times of emotional turmoil in many people. Also, relationships between some aspects of sleep (number of stage shifts) and personality in average length sleepers have been reported (Schubert, 1977).

Manic-depressive individuals also show changes in sleep that are consistent with these generalizations (Hartmann, 1973). A manic-depressive person shows dramatic swings in mood. At times they will be in a state of great elation and activity, and make many grandiose schemes for the future. Very quickly they will swing to being sad, withdrawn, and slow in thoughts and actions. These extremes are interspersed with periods of relative calm that are sometimes very long. In the manic phase, such individuals show a dramatically decreased need for sleep with no subsequent rebound or need to make up for lost sleep. In contrast, sleep needs increase during the depressed stage.

Sleep Deprivation

What are the consequences of going without sleep? Although the need for sleep is compelling, we can nevertheless, by will power, prevent its occurrence for a while. Sleep has been likened to a gentle tyrant in this regard (Webb, 1975). At other times, circumstances may prevent us from obtaining sleep even if the desire is there. Yet, except perhaps in children (Wolff & Money, 1973), lack of sleep in and of itself does not appear to result in long-term consequences (Kleitman, 1972). (In children, chronic, severe sleep loss may result in stunting of growth - see chapter 2.) Certainly, a lack of sleep does make people sleepy (Webb & Cartwright, 1978) and increase sleep efficiency during subsequent sleep (Levine, et al, 1988). The sleepiness caused by lack of sleep may result in severe secondary consequences, such as a car accident[2] or the loss of a job. For some others afflicted with sleep disorders, sleepiness can be an ongoing, continually devastating aspect of their lives (see chapter 9). Yet, for most people, the occasional sleepiness resulting from a lack of sleep seems a minor annoyance at most. Nevertheless, sleep researchers, through careful observation, have found subtle but measurable effects of sleep deprivation on the body, mind, and performance (Anch, et al, 1988; Borbély, 1986; Dinges, 1992; Hauri, 1979; Horn, 1988; Kleitman, 1972; Mendelson, 1987; Mikulincer, Babkoff, Caspy, & Sing, 1989; Webb & Cartwright, 1978).

The changes in the body during sleep deprivation include more catabolic than anabolic process (that is, more using up of bodily resources and breakdown of body tissues), accompanied by an increase in energy demands and a more voracious appetite. Also noticeable is a fall in body temperature (by about a half degree Celsius), together with efforts by the body to cut back on heat loss by decreasing sweating and decreasing the amount of blood flowing through the skin. The response threshold of the respiratory system to the level of oxygen in the blood decreases, while the response to carbon dioxide levels increases. Slight decreases in immune system functioning have been observed. And many sleep deprived subjects complain of heart palpitations, itchy eyes, and slight loss of strength and energy.

Some changes in the functioning of the nervous system have been observed during sleep deprivation. Disturbances of the nervous systems are evidenced by shakiness, problems focusing the eyes, greater sensitivity to pain, and (Thomas, Sing, Belenky, Shepanek,

---

[2]While there is no doubt that lack of sleep results in accidents at home, on the job, and in transportation, there is no accurate data about their prevalence (Lauber & Kayten, 1988). In the absence of such hard facts, too many myths prevail and find their way into federal regulations.

Thorne, McCann, Penetar, Fertig, & Redmond, 1990) changes in certain brain waves. Other changes include weakness in neck muscle flexion, tremors, jumpy eyeballs, and more frequent seizures in epileptics. Brain glucose utilization (a measure of brain activity) may decrease 14% overall after two days of sleep deprivation, with even more pronounced decreases in the limbic system (see chapter 2) which is important for many emotional and short term memory behaviors (Thomas et al, 1989). (Also see discussion in chapter 9 of the research by Rechtschaffen and colleagues for the effects of several weeks of sleep deprivation on rats.)

Although severe psychological disturbances as a result of sleep deprivation are rare (Anch et al 1988), there are, nevertheless, effects on the mind and behavior. Many sleep deprived people are "serious, listless, and grim" (Hauri, 1979, p 254) as well as appearing irritable and aggressive (both of which may result as much from the stress of sleep deprivation as the loss of sleep itself). Also occurring is a loss of spontaneity, and feeling "washed-out, depleted, and without reserves" (Hauri, 1979, p. 254). These effects are worse when an individual would normally be sleeping. Others report feelings of paranoia, disorientation, and occasional periods of loss of control of emotion. In addition, sleep deprived people may experience a decrease in ego functioning, characterized by a reduction in social adaptation, less tolerance, more immaturity, and making more basic demands.

If the deprivation continues into a second and a third night, people may become more and more indifferent and apathetic, yet become irritable if disturbed. They show no initiative. Their mood swings may become dramatic and sudden. Staying awake requires almost constant activity. Illusionations and actual hallucinations are more frequent. One that is often experienced is the "hat phenomenon": the sensation of a ring of pressure around the forehead, such as a hat might produce.

After four continuous days of no sleep, people may become delusional. They may believe that other people are doing things to them or are plotting against them. Eventually, they may even feel "depersonalized" (loss of self in relation to the normal world). It is easy to see why sleep deprivation is often a part of the "brain washing" procedure used on political prisoners. (Deprivation of other drive states such as starvation, thirst, salt, and even sensory stimuli, can also produce similar, severe changes in psychological states [Meddis, 1979].) The resistance to such effects depends on psychological stability prior to the deprivation.

A large number of studies attest to the negative effects of lack of sleep on performance. The negative effects of sleep loss on performance are most likely when the environment is isolated and monotonous, the task is long and without feedback, and the person is not intrinsically interested. Difficulties with concentration are commonly reported, although motivation is not always reduced. Problems on psychomotor (thinking and decision making which lead to movements to execute these decisions) tasks are among the most consistent effects of sleep deprivation (Anch et al 1988). This is especially true for longer, repetitive tasks administered when one is normally sleeping (see the next chapter on circadian rhythms). But deficits can also occur on very short-duration tasks that require great attention and high response rate. Nevertheless, (Horne, 1988) short tasks can be done fairly normally and extra motivation can help maintain performance during 1 1/2 to 2 days of deprivation (see also Dinges, 1989).

On many, many performance tasks, errors during sleep deprivation appear to be due to LAPSES in responding because of the heightened drive to sleep, which results in the occurrence of **microsleeps** (Dinges 1989; Horne, 1988; MacLean, Reiz, Austin, Coulter, Brunet, & Knowles, 1990) (Microsleeps are short, 1 to 10 seconds, dips into stage 1.) During a microsleep, a person stops whatever they may be doing and stares off into space. Lapses due to microsleeps are especially prevalent during long, monotonous, relatively simple tasks in which a person has to respond to a stimulus such as steering a car around a curve on an interstate. Such tasks require continuous attention and give little feedback with few incentives. In contrast, decrements in performance are less in shorter tasks where the person controls the pace, such as dialing a telephone and tasks which require memory.

The lapse hypothesis does not account for all decrements in performance following sleep deprivation. There is also evidence for a genuine decrease in perceptual, cognitive, and psychomotor CAPACITY (Dinges 1989; Hauri, 1979; Horne, 1988; MacLean, 1990) even on some short (10 minutes or so) simple tasks (i.e.. reaction time). A decrease of alertness, short of microsleeps, may also affect performance (Thomas,1990) The effects of lack of sleep on performance are not like a battery running down, but more like what can happen to an overworked automobile engine. (Dinges & Powell, 1989; Horne, 1988). First, a spark plug may occasionally miss fire, causing the engine to sputter occasionally. This is equivalent to occasional lapses due to microsleeps (Dinges, 1989). But even between the misfirings, the engine loses some peak horsepower, just as sleep deprived people show a reduction in optimal performance capability. Early on, these engine deficits can be somewhat compensated for by gradually increasing pressure on the accelerator, just as a person can reduce the effects of sleep deprevation by extra effort and motivation, but eventually even this does not help compensate much. Revving the engine occasionally may help at first, just like stretching or splashing cold water on your face helps. But the engine becomes less and less effective as time goes on. Eventually, even revving or stretching cease to be very effective.

What about more vigorous tasks following sleep deprivation? There are no *actual* changes in exercise Endurance, and peak performance levels (Horne, 1988). However, during measurement trials, subjects incorrectly Felt exhausted up to 10% sooner and incorrectly Felt they were exercising harder! This effect increased up to 20% after the second night. Even after the third consecutive night of sleep deprivation, no actual change in endurance and peak performance levels could be noted.

Many of these effects (mental, physical, and performance) increase in intensity, with continuing sleep deprivation, for 2 to 5 days (Anch et al 1988; Dinges, 1989: Horne, 1988). Thereafter, some continue to get worse, others remain level, while others seem to improve. Those that improve may do so because of the added effects of more and more frequent microsleeps after 40 continuous hours without sleep (the start of the second missed sleep period). At this time, microsleeps are unavoidable without stimulants (Dinges, 1989). Also, the effects are often worse during the time that one would typically be asleep (Dinges, 1989; Horne, 1988).

Recovery from sleep deprivation appears to be relatively quick and easy (Hartmann, 1973) and only about one third (Horne, 1988) to one half of the total lost sleep time needs to be made up. Part of the reason for this is that there is greater INTENSITY of SWS sleep, more so than greater duration. SWS is recovered before REM, most of it in the first cycle (Feinberg, 1989). REM is recovered by an increase in length of time in this stage and may not be completed until the second night (Horne, 1988). Following 1 or 2 sleepless nights, almost all of the lost SWS is recovered, but only about half of the REM (Horne, 1988). With more sleep deprivation, the percent of all sleep stages that are recovered declines (Meddis, 1979). Recovery sleep appears to be a better quality sleep, as indicated by improved sleep continuity (Kupfer & Reynolds, 1989) and higher arousal threshold (Carskadon & Dement, 1989).

Normal levels of sleepiness (as measured by the MSLT[3] return after the second recovery night (Anch et al, 1988). Even after very

---

[3] *The Multiple Sleep Latency Test (MSLT).* Before proceeding we need to introduce a very important test of sleepiness called the Multiple Sleep Latency Test (Carskadon & Dement, 1987). For this test, a person is prepared as they would be for an overnight polysomnogram (and in fact the night of sleep is usually recorded). Then the person is given 4 to 6 20-minute opportunities to fall asleep spaced two hours apart during the day, the first typically starting at 9:00 or 10:00 p.m.. Latency to sleep onset (defined as three consecutive epochs of stage 1 or any epoch of stage 2, delta, or REM) is assessed. Sometimes the person is allowed to obtain up to 10 minutes of sleep while other times the person is awakened as soon as sleep onset is noted. The data are the average (mean) of all the sleep latencies, but the individual nap latencies across the day may also be plotted to give a profile of daytime sleepiness.

This test, aptly called the Multiple Sleep Latency Test, or MSLT, is a direct measure of sleepiness (i.e.. the ability to fall asleep). A mean latency of 5 minutes or less is considered severe (pathological) sleepiness, 5 to 10 minutes moderate sleepiness, 10 to 15 minutes mild sleepiness, and greater than 15 minutes average sleepiness (ICSD, 1990). The MSLT is a more subtle test of sleep need than are performance tests. When pathological sleepiness is indicated, performance on many tasks is impaired (Carskadon, 1990a), but performance may not be affected when the MSLT shows the presence of borderline sleepiness. Another indication that the MSLT is a direct measure of sleepiness is the influence of sleep deprivation on it (Rosenthal et al, 1991). The more sleep missed on the prior night, the lower the MSLT score. Also, the lower the MSLT score, the more "recovery" sleep the next night.

An important variant of the MSLT is the Maintenance of Wakefulness Test (MWT) (Mitler, Guyavarity, & Browman, 1982; Poceta, Ho, Jeong, & Mitler, 1990). The MWT is similar to the MSLT in many respects except that during the MSLT the person is lying in bed in a quiet, darkened room and is instructed to close their eyes, lie quietly, and try to fall asleep. During the MWT the person is semi-recumbent on a bed, and is instructed to remain awake but not to use extraordinary methods to do so (such as biting the tongue). Each MWT trial lasts 40 minutes.

The MSLT is considered to be a measure of the physiological need or drive to sleep. The MWT is said to measure the ability (or lack of ability) to stay awake. Put another way, the MWT measures the likelihood of sleep BEHAVIOR (Anch et al., 1988). The ability to stay awake is a function of long sleep deprivation, psychological performance and other behaviors are back to normal after only one to three recovery nights, even though some recovery of SWS and REM may be continuing for up to five to six nights (Horne, 1983c).

Recent reports have related the beneficial effects of naps during or before sleep deprivation, (Bonnet, 1990; Dinges, Orne, Whitehouse, & Orne, 1987; Walsh et al., 1990). A nap taken anytime during sleep deprivation improved subsequent performance, but resulted in no change in subjective sleepiness (which is opposite of the effect of naps taken following normal sleep). However, naps taken earlier in the deprivation period, or even prior to it, produce better and longer lasting effects on performance. The longer the nap, the greater the benefit. It should be emphasized that the naps reduce, but do not totally eliminate, the effects of sleep loss. Also interesting is the fact that the expectation of an impending nap can also cause a temporary increase in performance. (Caffeine has been shown to have an even more beneficial effect than naps during sleep deprivation - see chapter 2.)

A caution needs to be extended here (Rechtschaffen, 1979). Studies of the effects of sleep deprivation are correlational, and correlations do not necessarily reflect causation. The procedure used to deprive sleep, rather than the deprivation itself, may result in the observed changes. Also, the procedures could disrupt the circadian rhythms (see chapter 4), which may have more of an effect than loss of sleep itself. Research has shown that small disruptions of circadian rhythms can effect mood and performance (see chapter 4). Also, the effects of sleep deprivation may be more appropriately viewed as homeostatic, compensatory reactions, rather than deficits. [That is, the fatigue that occurs may not be the *result* of the loss of sleep, but the *means* by which the body encourages a person to the sleep when sleep is necessary for other purposes (see chapter 9).] Improved performance following sleep may occur because sleep preparatory responses no longer compete with other responses. And extra or improved sleep following loss of sleep may not indicate an increase in the need for sleep, as much as more efficient mechanisms of sleep production.

---

sleepiness, but also the interaction of sleepiness with environmental factors (see below). The correlation between MSLT & MWT is 0.41 (Savgal, Thomas, & Mitler, 1992), suggesting that while sleepiness is important in ability to stay awake, other factors are also very important.

Deprivation of Selected Stages of Sleep

REM. In the laboratory it is possible to prevent specific stages of sleep from occurring to assess the effects of their deprivation. REM sleep is prevented by awakening the sleeper every time the polysomnogram shows that they are entering REM. In this situation, the sleeper is allowed to obtain all the NREM sleep that they desire - only REM is prevented. (In practice, it is impossible to prevent all of REM from occurring since a small portion occurs prior to the awakening. Likewise, it is impossible to deprive a person of REM without somewhat affecting other stages of sleep. Stage 2 is also decreased by this procedure, delta sleep is unaffected, but stage 1 increases [Agnew, Webb, & Williams, 1967; Horne, 1988]).

The original studies - and these were among the earliest laboratory sleep studies performed - suggested that severe mental disorder would result if REM deprivation lasted several days (Hartmann, 1973). Without REM, a person would become a paranoid schizophrenic. Less severe deprivation was reported to result in irritability, poor social interactions, agitation, and increased impulsivity. The results were interpreted at that time as showing the need to dream in order to maintain mental stability, since it was believed that dreams occurred only in REM (Cartwright, 1978).

Both the results and their interpretation have been subsequently modified (Hartmann, 1973). First, mental disorder is not the inevitable outcome of even severe REM deprivation. A number of volunteers have been deprived of REM for several days with no lasting effects. The procedure is stressful, however, and, like any other stress, may cause an unstable person to manifest a behavioral disorder, sometimes severe. Apparently, that is what happened in the subjects who first underwent REM deprivation (Freeman, 1972). Second, it is now known that dreaming is not always confined to REM, but may also occur in NREM (see Chapter 5). Thus, any deficits seen in behavior following REM deprivation cannot unequivocally be attributed to the loss of dreaming.

One of the major effects of REM deprivation is an increase in the number of attempts to start REM during the sleep period. Another is a decrease in the length of the time between these attempts. These effects have been given the name "REM pressure." REM pressure builds with the duration of the deprivation procedure until a person may make a dozen attempts per hour to initiate REM! In one REM deprivation project in which I participated, I had to awaken the subject 6 times between the hours of 3 and 4:30 in the morning. During that time he was awake a total of thirty minutes and asleep 60 minutes. I found that it was difficult at that time of the morning to constantly watch the moving polysomnogram to try to spot the first signs of REM, and when REM did reappear, to believe that it was happening again so soon!

Subsequent uninterrupted sleep also shows REM pressure effects in that the percent of REM is increased, the REM cycle length is decreased, and the "density" of eye movements is greater (that is, there are more eye movements per minute than normally occur). This entire pattern is called REM rebound (Cohen, 1979). So strong is the REM rebound effect that it will occur several nights later if extra REM is prevented until then (Koulack, 1991).

The effects of REM deprivation can also be seen during subsequent waking hours, but they may be subtle (Dement, 1978). There are changes in emotion. The person is more animated and activated. This effect is sometimes used to help treat severely depressed individuals when other treatments fail (Cartwright, 1977; Vogel, 1979). In fact, the person whom I helped deprive of REM was undergoing such treatment. Also noted have been increases in appetite and food consumption, more interest in sex, greater animation and activation, and more irritability and aggression (Horne, 1983c; Mendelson, 1987).

Effects on other aspects of behavior have been noted as well. REM deprivation has also been reported to interfere with memory (McGaugh, Jensen, & Martinez, 1979). Humans, as well as animals, experience some reduction in the ability to memorize new things as a result of REM deprivation. Even when REM deprivation follows learning attempts, a reduction of retention may occur. These effects appear to be more apparent when the material to be learned has emotional importance to the subject.

Finally, changes have been noted in brain functioning as a result of REM deprivation. The cerebral cortex is more excited.

SWS. SWS can also be selectively blocked in the laboratory, but the procedure is different from REM deprivation (Agnew et al, 1967; Webb, 1973). Whenever the chart indicates that SWS is about to begin, a tone is sounded that is not loud enough to awaken the person, but is loud enough to drive sleep back to stage 2 or 1. Depriving people of NREM is more difficult. It takes about six times as many sleep interruptions to deprive a person of SWS than REM (Anch et al,

1988). (Even then, SWS is not totally eliminated, but it is substantially reduced. REM sleep is not affected by this procedure but stage 2 increases).

SWS deprivation results in SWS pressure. This is shown both by the increase in the number of attempts to initiate SWS during sleep and by the increase in SWS following return to undisturbed sleep on the subsequent night. The recovery occurs by a greater intensity of delta waves and/or by longer duration of SWS (Gillberg, Anderzén, & Åkerstadt, 1991). SWS recovery appears to be accomplished in one night (Anch et al 1988).

SWS-deprived individuals do not consistently report any behavioral problems; rather they complain about body problems. They say that they feel lethargic and depressed. They also complain of muscle aches. As a result, they tend to act more subdued and withdrawn.

Stages 1 and 2. It is not yet possible to deprive people of only stage 2 or stage 1 sleep, since these stages normally precede other stages of sleep. Depriving a people of these stages would necessarily deprive them of both SWS and REM. Thus, little is known about the importance of these stages of sleep.

Partial Sleep Deprivation

Far more common than totally sleepless nights or sleep without REM or SWS, is a night of shortened sleep. What are the effects of this kind of sleep deprivation? In effect, they clip off the end of sleep, which reduces mainly REM and stage 2, but the amount of SWS sleep is essentially unchanged unless the sleep period is severely curtailed. The result is a direct, but not linear, relationship between the amount of sleep obtained and sleepiness (as measured by MSLT) (Anch et al, 1988). This can best be seen by examining the results of a study by Dement & Carskadon (1981).

In this experiment, subjects slept on two successive nights for various lengths of time, ranging from 9 hours (extended sleep) to no sleep at all (total sleep deprivation) with MSLT's following each night. The averaged results of the second day are shown in Figure 2-2Four things are apparent in these data. First, overall sleep onset is more rapid, as sleep is more restricted. Second, the "mid afternoon dip" (see Chapter 4) in sleepiness persists, except in the totally sleep deprived subjects. (This may be a "basement effect", since sleep latencies at all

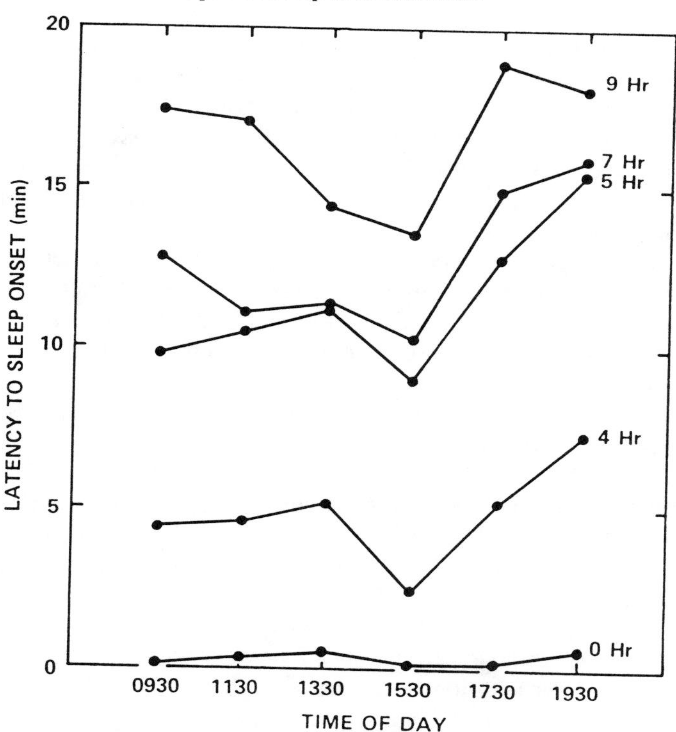

Figure 2-2. Latency to sleep onset (MSLT) in young adults on the second day of various nocturnal sleep time conditions. Individual subjects in the various conditions differed, and the numbers per condition were 9 h, $n = 20$; 7 h, $n = 14$; 5 h, $n = 10$; 4 h, $n = 13$; 0 h, $n = 6$. Data from the second day only are shown. From Roth, Roerhs, Carskadon, & Dement, 1989. Used with permission.

times were almost zero). Third, the sleepiness resulting from mild sleep restrictions has a proportionately greater effect in the morning hours. This is seen by comparing the slope of the curves during the morning hours for the 9 and 7 hour groups to that of the other groups. Fourth and finally, there is a much greater drop in sleep latencies between the five hour and four hour groups than between the nine and seven and the seven and five hour groups. That is, although the four hour group is getting only 1 hour of sleep less per night than the five hour group, they are dramatically sleepier.

Performance measures following nights of partial sleep have shown few deficits, even if sleep is curtailed by one third (Anch et al, 1988). Except for occasional decrements in performance on a long, boring task over which the person has no control (for example, 30 minutes of staring at a radar screen looking for infrequent, unusual occurrences), one night of sleep restriction seems to have little effect on performance the next day.

Many people also experience successive nights of shortened sleep because of the demands of work, school, and social life (Tepas & Papkin, 1989), as well as choice and distractions (such as TV and alarm clocks). In fact, most people are thought to be chronically, partially sleep deprived (Dement & Carskadon, 1981; Webb & Agnew, 1975). Researchers cite the following evidence: 1) A comparison of the sleep of adolescents in 1963 with those in 1910-11 (a reduction in total sleep time of 1 1/2 hours). 2) The tendency of people to "sleep - in" on weekends and holidays (although this may be like eating - given an abundance of food we eat too much and hence we may get "sleep fat"). 3) When the average 7.5 hour sleeper is allowed to sleep in the lab as much, and whenever they want, total sleep time increases to over 9.6 hours. 4) MSLT latencies increase (reflecting less sleepiness) if the average 7.5 hour sleeper gets 8.5 hours of sleep and continues to do so for three additional successive nights. In addition, there is evidence from circadian rhythms studies (see chapter 4) that humans are biologically 25 hour organisms forced to live in a 24 hour world - usually at the expense of sleep. Dement & Carskadon conclude that people may be better off and get more done (more efficiently) when they are awake less and sleep more.

What does research show about the effects of accumulated partial sleep deprivation? An experiment conducted by Dement and Carskadon, (1981; see also Carskadon & Dement, 1981) is illustrative. The subjects were allowed only five hours of sleep over seven consecutive nychthemerons, As noted in similar studies, stage 2 and REM were significantly reduced, but SWS was not reduced. In addition, stage 1 and wake after sleep onset were reduced, indicating improved quality of sleep. MSLTs were done each day to assess sleepiness. The average sleep latencies from all the subjects are shown in Figure 2-3. (Individual subjects showed the same trends, but with noticeable individual differences.) Three things can be noted in this figure. First, the subjects got sleepier as the experiment progressed. Second, the mid-afternoon heightened sleepiness (see Chapter 4) is

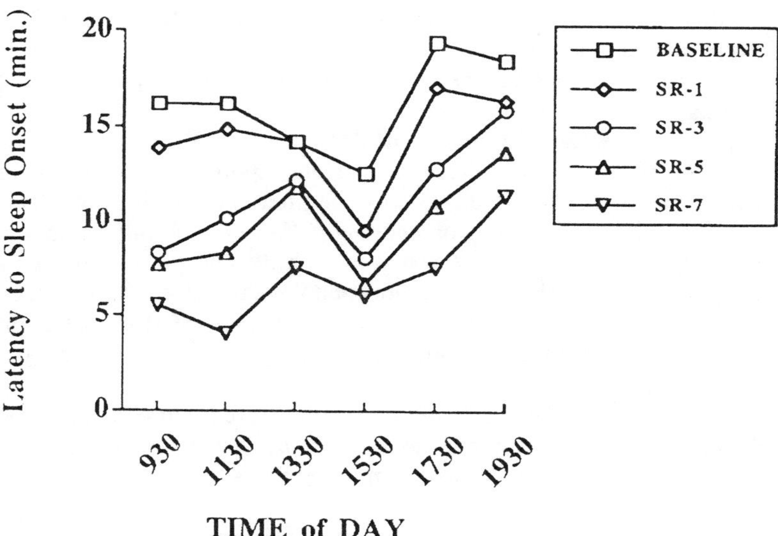

Figure 2-3. Average daily MSLT scores for young adults whose nocturnal sleep was restricted to 5 hrs on 7 consecutive nights. Baseline or predeprivation condition is indicated with a "B." Days 1, 3, 5, and 7 represent days during the sleep restriction condition. Figure kindly provided by Mary A. Carskadon from data from Dement & Carskadon (1981).

present from the very start through the very end of the experiment. Third, the successive increase in sleepiness was greater in the morning hours than during other times of the day. When asked, the subjects said that they felt fatigued. However, no effects could be consistently seen in behavior or mood.

Recovery sleep was studied in some of these subjects after two nights of 10 hours in bed. REM rebound was noted during the first recovery night, but sleep in the second night was like the sleep prior to deprivation. This suggests REM pressure was building because of the sleep restriction. Daytime sleepiness also returned to baseline levels after the first recovery night.

What are the effects of sleep deprivation outside of the lab? Mary Carskadon (1987) presented a summary of a number of field studies on children and preadolescents. Sleepy children behave differently than sleepy adults. They may fall asleep in a sedentary setting (such as riding in a car) but be absolute "monsters" in an active, arousing setting.

In a survey of 272 high school students, 2/3 reported having problems with sleepiness. Thirteen percent reported falling asleep in school in the mornings and 23% in the afternoons. More problems were reported when reading or studying (48% report falling asleep and 32% report struggling to stay awake). Thirty one percent say they struggle to stay awake during exams and 4% fall asleep during them. Significantly, students reporting six or fewer hours of sleep per night contribute more to these statistics than those getting seven or more per night.

Carskadon has studied college students even more extensively. Beginning with a survey question, "What do you do when sleepy in class?" she found that students (from most to least common):

Prop head in hand

Slouch with head on back of chair

Squirm in seat

Prop feet on chair in front of them

Put head on desk

Stand up and move.

Next, she hid cameras in classrooms and observed the frequencies of these behaviors. On Mondays, an average 8% of students showed one or more of these behaviors. This increased to an average 12% on Fridays. During the third week of the semester, the average was 4%, increasing to an average of 10% on week nine. Finally, students (about 300) were again surveyed but in more detail. They were asked about behaviors when sleepy, when alert, or when neither sleepy or alert. Some behaviors are much more frequent when sleepy, others when alert, and still others in both states.

The effect of sleep deprivation has also been studied in young adults in a military setting (Anch et al, 1988.) Sleep deprivation in this setting has been shown to have the least effect on tasks requiring manual effort, but the greatest negative effects on tasks requiring vigilance and thinking (diminished by up to 50% during the first four days). All performance deficits recovered after 3 recovery days. A study of US. Army Ranger trainees is an example (Penetar, Redmond, & Belenky, 1989). During such training, the soldiers averaged 3.2 hours of sleep per night for the 8- week training period. During later phases of the training, the instructors have often noted what they call "droning" - the soldiers were unresponsive and were unable to process information.

Of course, soldiers in such situations are also exercising more than normally, experiencing more intense and varied sensory stimuli, and are experiencing more stress, in addition to a loss of sleep, which may have contributed to their behavioral symptoms. In an interesting series of experiments, Horne (1988) found that varying the amount of physical exercise of sleep deprived subjects had no effect, better or worse, on any observed deficits. However, increasing the variety and intensity of the sensory stimuli (by filling the days and nights of sleep deprived subjects with trips to zoos, movies, etc.) caused them to feel sleepier, perform worse on tests, and show more rebound of SWS.

Many times the question is asked, "Can I learn to sleep less?" Many college students have tried to do this over the years, but it is difficult to know how successful they have been. Several systematic studies of shortening sleep have been reported - all with similar results (Horne, 1988). Volunteers decreased their sleep 1/2 or 1 hour every few weeks. After several weeks to several months, the subjects were to maintain this lower level for a few months before returning to whatever amount of sleep they desired. Initially, following each reduction, the subjects reported feeling sleepy, but this passed after a few days. When sleep had been reduced by a total of 1 1/2 to 2 hours, the subjects began to complain about difficulties waking up. Performance was frequently measured, but there were no signs of decrements. The pattern of sleep in the subjects changed. The amount of REM and stage 2 declined greatly, but SWS remained stable or, in some cases, actually increased a bit. Stage 1 and wake during sleep declined somewhat. In some cases, REM sleep time was down to 1/3 of original levels. In simple terms, the end of their night of sleep was clipped off, leaving them only to 3 REM cycles. Sleep latencies also decreased, and sleep efficiency increased. These last two observations suggest that the sleep was of better quality. In some of the studies, the sleep of the subjects was again assessed several weeks after the experiment ended. At this time, they were still sleeping less than before the experiment by an hour or more.

It must be concluded that people can learn to sleep less (Horne, 1988). An hour or two reduction was the common result in these studies, but more than this was not possible. Horne (1988) interprets this to mean people can eliminate their "optional" sleep but require their "core" sleep (see chapter 10). It also must be emphasized that this took several weeks of adhering to rigid sleep schedules every day of the week, no (or discouraged) napping (although some napping and oversleeping occurred that may have helped the subjects tolerate this procedure [(Carskadon & Dement, 1981]), and normal use of caffeine. Also, the subjects were getting a lot of support and attention from the experimenters. They also had to endure periods of sleepiness and difficulty arising in the morning. Could the same results be obtained by persons not involved in an experiment, especially if they were not as rigid in adhering to the schedule (such as napping or sleeping in on weekends)? This remains to be determined.

(As an interesting footnote, one experimenter asked his subjects what they did with the extra time awake to spend on specific endeavors. But in the end, most subjects admitted that the extra wake time was wasted on nothing important. This led the researcher to speculate, "maybe long sleepers are efficient people, able to do a day's work quickly and then have more time to sleep!" [Horne, 1988, p. 193].)

Recent observations (Roehrs, Vogel, Claiborue, Lamphere, Bohannon, & Roth, 1990; Rosenthal et al, 1992; Rosenthal, Roehrs, Kreslevska, Rosen, Sicklesteel, & Roth, 1992) lead me to caution you against trying to shorten your sleep time. These researchers compared young, healthy adults who have short MSLTs (less than 7 minutes) - called "sleepy normals" - to similar adults with normal MSLTs (greater than 16 minutes) - called "alert normals." The sleepy normals had higher sleep efficiencies, shorter sleep latencies, fewer awakenings, were more difficult to awaken, returned to sleep faster if awakened, and could easily fall asleep several hours before their typical bedtime -all signs of sleep debt. When alert normals were sleep deprived for 36 hours, they resembled the sleepy normals on these measures. The sleepy normals were apparently voluntarily restricting their sleep, and thus had accumulated considerable sleep debt. As indicated above, accumulated sleep debt can be uncomfortable, can reduce accuracy, and is potentially dangerous when doing extended driving.

Extended Sleep

Most people can easily extend their daily sleep by about 1 1/2 to 2 hours (some up to 4 1/2 to 5 1/2) via oversleeping and naps. Extending beyond this is difficult because of rising circadian body temperatures (see chapter 4). The efficiency of this extended sleep is less than that of normal length sleep. Such extended sleep contains little delta sleep, mainly stage 2 with 25 to 30% of REM, but shorter and more frequent REM periods. Interestingly, if sleep is extended beyond 12 hours, there is a return of some SWS in short 15-20 min. episodes (Mendelson, 1987; Horne, 1988). After about a week of extended sleep, sleepiness goes away (Horne, 1983; 1988).

Just a single night of 2 - 3 hours of extra (but not debt recovery) sleep lowers efficiency the next day (Anch et al, 1988; Dinges, 1989), resulting in an increase in reaction time, more errors committed during a vigilance task, depressed affect, impaired thinking, irritability, and increased sleepiness. These effects of extended sleep have been called the Rip Van Winkel effect and are possibly due to the extra REM sleep, since REM sleep seems to have a modulating effect on affect (see chapter 10). These effects are not seen if you get one extra hour of sleep per night for four nights.

Sleepiness

Dave Dinges (1987) of the University of Pennsylvania recently elaborated the factors that are a part of a subjective sense of sleepiness. His list includes:

1.Time. Amount of prior wakefulness and the current phase of the body's circadian sleep/wake rhythm (see Chapter 4) are important determiners of sleepiness..

2. Sleep. Both too little and too much prior sleep can make a person sleepy.

3. Age. Older people generally sleep less well, but young adults report more sleepiness (Addison, Thorpy, & Roth, 1987), probably due to life style.

4. Health. Illness causes sleepiness (see chapter 2).

5. Recreational drug use.

6. Environment/Context. Heavy meals, warm rooms, boring lectures, driving through Kansas, etc. can result in feeling sleepy. However, expectations, environmental stimulation, novelty, and so on can cause a person to feel less sleepy.

Most important, however, is the interaction between endogenous factors (such as sleep deprivation and circadian rhythms) and current environment. As the need of the body for sleep rises, the influence of the environmental factors on sleepiness becomes greater. Only sleep deprived students fall asleep during boring lectures, but almost nobody falls asleep watching an exciting basketball game (see also chapter 10). As Sterman and Shouse(1985) have stated, sleep may be "responsive to both internal necessity and to external encouragement." However, subjective evaluations of sleepiness do not show any relationship to performance on tasks, sleep latency, or brain activity (Broughton, 1987).

Napping

Napping has jokingly been called any rest period up to 20 minutes long involving unconsciousness but no pajamas (Webb, 1981). What is known about napping? Is it just for children? Is it a problem in adults, or is it beneficial for them, too?

We tend, in our culture, to think of sleep occurring in one continuous period each nychthemeron. We feel this pattern is normal, natural, and beneficial. Yet non-napping may be considered the exception rather than the rule in most humans and animals. In other cultures, a daily nap such as the Mexican siesta is considered appropriate and necessary. In such cultures, 2/3 of young adults nap at least once a week with 30% taking over 4 naps per week whereas 23% are non-nappers (Dinges, 1989). In the United States, 50-85% of college students take several naps per week. (Most of the rest wish they could, but report not having enough time!) Naps are common among US. adults with variable or irregular work/rest schedules such as shiftworkers, airline flight crews, long haul truck drivers, and so on (Dinges, 1989). On the other hand, most non-napping is due to the demands of work schedules or other aspects of our society (Webb, 1975).

Why do people nap? There appear to be five contributing factors (Dinges, 1989; Webb, 1981): **compensatory** - "catching up" on lost sleep; **environmental** - caused by events from outside a person's body; **biological rhythm** - another example of the influence of the circadian rhythms on the body (which are discussed later in chapter 4); **recreational** - napping for the pure pleasure of it; and **anticipatory** - napping prior to a long work period or sleep deprivation.

Compensatory napping is most frequent following a night of shortened sleep or in shift workers. The recuperative value of a nap depends on the amount of prior wakefulness, the timing of the nap (early afternoon is best), and its duration (Anch et al 1988). The amount of sleep deprivation and the presence of illness are two additional factors. However, the improvement in alertness as a result of a nap may not be apparent to the napper (Connell, Dinges, Rosekind, Gregory, Roundtree, & Graeber, 1991). Naps taken in the midst of sleep deprivation may be helpful in improving performance during the deprivation, and napping early in the deprivation period are best. Although performance improves with such naps, feelings of sleepiness are unchanged.

Environmental napping occurs more in people who live in a hostile environment, especially one in which very hot afternoons occur. Societal and social demands are also a part of the environmental factor. For example, most employees cannot nap on the job. Environmental napping accounts for weekend napping in the US. and other industrialized countries. Adults tend to become sleepy during the early afternoon (Carskadon & Dement, 1987), and the urge to nap is often greatest at this time. Naps are usually best (more efficient, contain significant SWS, and increase subsequent alertness) during this time (Lavie, 1989).

Recreational nappers look forward to their naps and enjoy them emensely. Recreational nappers report they can sleep "anytime, anywhere."

Anticipatory naps have been shown to improve alertness during subsequent sleep deprivation in the lab (Rosa & Bonnet, 1991), but their value has been questioned in real world settings and in some cases they were found to be detrimental for night shift workers (Rosa, 1990).

Undoubtedly, any nap may be influenced by more than one factor. Consider the napping of college students in the classroom; frequently compensatory, certainly environmental, influenced by biological rhythms, sometimes anticipatory, and mainly recreational!

The stages of sleep during naps tend to resemble those during night sleep (Hume, 1987). Delta sleep usually precedes REM, but occasionally sleep-onset REM naps do occur. (If they are frequent, they indicate a condition known as Narcolepsy - see chapter 9.) The likelihood and duration of REM, on the other hand, seem to be more determined by when the nap occurs in the circadian cycle (see Chapter 4). Thus, REM is more likely and more prevalent during morning naps. (Horne, 1983c).

The average nap is 1 1/4 hours in length, seldom less than 15 minutes or longer than 2 hours (Dinges, 1989). Naps usually do not shorten the sleep during the following night, except in some elderly persons (Horne 1983;1988). Nor does a nap containing REM sleep diminish the amount of REM the subsequent night. In contrast, if SWS occurs during nap, then the amount of SWS the following night is correspondingly diminished.

Some people do not like to nap because of unpleasant after effects (C. Moorcroft, personal communication; also Horne, 1988). Most people will experience some degree of "sleep inertia" (see chapter 10) lasting for about 30 minutes (Dinges et al, 1987) during which time their performance will be sub-par. The longer the nap, the greater the sleep inertia, but after the inertia wears off, the benefits from the nap emerge (Stampi, Broughton, Mullington, & Rivers, 1989).

Overall, naps may be good and beneficial, but may be best avoided by some elderly and insomniacs when the naps result in difficulty sleeping the following night (Anch 1988). Too much napping may also interfere with normal setting of the circadian rhythm (see chapters 4 and 9). Also, naps used in place of a single period of nocturnal sleep (such as might be done by shift workers) are not as efficient when compared to a single, consolidated, nocturnal sleep period.

Good Sleep

In a recent survey of the general public (Addison, Thorpy, & Roth, 1987), only 29% of people said they felt they had no problem with their sleep. The others complained about being awake too much after falling asleep, or having trouble even getting to sleep, difficulty waking up in the morning, and being sleepy during the day. Good sleep, it seems, is not as prevalent as poor sleep.

What then constitutes good sleep? First and foremost, good sleep is a subjective feeling (Spiegel, 1981). While it is possible to identify some poor sleepers using the polysomnogram, others who identify themselves as poor sleepers are indistinguishable from good sleepers (Johnson & Spinweber, 1983). For this reason, the following is only a partial explanation of good versus poor sleep - a beginning of understanding - that emerges from studies of good versus poor sleepers and good versus poor nights of sleep in the same person (Anch et al, 1988; Borbély, 1986; Bonnet & Johnson, 1978; Cartwright, 1978; Hobson, Prokop, & Spagna, 1978; Johnson, Church, Scales, & Rossiter, 1978; Johnson & Spinweber, 1983; Prinz, 1980; Rechtschaffen, Bliwise, Lichtman, & Pivik, 1978; Spiegel, 1981; Viot-Blanc, Benoit, Pailhous, & Bouard, 1987.)

Several of the things that have been identified as related to poor sleep are as follows: First, poor sleep is sometimes related to falling asleep more slowly or less easily. Second, some studies show higher body temperatures prior to and during sleep in poor sleepers. Also, higher heart rates and GSR have been observed during poor sleep. Third, lack of continuity of sleep is apparent in poor sleep.

Poor sleep seems to be more easily disrupted by noises and other stimuli. There may be more awakenings and longer time awake, with more stage shifts and body movements. Related to this is more stage 1, less REM, and maybe less SWS. As a result, sleep efficiency (see chapter 1) is lower. These things all may be summarized as less SLEEP CONTINUITY or, said another way, more SLEEP FRAGMENTATION. Indeed, sleep continuity is beginning to be recognized as one of the most important contributors to sleep quality.

Researchers at Henry Ford Hospital in Detroit and the Loma Linda (California) VA. Hospital have recently attempted to specify what it is about sleep fragmentation that results in subsequent daytime sleepiness (Bonnet, 1986; Downey & Bonnet, 1987; Stepanski, Lemphere, Bodin, Zorick, & Roth, 1984). In studies of very sleepy patients, the number of arousals during sleep (rather than the amount of sleep or changes in sleep stages) was seen to relate significantly to daytime sleepiness. Based on this observation, a sleep lab experiment was conducted with normal sleepers who had their sleep briefly, but frequently, punctuated by arousing noises. Although the arousals were so brief (2 to 10 seconds of stage change) that the typical sleep stages and lengths were unaffected, subjects reported substantial sleepiness the next morning if the arousals had occurred about once per minute. Disrupting sleep every 5 minutes had little effect. Thus, a poor night of sleep is related to the frequent disruption of sleep continuity more than anything else. Other studies have suggested that poor mood in the morning is related to another factor - lack of adequate REM. Length of sleep (total sleep time) is only mildly related to quality of sleep if at all. Unrelated to sleep quality is REM/NREM cycle length.

Personal characteristics related to poor sleep include poorer sleep habits, especially irregular bed and arise times (see chapter 9). Poor sleepers also have poorer moods and worse coping skills. People complaining of poor sleep also report more nightmares, trouble getting up in the morning, more fatigue and less vigor, more confusion upon awakening, more tension, and generally do not feel good. Highly neurotic or highly extroverted men often say they are poor sleepers. Otherwise, no consistent personality traits have been related to poor sleep. Poor sleep has not been shown to result in performance task decrements, but has been related to less success in careers.

While many people have an occasional night of poor sleep, others seem to have a predisposition toward poor sleep (see chapters 9 & 11). We tend to assume that good sleep results in alertness the next day, whereas poor sleep results in sleepiness the next day. However, Lavie (1989) presents evidence to suggest that some people are basically sleepy and others basically alert. Sleepy people may fall asleep easily at night but have difficulty staying awake during the day, whereas alert people cannot easily fall asleep but have little trouble staying awake. Further, he maintains that the characteristics of being sleepy or alert may be stable in individuals.

What kinds of things may cause a person to have a poor night of sleep? Certainly, psychological stress may have an effect. Such stress can result from something very good, as well as from something very bad. Furthermore, it can result from something that has already happened (usually during the preceding day) or in anticipation of something (like a wedding or court appearance). Stress may reduce the quality of sleep by causing more nighttime arousals, decreasing SWS, and disturbing REM. Anxiety may increase sleep latency (Ware, 1988).

Environmental stresses can also be important. Noise is the most obvious and has been shown (even if a person is adapted to it) to lighten and disrupt sleep, even if the person does not wake up (Nakagawa, 1987). People find that noise tends to disrupt their sleep more as they get older. Research also shows that sleeping with someone results in less delta sleep (probably due to arousal when the sleeping partner moves) but slightly more REM. Weather and exercise may also have both positive and negative effects on sleep (see chapter 2).

Depth of Sleep

Which sleep stage is the deepest? When we are awakened from sleep, sometimes it is very easy to regain full consciousness. But at other times, waking up is slow and difficult. In the latter case, we say we were very soundly asleep or in a deep sleep. It seems like it should be easy to determine which stage of sleep is the deepest, but it is not.

In the laboratory, depth of sleep is determined by the degree of loudness of a noise necessary to awaken the sleeper. Increasingly louder noise is needed to awaken a sleeper going from stage 1 to stage 4 with REM being like 4 (Horne, 1988) (except in the cat,which requires more noise in REM than even stage 4 to awaken it [Freemon, 1972].) But it also depends on just what noise is being used. We awaken, for instance, much more easily and faster to someone barely saying our name than to someone shouting other names. In this case, REM is like stage 2. Or there is the example of a mother sleeping through the roar of city noises but awakening at the first cry of her baby (Anch et al, 1988). (Except in our family - I was the one who woke to the baby's cry, but since my wife was nursing, there was nothing I could do but awaken her!) When awakened out of SWS, people show signs that do not occur when awakened out of other stages such as grogginess, confusion, slurry speech, reduced responsiveness to stimuli, and no later memory of the awakening (Anch et al, 1988). REM is about like stage 2 on this scale. In contrast, if we use muscle relaxation as the indicator of depth of sleep, then REM with its muscle paralysis is the deepest stage of sleep.

Perhaps, then, the question is too simple (Dement & Mitler, 1974). It assumes a continuum in which various degrees of wakefulness (hyperactive - alert - drowsy) continue into various degrees of sleep (light - moderate - heavy) in a straight line. Rather, it appears we should think of three different states - wakefulness, REM, and NREM - each with its own characteristics. Rather than being like a continuous hallway which is very bright at one end and very dark at the other, the states of sleep and wakefulness are more like separate rooms in a house - each room with its own furnishings and functions.

CONCLUSION

In this chapter we have explored things that affect and are affected by sleep. In more technical terms, sleep can be viewed as both a dependent and independent variable. Sleep is both affected by the prior period of wakefulness (as well as the amount and quality of prior sleep), but sleep amount and quality also affect the subsequent period of wakefulness (as well as subsequent sleep).

Sleep as a dependent variable can best be seen in the relationship between prior wakefulness and SWS. The longer we are awake, the greater the duration and intensity of the subsequent SWS. Furthermore, what is done during that wakefulness also has an influence on the amount of subsequent SWS. Length of prior wakefulness also has an influence on how quickly we fall asleep.

Sleep as an independent variable is best seen in the influence of insufficient or fragmented sleep on the subsequent waking period. Level of alertness is very much related to quantity and quality of prior sleep. Mood is also affected. The effect of prior sleep on performance is not as direct and simple, but prior sleep is, nevertheless, sometimes a factor, especially for long, repetitive tasks in which we have to make responses to stimuli.

But it is also evident that sleep is a biological need - a drive. All people need at least some sleep on a regular basis, but the amount that is needed is strongly influenced by genetics. If the needed sleep is not obtained one night, then it needs to be made up (at least in part) on a subsequent night. This is true not only for total sleep, but also its substages of REM and SWS.

All of this leads us to conclude that sleep is homeostatic. Although it is not clear what is being regulated (see chapter 11), sleep can be considered homeostatic since the body attempts to regularly get a certain amount, and too little, or even too much, has negative consequences.

Chapter 4

Sleep as Rhythmic

Circadian Rhythms

Regular variations every nycthemeron have been observed in almost every aspect of physiology in both plants and animals. Many of these physiological rhythms of the body influence or are influenced by sleep (Carskadon, 1993; Coleman, 1986; Hume, 1983; Kalat, 1992). These dozens of rhythms are known collectively as circadian rhythms (circa = about; dian = a day). Things such as the levels of many hormones in the blood show a distinct peak and valley each day (see Chapter 2). Other chemicals in the body, likewise, show such fluctuations as do reflexes, mood, and many other kinds of processes that can be measured. Body temperature is the most obvious, fluctuating about 1°F everyday. For people accustomed to sleeping at night, body temperature is highest at about 8 p.m. and lowest during sleep, between 3 to 5 am. While sleep itself contributes to this drop in temperature, most of it persists even if a person remains awake. This helps account for the fact that when people stay up all night they feel coldest in the early morning, even if the temperature in the room is unchanged.

For most functions, the circadian cycle is slightly greater than 24 hours. Typically, however, the various functions all stay in phase with one another. That is, their peaks and valleys tend to happen at the same time relative to one another. Or to think of it another way, the near 24 hour rhythms of the various functions become interlocked into exactly 24 hour cycles. For example, every day, when body temperature starts dropping, growth hormone reaches a peak. The clock for these rhythms appears to be some internal physiological process (or processes) acquired genetically.[1]

How does this rhythm synchronization happen? The process is called entrainment and is caused by some regularly occurring event external to the body called a zeitgeber (German for "time giver") (Coleman, 1986). Think of a watch repair store with dozens of clocks and watches all continuously running. Some are a bit fast, others a bit slow, so every morning when the watchmaker arrives, he acts as a zeitgeber by going around and setting each clock to the same time. The most important zeitgeber in humans is light following a period of darkness. Examples of other possible, but weaker, zeitgebers include warm days followed by cool nights, daily variations in radiation levels, social events such as mealtimes, and work and school schedules. For some functions, at least in some people, sleep-to-wake transitions appear to be important zeitgebers for entrainment. In the absence of zeitgebers, the various rhythmic processes of the body become desynchronized with one another and are said to be "free running."

Time-free lab experiments

Experiments at a special sleep laboratory in New York demonstrated some of these rhythms and what happens when entrainment cues are removed and the circadian rhythms are allowed to run free. In one such experiment, Dava Sobel, a New York Times reporter, spent 25 days and nights in this lab. It consisted of a suite of three soundproof, windowless rooms - a bedroom, a bathroom, and a living room. Next to these was a control room in which a technician was always present. There was nothing in the suite by which Ms. Sobel could tell the time or even the day - no TV., radio, phone, or paper. The technicians were carefully trained to never say "Good afternoon",or "How are you this evening?" They even worked varying shifts so she could not determine who came in at night, for example.

[1]Be aware that these phenomena have been scientifically established; a pseudo-science called bio-rhythms is totally unrelated and has failed to be validated by scientific means.

The male technicians even had to shave before coming into Sobel's presence! (Her reports of this experience can be found in the *NY Times* of June and July, 1980.)

Ms. Sobel, like other subjects before and after her, had many of her physiological and psychological processes checked numerous times per day while living in the lab. Her temperature, blood hormones, and urine were often sampled. She frequently had to fill out alertness scales, take performance tests, and, before retiring, complete a bedtime questionnaire. She carried an activity monitor on her. Closed circuit TV gave the technicians a view of her activities. And, of course, her sleep was recorded in the standard laboratory way.

For two weeks, Ms. Sobel was allowed to go to sleep and awaken when she pleased. What happened during this time is typical of the many subjects, each paid $200.00 per week, who preceded her. She tended to go to bed later each night and arise 1 hour later each subsequent morning, thus maintaining a 25 hour day. She spent 30% of her time asleep (ranging from 5h 57m to 10h 45m per sleep period) and the percent of time spent in each of the sleep stages was typical for her age (see Chapter 1).

Other things began to deviate from what is typical in the normal 24 hour world. Her body temperature cycled every 24 1/2 hours. Since her sleep/wake time was about 25 hours in length, these two rhythms became "uncoupled." As mentioned above, normally body temperature reaches its low point several hours after going to bed. Ms. Sobel's temperature often began to drop before going to sleep, reaching a low point shortly thereafter, then climbing during the rest of her sleep time. On days when her temperature was high when retiring, she tended to sleep much longer than when falling asleep with a low temperature. She tended to awaken when her temperature rose. On days when she fell asleep near the low of her temperature cycle, she also had more REM sleep in the early part of the sleep period than is typical and frequently went directly into REM at the onset of sleep. Yet, the total amount of REM and its percent of the total sleep time remained unchanged. Likewise, there was no change in SWS nor in the REM/NREM cycle length.

The rhythm of cortísol secretion, a hormone produced by the adrenal gland, also became uncoupled. It is normally secreted in large amounts near the end of a sleep period (see Chapter 2). By Ms. Sobel's 25th day this outpouring of cortisol occurred several hours prior to sleep.

At the end of the experiment, Ms. Sobel was sleeping in the afternoon of the real world. When released into that world, she felt disoriented - somewhat like in jet lag. It took her 10 days to return to her normal nocturnal sleep pattern. Even then she still complained of being hypersensitive, unable to make decisions quickly, and lacking energy. Others who have continued in isolated sleep labs for much longer periods have experienced even longer sleep/wake cycles. "Nychthemerons" of 50 hours in length (but still with an average 30% spent in sleep) have been observed, but not if subjects are encouraged to take naps in addition to their longer periods of sleep (Carskadon, 1993).

You may be asking, as Ms. Sobel did, "Why do the rhythms of the body differ from those of our 24 hour world?" The key to the answer is flexibility. If we were locked into 24 hour rhythms, we could never adapt to changing conditions such as those that occur during long distance travel or shift work. We would be locked into the cycle we were born with regardless of whether or not it coincided with the day/night cycle of our part of the world, our society, and even our family. Having such flexibility is not without cost, however, because we may suffer from jet lag, the effects of shift work, and, for some, more serious problems (see Chapter 9 on sleep disorders).

To find out just how flexible people can be, other experiments were done in these isolated sleep labs (Coleman, 1986). In these experiments, the occurrences of zeitgebers were artificially manipulated to see if people could follow days shorter or longer than 24 hours. In one such experiment, the room had a clock on the wall, but it gradually sped up or slowed down until a shorter or longer day occurred. When the clock completed 24 hours in 23 real hours, the subjects followed it well, maintaining normal (according to the clock) sleep and wake periods. They showed no ill effects. Likewise, if the clock took up to 27 actual hours to complete its 24 hours, the subjects followed it easily. However, faster or slower clocks than these were not followed, and people in these cases tended to maintain a real 25 hour schedule regardless of what the clock said. Thus, our daily sleep/wake rhythms can vary a bit but not by much, and it is easier to maintain a day longer than 24 hours than one shorter. As we shall see, this turns out to be important with regard to jet lag, shiftwork, and sleep disorders.

Effects of circadian rhythms

But our inborn circadian sleep/wake rhythm can have other consequences for us (Coleman, 1986). Our alertness and ability to perform well are affected by this rhythm. For example, truck accidents involving no other vehicle are 7 times more prevalent between midnight and 8 am, with an even greater peak between 3 and 6 am. This occurs even though there are fewer trucks on the road at this time. The most likely cause is "dozing off at the wheel."

During an experiment involving night driving on country roads as well as monotonous freeways, electrodes recorded the brain waves and eye blinks of the drivers. The scientists conducting the experiment were surprised to see 20 minute periods or so of no eye blinks and sleep-like EEG. Since no accidents occurred, it was assumed that the driver had his eyes open and was controlling the car although "asleep!" Such a state has been called **automatic behavior**; the brain is asleep but low-level behavior continues. It is thought to be a dangerous state because the brain does not anticipate and prepare for potential problems. It has to awaken first and then respond; by then, as in some driving situations, it may be too late.

Automatic behavior is not unique to automobile driving. Sixty-five percent of Swedish train drivers fell asleep (as determined by EEG and EOG criteria) sometime during a 212-mile night run, whereas "only" thirteen percent did so during the same day-run. Nurses have reported "night-shift" paralysis. This is the inability to make gross body movements and a sense of paralysis while writing or reading. Sometimes they are unable to get up and do their jobs for several minutes. Night-shift computer operators have been reported to run the same data analysis program over and over again resulting in expensive waste.

It is not unusual for students to "pull an all-nighter." What should you expect when you stay up all night? First, it's not easy. You have to fight off sleep almost constantly, especially between 3 and 6 am. And you feel cold during those hours. Concentration is much more difficult and mechanical mistakes (such as when typing) are more frequent. But when morning finally arrives, you "get your second wind" and don't feel so tired (although still more tired than if you had slept all night). If you take an early morning exam and then (finally) go to bed, you may have trouble falling asleep. You will also probably wake up frequently or too soon and, in the end, get only 1/2 to 2/3 of your normal sleep. Even the sleep you do get does not seem like very "deep" sleep. Such experiences show that when you try to manipulate sleep it will yield, but it applies counter pressure. (From what was said previously in the chapter, what else do you think happens to your sleep under these conditions that you may be less aware of?)

Other aspects of the circadian sleep/wake cycle have been noted (Moorcroft and Clothier, 1987). The length of the free-running sleep/wake cycle appears to get shorter with aging but, whatever the cycle, the ratio of sleep to wake time stays relatively constant at 30%. The free-running sleep-wake cycle in females averages about 1/2 hour less than in males while free running, yet females average 18% more sleep than males. In some cases, when sleep continued for 14 to 16 hours, SWS begins to occur again. Under free-running conditions, humans are capable of maintaining a stable average circadian rhythm over the long run; that is, any deviation from the individual's pattern is compensated for in the next few cycles. Furthermore, under these conditions, the length of wakefulness influences the length of the subsequent sleep,and, to a lesser degree, the length of sleep influences the length of subsequent wakefulness.

Circadian Body Temperature Effects on Sleep

The length of our sleep is partially dependent on the circadian rhythm of our body temperature (Carskadon, 1993; Horne, 1983b; 1988). Sleep tends to terminate when our bodies are warming (Zulley, Wever & Aschoff, 1981). This is best seen in free-running subjects sleeping in an environment free from time-cues . Sleep is extremely long when initiated at the peak of nycthemeral body temperature but is much shorter (and not too much different from normal sleep length) when sleep is initiated at the nadir of body temperature or when just beginning to rise. Also, the termination of many sleep episodes occurs during the rise of body temperature (especially sleep initiated during body temperature peak, fall, and nadir) regardless of the length of the sleep. The circadian rhythm of our body temperature has another effect on sleep (Czeisler and Allan, 1988; Zulley, Wever, and Aschoff, 1981). In subjects with synchronized sleep/wake and body temperature rhythms, sleep onset is much more likely to be *initiated* when body temperature is getting close to or is at its nadir. There are exception to these relationships that can occasionally be observed, indicating that temperature does not have complete control over sleep length.

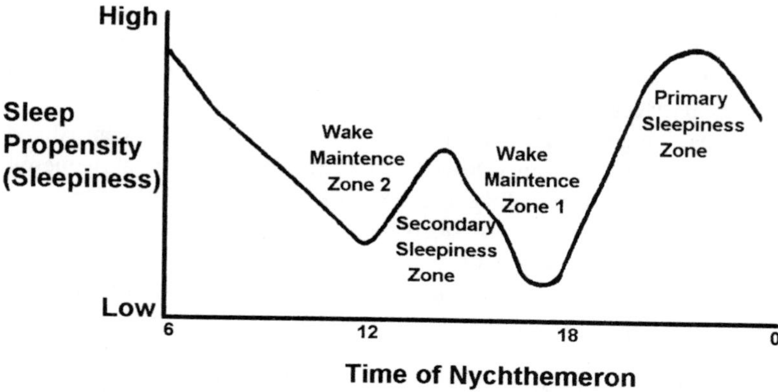

Figure 4-1. Typical sleepiness and wake maintenance zones during the nychthemeron.

An additional factor comes into play here. There is some indication that the placement of the peak and slope of the rise in the circadian temperature cycle change with the season. Earlier peaking and more rapid rise occur in the summer, leading to the speculation that it may not be possible to extend sleep as much in the summer as in winter (Horne, 1988).

Sleepiness/Wake Zones

During each nychthemeron,there are two periods of time when a person is more likely to fall asleep and two periods when a person is most awake and finds it more difficult to fall asleep (Dinges, 1989; Lavie, 1989; Strogatz, 1986; Morris, Lack, & Dawson, 1990). Figure 4-1 shows these periods for an average young adult with a bedtime at midnight. (The curve is typically shifted an hour or so left for morning types and others going to bed earlier than midnight, but typically is shifted to the right an hour or so for evening types and others with a later bedtime.) The PRIMARY SLEEPINESS ZONE (also known as the Primary Sleep Gate or Sleep Onset Zone) is the longest and strongest period of sleepiness. It begins at about the typical bedtime and lasts several hours. The SECONDARY SLEEPINESS ZONE occurs during the mid-afternoon, is not as intense, and lasts about two hours. There also appears to be two WAKE MAINTENANCE ZONES (also called the Forbidden Zones of Sleep). Wake Maintenance Zone 1 begins a few hours prior to sleep and lasts for a couple of hours. The weaker Wake Maintenance Zone 2 occurs for a few hours prior to the secondary sleepiness zone.

Dave Dinges of the University of Pennsylvania has conceptualized these zones another way (Dinges, 1989). He divides the nychthemeron into four equal zones. Zone I (approximately 100 to 700 hours) is a time of high probability of sleep onset and low probability of sleep offset. The main, longest block of sleep typically occurs during this zone. Zone II (700 to 1300 hours) is a time of low probability of sleep onset and high probability of sleep offset. Zone III (1300 to 1900 hours) has a high probability of sleep onset and a high probability of sleep offset. This is siesta or nap time - that is, time for a bout of short sleep. Zone IV (1900 to 100) hours has a low probability of sleep onset and a low probability of sleep offset.

It is important to note that preadolescents do not have a secondary sleepiness zone, but they sleep more deeply during the primary sleepiness zone at night.

The existence of these zones has been demonstrated through several experiments using various research procedures including sleep and nap logs, prolonged MSLT studies, and measurement of sleep onsets and durations in subjects free-running in time free environments (see later in this chapter). However, all of these zones may be best demonstrated in experiments using ultra-short sleep-wake schedules. Lavie (1986), for example, had subjects live on 20 minute sleep-wake cycles. They were required to be awake for 13 minutes followed by 7 minutes of opportunity to sleep for 24 or 36 continuous hours - sometimes following a night of sleep deprivation. In all cases, the subjects obtained much more sleep during certain parts of the nycthemeron and very little during other parts. The former are the sleepiness zones and the latter the wake maintenance zones. Sleep deprivation was found to change the intensity of the zones, (weakening wake maintenance zones and strengthening the primary sleepiness zones) but not their timing.

Morning Larks and Night Owls

One morning while I was in college, a "night owl" friend of mine dragged himself out of bed after yet another short night of sleep. He was wandering down the dorm hall to the bathroom in a haze in an effort to get ready for his morning classes. Suddenly, another dorm resident, a "morning lark," toothbrush in hand, cheerily said, "HI, JACK. GREAT MORNING, ISN'T IT?" whereupon Jack turned around and went back to bed.

Are there differences between morning larks and night owls? If so, what are the differences? And are people created morning larks or night owls (or neither type), or do they become that way out of habit? These questions have been studied in six different countries (Sweden, U.S.A., France, Italy, Netherlands, and Japan) with surprising cross-cultural agreement (Foret, Toaron, Beroit, and Bouard, 1985; Ishibara, Miyasita, Inyami, Fukuda, and Miyata, 1987).

Yes, there are differences between night owls and morning larks (more properly designated evening types and morning types or ET and MT, respectfully) as shown by both surveys and polysomnographic studies. Most people are neither type (NT) - somewhere between the extremes. MTs sleep better than ETs as shown by shorter average sleep latencies, are in a better mood upon arising, feel that they got an adequate amount of sleep, and feel more mentally efficient. ETs have metabolic and performance peaks later in the day than MTs (Hauri, 1982). But even more important than these differences in quality of sleep are measures of irregularity (or flexibility depending on your viewpoint). ETs go to bed later (by an hour or more), get up later (again by an hour or more), and vary more from night to night in sleep length. On the average, however, they obtain the same amount of sleep as the MTs. These differences are even more exaggerated on non-work or non-school nights, with MTs going to bed 1 hour later but ETs 2 hours later, MTs getting up about 1 hour later but ETs 2 or 3 hours later, and MTs getting 1 hour more sleep than on work or school nights, but ETs almost 2 hours more. ETs average more "all-nighters" and take longer and more frequent naps than MTs.

There is little difference between the types on polysomnographic measures except for a shorter than average REM latency (the time from sleep onset until the start of the first REM period) in MTs and a longer REM latency in ETs. However, both are still within normal limits. No physiological differences between the groups have been demonstrated. ETs tend to fall asleep either quickly (within 10 minutes) or lie awake for a long time (30 or more minutes), but there is no such division within the MT group who usually fall asleep within 20 minutes. Although the MTs show a peak of alertness 2 hours earlier and a peak of temperature 1 hour earlier than ETs, there is no consistent difference in actual performance between MTs and ETs at any time during the day. The difference in temperature peaks parallels the difference in arousal times between the two groups. Just as ETs go to bed an hour later than the MTs, so too does their temperature peak an hour later than that of the MTs.

If suddenly forced to adopt bed times and arising times of the other type, neither ETs or MTs sleep well. If allowed to sleep in the morning after a night without sleep, MTs have less REM and more wake-ups than ETs or NTs. In an experiment (Clodore, Foret, and Benoit, 1987) both MTs and ETs were awakened 2 hours earlier than usual. The subjective alertness of the MTs was higher than usual 2 to 4 hours later but not changed in ETs. When given a chance to nap at 10 am, more MTs (40%) fell asleep than ETs (12.5%). In a related experiment, NTs were similarly awakened 2 hours earlier. Their subjective alertness was less than typical a few hours later and it was easier for them to nap at that time (Foret and Petit, 1987).

In one study of people who were the same age, workers were found more likely to be MTs than students, suggesting that sleep/work habits are important in producing morning or evening types of people. On the other hand, the workers expressed a preference to be other than what they were, suggesting many more of them were going against a natural, inherited predisposition. However, as people get older they tend to become more and more like MTs, suggesting that people can and do change (Moorcroft and Clothier, 1987).

Several simple paper and pencil tests are available to determine if a person is a MT, ET, or NT. Results of these tests correlate with measures such as body temperature peaks (Carskadon, 1993). The newest by Smith, Reilly, and Midkiff (1989) was derived from three of the previous tests using statistical techniques to pick out the best questions. Most of its questions are from the Horne and Östberg (1976) scale. It consists of questions about what time of day you feel best, what time of day you prefer to do things, and what you would be like at other times of the day.

Timing of Sleep

What are the effects of changing the time when you go to bed? Such occurrences are not uncommon in the modern world with changing shift work and jet travel. For example, it has been estimated that

20% of US. workers are on shift schedules. Sleep attempted during usual waking hours results in more arousals, less stage 2, less REM, shorter REM latency, and often shorter total time asleep (Anch et al, 1988). Performance during normal sleep time is greatly reduced, especially for long, repetitive, and uninteresting tasks. More industrial accidents occur during such times. Although the body can adapt, it does take several weeks when switching from nighttime sleeping to daytime sleeping. (Interestingly, when shifting back to night time sleeping, the switch takes place in a much shorter period of time - several days.)

Jet Lag. Eastern Airlines flight 212 from Charleston to Charlotte, N.C. crashed on the morning of September 11, 1974. Captain James Reeves, 3 other crew members, and all 68 passengers aboard were killed. Subsequent investigation blamed the crash on pilot error - pilot and crew were not paying attention to their altitude. Why did this happen? We will never know for sure, but fatigue from shifting schedules was strongly suspected. The pilot's schedule during the week before that crash started with getting up at 4:15 a.m. to make five flights, then 4:45 p.m. the next day to make three flights, followed by 3:30 p.m. for another four flights. The fifth day he arose at 6:45 a.m. for four flights, then had a day off. The day before the crash he got up at 7 am, followed by a 3:30 a.m. arising on the crash day. One half hour prior to the crash, a tape recording of a conversation with a control tower has the pilot saying, "Rest. That's what I need is rest. I don't need all of this damned flying."

Captain Reeves chose that schedule, preferring to do most of his flying early in the month in order to have the rest of it off. This was in perfect accord with FAA rules which, at the time, required at least 10 continuous hours of rest per day. These rules, unchanged since 1934, were aimed at preventing fatigue from long work shifts. However, they do not take into account the recent knowledge that *when* a pilot rests is as important as how long. Varying sleep schedules using these rules upset the important coordinated circadian rhythms of the body and also results in fatigue. The body is not a battery that runs down and can be recharged at any time. Rather it is more like a complicated machine that needs regularly scheduled periods of maintenance, repair, and adjustment in order to function well.

Flight 212 is not the only example of a crash which was possibly caused by circadian rhythm disruption. The crash of a Western Airlines jet on the early morning of Oct. 31, 1979 in Mexico City occurred when the fatigued pilot attempted to land on runway 23-left instead of 23-right. A Pan Am jet went down in the South Pacific in April 1974 following several days of international flying by the pilot which required erratic sleep scheduling. Sixty percent of flying accidents are attributed to pilot error. Furthermore, pilots report that, although against the rules, napping and falling asleep in the cockpit are not unusual, especially during night and early morning flights.

Until the twentieth century, travel never had much of an effect on our circadian rhythm of sleep. Travel was slow enough that the body could readjust the phase of its circadian rhythms to local conditions when a person lived on a 22 to 23 hour daily schedule going east or 25 to 26 hour schedule going west. Rapid aircraft have changed all that. Today you can travel through several time zones on one eight hour flight; your body cannot keep up with that.

Symptoms of jet lag (Carskadon, 1993; Kryger, Roth, & Dement, 1989) include disorientation, fatigue, decreased performance and concentration, insomnia, excessive sleepiness, muscle aches, and disruption of appetite and digestion. Polysomnographic studies of sleep during jet lag following westward flight show a decrease in REM latency and more REM early in the night. SWS tends to be displaced toward the second half of the night. Phase shifts of many of the chemical rhythms of the body have also been reported (see Chapter 2 for a discussion of normal circadian rhythms of the biochemistry of the body).

Studies of jet lag have shown several interesting things (Carskadon, 1993; Coleman, 1986; Lamberg, 1984). Jet lag results from the zeitgebers of the destination assaulting the body with information that is too discrepant from its internal phase of circadian rhythms. The cause is not solely the fatigue of travel but also the number of time zone changes, the rate of these changes, and their direction. Travel of even 10 or more hours to the north or south does not produce jet lag, but travel of only a few hours to the east or west will. Flights near the equator result in less severe jet lag than those nearer the poles, since one changes time zones less rapidly. However, the time of day when a person travels is not a factor.

There is less of an effect when traveling to the west than to the east. This is true regardless of whether one is leaving or coming home. When going west we have to phase delay (lengthen days) which is easier, since our internal rhythm is longer than 24 hours. When going east we have to phase advance (set the clock ahead and thus shorten days) which is in the opposite direction of our internal tendency and thus more difficult. Some reports show that recovery from jet lag following travel to the east takes 50 to 100 percent longer than equally distant travel going toward the west. Complete recovery may take up to 18 days for 6 time zones, but a good rule of thumb for the majority of recovery is one day of recovery for each time zone. Some people have found it easier to adjust to eastbound travel over six time zones by gradually phase delaying by 18 hours rather than phase advancing by 6 hours. (Both would get you to the same local time since this approach is equivalent to gradually setting your watch ahead by 18 hours instead of back by 6 hours in order to have it read the local time.

There are differences between individuals, also. Twenty five to 30% of people are minimally affected by jet lag and an equal percent are highly susceptible. Older people suffer from jet lag more than younger people, with 40 years of age being the turning point. Morning larks are affected more than night owls. Personality may also be important; introverts and "neurotics" adjust more slowly to jet lag. Insomniacs also have more trouble with jet lag. People who fly regularly are not immune. The incidence of insomnia and fatigue is higher for flight crews than the general population. Eighty-seven percent of flying airline personnel report disturbed sleep. They also report above average frequency of gastrointestinal disorders and general nervousness.

Some other countries - Britain, Germany, and the Scandinavian countries for example - do take the body time of the pilots into account when scheduling their flights. Britain, for instance, requires a 32 hour break in every seven-day sequence of flying, with at least 2 spans between 10 p.m. and 8 am. Also, British pilots are required to return home 3 days out of every 14 to get good sleep at night.

There are several ways that jet lag can be combated. These are only general principles, some of which are logical, others of which have come out of scientific labs. An individual can choose which ones to use, depending on the circumstances:

1. **Stay on Home Time** (Coleman, 1986). If you will not be in any one time zone for more than a few days, do not even try to adapt to local time. Keep a watch set for your home time and eat and sleep at times that you would at home.

2. **Synchronize to Your Destination Before Your Trip**. Gradually phase delay by 2 or 3 hours per day (or phase advance by

1 hour per day) until you are eating and sleeping on the schedule of your destination. You may have to pick your flight carefully to do this so that you are flying during your wake time. This approach has been successfully used by athletic teams participating in international competition but has not been adequately validated using scientific methods.

3. **Use the Jet-Lag Diet** (Ehret & Scanlon, 1983). This approach is advocated by Charles Ehret of the Argonne National Laboratory near Chicago. (In fact, he will send you a wallet-size card summarizing the diet if you send a stamped self-addressed envelope to Anti-Jet Lag Diet, OPA, Argonne National Laboratory, 9700 S. Cass Avenue, Argonne, IL 60439). It is based on generalizations from animal work that show: a) eating on an empty stomach can act as a zeitgeber; b) proteins promote wake, carbohydrates promote sleep; c) caffeine, in addition to its general arousal effects, can speed up or slow down the bodies clock if taken only in the morning or evening, respectfully. However, convincing direct scientific validation in humans remains to be done.

You start your diet four days before your trip. Feast on day one on a high-protein breakfast and lunch, then have a high-carbohydrate dinner. Fast on day two on light meals (salads, soups, fruits). Feast again on day three, and fast on day four. Break the final fast at your destination breakfast time. On the first three days drink caffeinated beverages only between 3 and 5 P.M. On the final day, drink them in the morning only if going west, and only between 6 and 10 P.M. if going east.

A simpler version attributed to Stephen F. Forsyth, president of the Forsyth Travel Library (*Des Moines Register, February 21, 1993*) also includes several steps. On the day before the flight, eat a full, balanced dinner with lots of carbohydrates, such as spaghetti. On the day of the flight, avoid all food and caffeine. Do drink a lot of water and fruit juice. Break this fast with the breakfast snack typically provided just before the flight lands in Europe. Once on the ground, have a big breakfast as soon as you can.

4. **Arrive Early.** Add two or three days to your travel plans with the idea that they will allow time for your body to adjust before you do anything important.

5. **Synchronize Quickly to the New Environment**. Eat and sleep according to local time. Avoid napping. Get out and be active and with other people during local waking hours.

6. **Other**. These may be used alone or in combination with the above:

a. **Sleeping Pills and Stimulants**. Short acting sleeping pills for the first few days may help reset your sleep times and caffeinated beverages your wake times. However, some research suggests that they only delay jet lag effects and not cure them. That is, they prolong the time required to get over jet lag. Other recent research shows that sleeping pills, alcohol, and travel can interact to produce several hours of memory loss and confusion (Morris & Estes, 1987). (Alcohol should never be taken with sleeping pills under any circumstances, but travelers, unfortunately, often do it anyway.)

b. **Avoid alcohol or carbonated beverages on the plane** (Lamberg, 1984). Water or fruit juices on the other hand should be drunk plentifully. Alcohol and dry cabin air tend to dehydrate you. Carbonated beverages may uncomfortably distend the abdomen. So drink plenty of non-alcoholic, non-carbonated beverages.

c. **Bright light.** Daylight or indoor light four times brighter than average can help shift circadian rhythms. Light in the morning seems to phase advance circadian rhythms and thus would be good for eastbound travel, while light in the evening appears to do the opposite and would be best for westbound travel.

d. **Melotonin** (a hormone from the pineal gland - see Chapter 2) has been used experimentally to treat jet lag. However, it has not yet been approved for this pending more research.

Shift Work. Just as the invention of the jet resulted in the modern circadian rhythm disorder of jet lag, the invention of the electric light is responsible for the prevalence of circadian rhythms disorders associated with shiftwork. However, the shift worker, unlike the sufferer from jet lag, is constantly opposing zeitgebers rather than adjusting to new ones. In the US., 26% of working males and 16% of working women rotate work schedules. Shift work causes sleep/wake problems for workers (Åkerstedt 1984; Coleman 1986; Lamberg 1985). But the problem with shiftwork is more than just a problem of the circadian timing of sleep/wake. It is also a problem of sleep itself and domestic/social disruptions (Monk, 1989).

Shift workers report problems with sleep more often than day-workers (62% vs. 20%) and for good reason. They have several fewer hours of total sleep time per week with less REM and stage 2. In addition, the amounts of REM and SWS are level throughout the sleep period rather than increasing and decreasing respectively, and the REM latency is short. Perhaps more important was the increase in disruption of sleep by numerous awakenings. Night shift with day sleep presented the most problems.

The number one complaint of shift workers was fatigue. They take up to five days a year off of work because of fatigue without illness. Half admit falling asleep on the job at least once a week, and 15% also had fallen asleep driving to and from work at least once in the last three months. They rated themselves least alert when on the job. Shiftworkers nap more than day-workers and drink more caffeinated beverages (as many as 10 cups of coffee per day). They also use more drugstore stimulants to stay awake and more alcohol and sleeping pills to sleep.

Shift work affects performance and health. Lowered efficiency and increased accidents are common. Shift workers express more dissatisfaction with their jobs and social life, and increased friction with other workers is common. Shift workers also have a higher percentage of health problems, especially involving the gastrointestinal system, such as gastric and peptic ulcers and gastritis. Newer research suggests some of these problems may be permanent in long term shift workers (Anch et al, 1988).

Like the problems of jet lag, shift work problems cannot be eliminated, but some things can be done to try to alleviate them (Anch et al, 1988). Some people can adapt to shift work reasonably well. Permanent night shift workers do not have as many complaints or problems as rotating shift workers do. And after changing to a new shift, workers show a slight but gradual improvement in successive sleep cycles. One problem is that most shift schedules are set up wrong. First, they shift in the wrong direction - against the body's natural tendency. The typical rotation is from days to nights to evenings to days and so on. A better rotation would be days to evenings to nights to days. But this alone is not enough. How quickly the worker rotates shifts is also a problem. The typical length on a shift is about seven days - not long enough to adapt, yet long enough to cause problems. American experts say that ten days on a shift is better, and three weeks is better yet. Workers can then anticipate the next shift by gradually phase advancing their sleep time, thus going smoothly from one phase to another. If this is not totally possible, even a few days phase advancement of about equal steps can be helpful. Some European experts recommend rapid shift rotation, such as 2 days on each shift before shifting to the next. This allows the person to maintain their normal circadian rhythms.

A change in shift schedules had significant results for one company in 1980 (Coleman, 1986). The Great Salt Minerals and Chemicals Corporation in Utah operates a plant to harvest and process potash. The 150 shift workers there had trouble sleeping, and management contacted the Stanford Sleep Clinic for help. The consultants from Stanford found that the typical weekly changing of shifts were going in the wrong direction - against the body's natural tendency. This schedule had been in use there since 1890. Following the suggestions of the consultants, the workers were phase delayed to the next shift every third week. Also, workers were taught to gradually delay their sleep in anticipation of the next shift change. Eventually (it took a while for the workers to learn the new schedule and come to like it), productivity improved by 20%. Job satisfaction was much higher, and the health of the employees improved. In short, everyone, both the company and its employees, gained.

Other considerations have also been found helpful. Employees can be selected that have a better tolerance for shift work. Night owls shift more easily than morning larks; so do other people who find they can sleep at unusual times. Extroverts also do better, and so do people with minimal daily temperature fluctuation. Finally, younger people generally are better able to tolerate shift work than older people.

Shift workers can do things for themselves to help tolerate their schedules. Spending leisure time after work before sleeping is preferable to sleeping right after work. Avoiding snacks but eating on a regular schedule helps. And avoiding overuse of caffeine is recommended.

Other sleep schedules problems. Other events of normal living can also disrupt our circadian rhythms. Irregular sleep periods, especially arousal times, may throw the cycles out of phase. This can be most severe in workers with frequently changing shifts such as the jet pilots discussed earlier. But, for some people, the pattern on weekends of simply staying up later, followed by sleeping in the next morning can be disruptive. By Sunday night, they have phase delayed their sleep time enough they are "Sunday night insomniacs" when they try to get to sleep at their normal time. They may spend much of the subsequent work week in a semi-fog while their rhythms gradually return to proper phase, only to be disrupted again the next weekend.

Even the relatively small phase changes that occur with the switch to and from daylight savings time have been found to have effects on people. Moving the clock ahead in the spring results in a phase advance for people (since it results in a 23 hour day). An 11% rise in traffic accidents was found to occur during the week following, and injuries and outpatient hospital visits are increased (Carskadon, 1993). People reported awakening feeling more tense and more drowsy than usual during that week. Moving the clock back one hour in the fall is a phase delay (25 hour day) and results in the opposite effects to some extent.

Most people maintain a relatively regular fixed time of arising (Webb, 1992) - that is good! A regular time of arousal appears to be the most important factor for keeping the many biological and physiological rhythms of the body in synchrony, which in turn results in people reporting feeling rested and good. Again, society appears to demand a regular arousal time due to regular schedules of the job, market place, school and family life. Also, the availability of cheap alarm clocks has long made a regular time of arousal possible. Most people are less regular about their times initiating sleep than arising (Webb, 1992). All the indications are that this irregularity is not particularly harmful as long as a person does not continually push back the time of retiring and thus accumulate sleep deprivation.

"Internal Alarm Clocks." There have been numerous anecdotal and several scientific reports of people being able to awaken themselves spontaneously without the use of alarm clocks or other outside influences (Kleitman, 1972). They simply decide what time they would like to awaken before retiring. Tony Griggs, Krista Hennager, and I set out to investigate this more fully. First, we did a random telephone survey of adults primarily in the upper midwest of the US. The 269 respondents represented a good cross section of ages, employment, and sex. To our surprise, the results broke down into approximate quarters (Hennager, Griggs, & Moorcroft, 1991). Slightly less than one fourth

of the respondents said they never use an alarm, regardless of when they have to awaken. Another quarter of the respondents reported that they regularly awaken before their alarm goes off. Another fourth report that they sometimes awaken before the alarm. The final fourth stated that they need an alarm to awaken them (and even then they have difficulty awakening). Thus, three quarters of those surveyed said they awaken spontaneously at least some of the time and half said they do so regularly. The proportion of people who do not need to rely on an alarm increases with age and was slightly greater in people whose sleep times are consistent from day to day.

While random phone surveys are enlightening, they are not flawless. They may not be truly representative since not everyone has a phone and access to the phone varies considerably between people. Secondly, the responses people give may not always be accurate. Sometimes people are not accurate in their responses; other times they may not be entirely truthful. Thus Krista Hennager and I undertook a subsequent study. Through newspaper ads, we recruited 15 people in the vicinity of Luther College who said they could awaken from sleep without an alarm. Each was instructed to fill out a form prior to going to bed indicating, among other things, intended arousal time. Upon awakening, they also recorded when they actually did get up. In order to objectively measure awakening time, each subject wore an actigraph[2] from just before they retired for the night until they were up and around the next morning. The results from three nights for each subject confirmed that these people actually could, and do, awaken when they intended to without an alarm clock or any other external influence. The overall average difference between actual and intended arousal time was +4.61 minutes (i.e., they overslept by 4 mintues, 37 seconds) after a full night of sleep. Most awakenings occured between 3 minutes before and 12 1/2 mintues after the intended time.

Awakening without an alarm clock is a bit easier if the arousal time is the same every morning, but for some people it works even for very unusual times. (Besides being a more pleasant way to wake up

---

[2]An actigraph is a motion sensor, about the size of a large watch that is worn on the wrist. When its stored memory of motion is read by a computer, a graph and statistics of the wearer's active and quiet periods can be generated. The unique characteristics of motion during wakefulness, even quiet, inactive wakefulness, help make sleep distinguishable.

than being startled by an alarm - usually during the best part of a dream - this phenomenon provides interesting implications about the functioning of the mind during sleep. Just what is the unconscious process of the mind that occurs to allow it to keep time accurately - often with an error of less than 5 minutes - and then be able to interrupt sleep and initiate wakefulness? We need to know more about this often unrecognized, yet powerful, potential of our minds.)

Ultradian Rhythms

While we are talking of rhythms, another kind deserves mentioning. Ultradian rhythms are less than a nychthemeron in length. One such rhythm already mentioned is the approximately 90 minute REM-NREM cycle during sleep. There is evidence that this 90 minute cycle may continue during wakefulness as the basic-rest-activity-cycle or BRAC (Kleitman, 1982), but it may not be as obvious or stable as the NREM/REM cycle (Carskadon, 1993). Since this 90 minute cycle seems to be a basic physiological constant whether asleep or awake, it has also been called the "biological hour" (Horne, 1988). The observations supporting the presence of a 90 minute cycle during wakefulness include: alternating highs and lows about every 90 minutes in the performance of tasks requiring concentration, fantasizing, waking gastric activity, heart rate at rest, eye movements, and sexual excitation (Schulz in Carskadon, 1993). Also, people tend to feel sleepier about every 90 minutes (Hume, 1983; several articles in Shulz and Lavie, 1985). Other ultradian rhythms include variations in EEG frequencies, eye movements, some illusions, oral food intake, and waking fantasy reports (McGinty & Drucker-Colin, 1982). The effects may be subtle, but they are real. Whether these are all a manifestation of one BRAC or of many different processes is unclear at this time.

Summary

Sleep is rhythmic. There are times during the nychthemeron that our bodies prefer to sleep and other times that they prefer to be awake.

These observations have led to the statement that (after Lauber & Kayton, 1988):

AN HOUR OF SLEEP ≠ AN HOUR OF SLEEP

Sleep is best at night (and to a lesser extent, at mid afternoon), and we seem unable to change this very easily (Anch et al, 1988; Mendelson, 1987). The rhythmic nature of sleep seems to depend a great deal on the circadian temperature rhythm of our body. We tend to fall asleep and sleep when body temperature is falling or low and tend to awaken and be awake when it is rising or high.

In addition, the alternation of NREM and REM is rhythmic, but this cycle is faster than the wake/sleep rhythm. However, the propensity for REM is circadian. The likelihood of having REM sleep is greater, REM duration is longer, and REM latency is shorter during the early morning hours (400 to 700 hours) and just the opposite is true in late afternoon into early evening.

But sleep is also homeostatic as detailed in the previous chapter. This is particularly true for SWS and fatigue. The longer we are awake, the greater the pressure to go to sleep and the greater the pressure to have SWS. (A similar pressure also builds to have REM sleep, but the SWS pressure appears to be stronger.) These pressures decrease in proportion to the amount of sleep subsequently obtained.

The rhythmic and homeostatic aspects of sleep do not always coexist with one another well. Or at least it is difficult to satisfy the rhythmic without interfering with the homeostatic and vice versa (Monk & Moline, 1988). If sleep totally acquiesces to the dictates of one, the other remains partially unsatisfied. It thus appears that sleep is a **cooperative compromise** between its rhythmic and its homeostatic pressures. (Sleep also has to compromise with environmental influences [e.g. light, noise, danger, food availability] and behavior [e.g. work and entertainment schedules].)

Conclusion: Models of Sleep/Wake

One way to represent the homeostatic and rhythmic influences on sleep is through modeling (Hobson, Lydic, & Baghdoyan, 1986; Mendelson, 1987). Models help summarize, explain, and integrate known facts. The best models incorporate the greatest number of facts using the smallest number of assumptions. Good models also make predictions that can serve as a basis for further experimentation. Models also can help test hypothesies. But there are pitfalls with models. First, they may tend to become reified. That is, the model becomes confused with reality and takes on a life of its own. It becomes what is real. Second, models may be so flexible that they can fit any data. When this is the case, the model is untestible. In time, the survival or demise of a model depends on how well it corresponds to all varieties of pertinent data (e.g., neurophysiological as well as behavioral) and how well it makes accurate predictions. In many cases, modifications are made to the model based on new data as long as the modifications do no serious damage to the fundamental structure of the model. In other cases, the model must be abandoned because of new discoveries.

The most widely accepted model encompassing both the rhythmic and homeostatic aspects of sleep is the "two process model" of Borbély (1982; 1984; 1986). Borbély theorizes that two processes regulate sleep (see Figure 4-2, top). One, which he calls process C, is a circadian oscillator. It can be thought of as the circadian rhythm of sleep propensity. It is in phase with the circadian variation in body temperature. (¢ in Figure 4-2 is the mirror image of process C. It is used rather than C to make the model easier to understand. ¢ can be thought of as the wake threshold, whose lowest point is maximal sleep propensity).

The other process that regulates sleep is a homeostatic process called process S whose strength declines exponentially during sleep and increases exponentially during wakefulness. It can be thought of as sleep propensity when awake and depth of sleep when asleep. It also roughly corresponds to fatigue and is a function of the intensity, as well as the duration, of brain activity during waking (Feinberg, 1989) and REM during sleep (Horne, 1988). Process S is like an hour glass whose proportion of sand above and below changes with time with a 90 minute half life. Process C is like an on-going clock that can be set by environmental forces. Process C seems to diminish with age. Process S can be measured by the intensity of delta waves contained within the sleep period, since it has been shown that the intensity of delta waves diminishes as sleep continues, but increases proportionately to the amount of prior wakefulness.

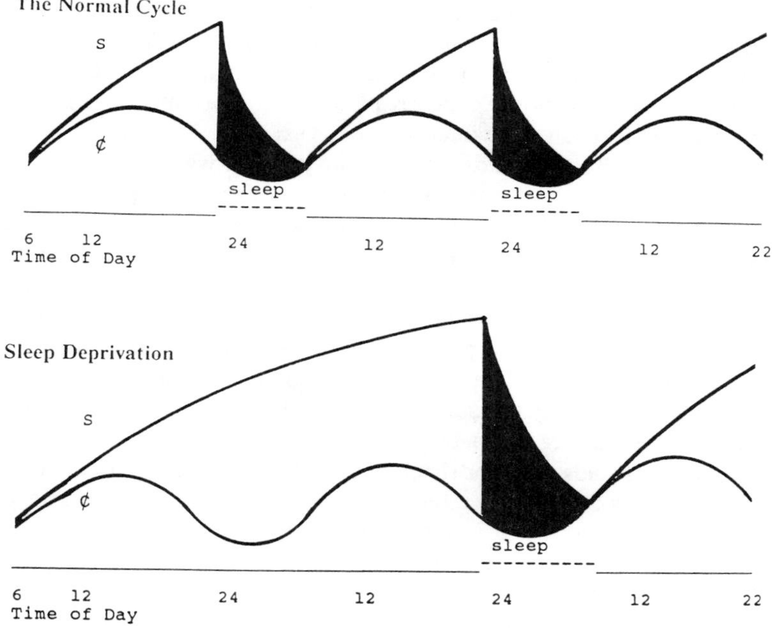

Figure 4-2. Borbély's model of the sleep/wake cycle. (Modified from Borbély, A A, 1982, A two process model of sleep regulation. *Human neurobiology, 1*, 195 - 204.)

Processes S and C combine to produce both the likelihood of sleep onset (or sleepiness) and the subsequent duration of sleep. Sleep propensity is the difference (or interval) between S and ¢ in Figure 4-2. Upon awakening, the curves are close together, and stay that way through the morning. The desire to sleep is small. Later, the interval becomes greater and greater reaching a maximum at bedtime. During sleep, the interval becomes progressively less, reaching zero at the time of awakening.

The lower part of Figure 4-2 shows what happens if a person does not sleep. Process S continues to rise and the interval between it and ¢ increases. However, a maximum interval is reached at about 4:00 a.m. From then on the interval lessens a bit (because of the circadian rise in process ¢) and the person feels less sleepy than before.

The large interval between the two curves after a night of sleep deprivation is seen in the lab by the intensity of SWS during the first

The large interval between the two curves after a night of sleep deprivation is seen in the lab by the intensity of SWS during the first part of the night. But process S declines exponentially. Thus, the length of sleep after sleep deprivation is only partially longer than normal, but is much more intense.

This model corresponds to both how you feel when staying up all night and how long you can sleep the next morning. If you can make it through the night without sleep, you feel like you are getting a "second wind" as morning arrives. However, should you go to sleep during the day, your sleep would be short and shallow, whereas your sleep the next night would be deeper, but only a bit longer. REM, in contrast, is relatively unaffected by prior sleep or wakefulness but shows a circadian rhythmicity. Thus, REM is strongly influenced by process C.

Borbély and collaborators have recently modified this model (Daan, Bearsma, & Borbély, 1984). They add the notion of dual parallel thresholds - one for sleep onset and one for waking from sleep. When process S rises above the sleep onset threshold, you fall asleep. On the other hand, when S falls below the waking threshold, you wake up. The levels of these thresholds vary regularly, each showing one peak and one low point every nychthemeron. The circadian variations in these thresholds are controlled by process C. Furthermore, the sleep onset threshold is always higher than the waking threshold. This model is analogous to a thermostat that turns off at a higher temperature than the temperature that turns it on. Also, like many modern heating systems, there is a night "cycle" with both on and off thresholds substantially lower at night. Additionally, either threshold can be affected by external conditions. For example, bedroom conditions conducive to sleep can lower the sleep-onset threshold. On the other hand, the sleep onset threshold can be willfully suspended for awhile, allowing S to increase well beyond its threshold limits.

Another version of this model (see Figure 4-3) combines it with the Hobson-McCarley model (see Chapter 2) to incorporate the ultradian NREM/REM cycle and the changing proportions of REM & NREM in successive cycles (after Achermann & Borbély, 1990; 1990; Borbély, 1982; Hobson et al, 1986). REM-ON is triggered when ¢ falls below a threshold (REM Threshold in Figure 4-3), thus REM is more likely to occur and be stronger during the night and early morning when sleep usually occurs. However, early in the night REM-OFF is strong, thus REM-ON is strongly inhibited by it. As the sleep period progresses, REM-OFF gets weaker (proportionally to the accumulation of SWS)

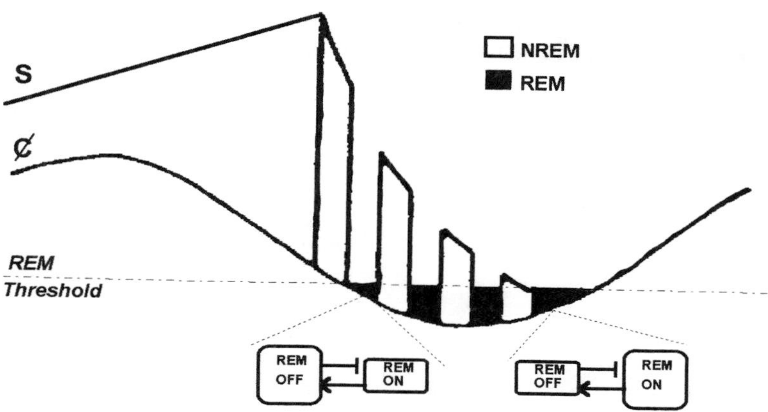

Figure 4-3. A hybrid model that combines the Borbély two process model with the Hobson-McCarley model to explain the increasing duration of REM with successive NREM-REM cycles. After Borbély, 1982 and Hobson, et al, 1986.

and thus more weakly inhibits REM-ON, allowing it to be active longer. Recall that this is precisely what happens during a typical night (see Chapter 1) - SWS predominates early in the night but quickly becomes less prevalent being replaced by longer and longer REM as sleep continues. The model also reflects the observation (Lavie, 1989) that the start of the first REM period is also dependent on the accumulation of a significant amount of SWS. The start of subsequent REM periods is independent of accumulated SWS; instead, they are regulated by the reciprocal interactions of the REM-ON and REM-OFF areas in the brain. Put another way, the timing of the first REM period is reset by SWS onset, but subsequent REM periods are controlled by an unentrained ultradian rhythm (Webb, 1987).

Several other models have been proposed to explain the circadian rhythms of sleep and related phenomena (Hobson et al, 1986; Mendelson, 1987; Strogatz, 1986; the entire issue 2 of the Journal of Sleep Research, volume 1, 1992). All of these models suggest one or more oscillators or timers that run continuously inside the body. These oscillators are strong enough to provide the near 24 hour intervals necessary for circadian rhythms, yet weak enough to be reset daily by necessary for circadian rhythms, yet weak enough to be reset daily by zeitgebers. The theories differ in the number of the oscillators, their nature, and their interactions with other factors.

Chapter 5

Sleep in Animals

Up to this point, we have been emphasizing sleep in humans. But obviously, humans are not the only inhabitants of this planet that sleep. Your pet dog or cat seems to spend a lot of time asleep, but what about your pet bird or fish? And now that you know how complex sleep is in humans, is it the same in all animals? Do all animals have REM sleep? Why do animals sleep? We will first review some examples of sleep characteristics in animals before attempting to answer these and related questions.

Grazing animals such as cows, sheep, deer, and horses spend little time asleep (as little as 2 hours out of every nychthemeron) (Webb, 1975), and the sleep they obtain occurs only in brief bursts, seemingly randomly scattered through day and night time. Little of the sleep that is obtained is REM. Animals in this group awaken to even the slightest stimulus and spend a great deal of time in a state called drowsiness (Meddis, 1983). Yet, elephants also get about 6 hours of sleep every nychthemeron, but in one consolidated period at night (Tobler, 1992).

The very small short-haired shrew obtains very little sleep; instead it spends most of its time gathering food in order to consume enough to survive (it must eat its own body weight each day) (Webb, 1975). Yet, the bat, similar in size and metabolism, sleeps 19 to 20 hours per nychthemeron (Meddis, 1975).

Cats and mice both sleep the same amount each nychthemeron - about 13 hours (Meddis, 1975).

A gorilla sleeps 14 hours out of every 24, as do ground squirrels in their burrows (Webb, 1975). Baboons sleep dusk to dawn in beds made high in trees but remain very alert during the day when foraging for food (Webb, 1975). Only a small percent of their sleep is spent in REM.

Possums sleep 19-20 hours per 24 in both REM and NREM (Rojas-Ramirez & Drucker-Colin, 1977). Moles spend 25% of their 8 nychthemeral hours of sleep in REM (Meddis, 1983), but the spiny anteater does not appear to have any REM sleep (Allison, Van Twyver & Goff, 1972). Other comparisons of the sleep states of mammals can be found in Table 3-1. AS per nychthemeron is rarely more than 1/3 that of QS per nychthemeron and about 1/4 of total sleep time.(Meddis, 1979).

Bull frogs may not sleep (at least very deeply), yet tree frogs do (Tauber, 1974). Reptiles such as turtles and snakes sleep but their EEG characteristics are not like those of mammals (Karmanova, 1982). Many fish have quiet periods spent in a specific location that seem to resemble many of the characteristics we identify with sleep (Hediger, 1983), yet other fish have to be in constant motion (Durie, 1981). Birds' sleep is very much like that of mammals with REM and NREM, yet their REM is of brief duration (measured in seconds) and occupies only about 5% of total sleep time (Karmanova. 1982).

Some animals sleep primarily during the nighttime (called a diurnal pattern) such as monkeys and humans. Others sleep primarily during daytime (nocturnal pattern) such as rats. Others divide their sleep into short periods throughout the entire nychthemeron (intermittent) such as cats and cattle. Finally, some are awake only at dawn and dusk (crepuscular) such as bats.

You probably found this list of sleep patterns in different animals interesting yet difficult to organize and put into perspective. You are not alone. Scientists have used two approaches in their attempts to make sense out of this welter of differences. One is to analyze the sleep in animals from an evolutionary standpoint. The other is to examine the functions that sleep serves in animals and how some functions may be more important to some animals than others. While both approaches provide some insight, each has its limitations.

Table 3-1 Comparison of the sleep/wake states in mammals

ANIMAL	STATES (% TIME/DAY)		
	Waking	Slow-Wave Sleep	REM Sleep
Cat	42.3	42.2	15.5
Fox	59.2	30.8	10.0
Dog (pointer)	66.2	30.0	3.0
Seal	55.7	33.5	10.7
Rabbit	50.0	48.0	2.0
Kangaroo rat	55.7	38.5	5.8
Rat	42.9	48.2	8.6
Cow	82.6	15.8	1.6
Opossum	19.2	76.7	4.1
Armadillo	28.0	59.0	13.0
Echidna	64.2	35.8	0
Squirrel monkey	17.0	59.3	22.9
Baboon	18.0	71.3	10.5
Human	60.6	32.8	6.6

(From Rojas-Ramirez & Drucker-Colin, 1977, Phylogenetic considerations between sleep and memory, in Drucker-Colin & McGaugh [Eds.], *The Neurobiology of Memory*, Orlando, Fla.: Academic Press. With permission.)

When trying to trace the evolution of animals, scientists rely on fossils. Fossils preserve the structure of species that no longer exist, but that gave rise (or were "ancestors") to currently living species. Comparisons of these preserved structures allows scientists to determine how appendages became wings in some animals and arms in others, for example. However, with regard to behaviors such as sleep, we have no fossilized evidence to study. All that is available is the diversity of sleep patterns among living species (Meddis, 1983). The best that can be done is to compare the patterns of sleep of currently living animals with evolutionary relationships among animals known from fossilized evidence, and then make the best of it. The assumption is that present-day animals sleep much like their ancestors millions of years ago. As we shall see, this has led to some disagreements and controversies, and even the assumption itself has been challenged (Foulkes, 1983).

The functional approach to sleep in animals is also imperfect. The functions of sleep are not satisfactorily known. (We will deal more with this in Chapter 11.) This makes studying and understanding animal sleep in terms of function difficult. Yet, the study of animal sleep increases our understanding of the functions of sleep. The analysis of sleep in animals, then, both contributes to the understanding of the function of sleep and suffers at the same time from a lack of knowledge of them.

But these are not the only problems involved with studying sleep in animals. The sheer number of living animals makes a comprehensive study almost impossible. There are about 5000 species of mammals, 9000 birds, 5300 reptiles, 3000 amphibians, and over 50,000 fish (Durie, 1981). The sleep of only a very small fraction has been studied, with twice as many studies in mammals as in all other animals combined (Carskadon, 1993). Even some of these studies have not always been done completely or adequately.

Even the studies that have been done are far from perfect. Most studies have been done in a lab or zoo (Meddis, 1983), thus the animals are out of their natural environment. Other variables such as environmental temperature, season of the year, diet, and so on have not been well studied or controlled (Campbell & Tobler, 1984). Behavioral criteria for describing sleep in non-mammals have not been adequately and consistently used, nor have tests of behavioral response thresholds, state reversibility, and sleep deprivation (Tobler, 1982). Any conclusions based on such inadequate sampling and experimental design must be very tentatively drawn indeed.

In the end, we are forced to make conclusions about sleep that may be similar to saying all reptiles have shells because we have only studied tortoises. However "science is a process of gradually diminishing deceptions" (Durie, 1981, p. 3), and we must start somewhere. For the rest of this chapter, we will proceed by making comparisons and conclusions, as if virtually everything about animal sleep is known, yet in the end we will realize that further study and discovery may soon change these pronouncements in their details or generalizations. For the moment at least, "the sleep researcher is obliged to live with an uncomfortably large amount of scientific uncertainty" (Tauber, 1974, p 140).

Defining Sleep in Animals

What do you look for when studying sleep in animals? Some researchers have said (or more often assumed) that you use the same criteria that you use to define sleep in humans - EEG, EOG, and EMG. But what do you do if you have an animal that cannot move its eyes (such as some owls)? Or animals that never relax their neck muscles (such as some perching birds)? Or animals whose brains are not advanced enough to show certain brain waves (such as reptiles)? Do you exclude these animals from consideration of having sleep? Many animal researchers have said, "No." Durie (1981), for example, has said that the study of sleep has become too anthropomorphic by maintaining that the essence of sleep is what can be seen in humans. Animals, he continues, are free to express sleep in any way advantageous to them and, thus, we must be more flexible when establishing our criteria for sleep. For example, the EEG aspects of sleep typical of mammals seem to have occurred rather late in evolution (Tauber, 1984). Reliance on behavioral signs supplemented by physiological indicators of sleep may be more realistic in this endeavor until EEG criteria are developed for lower animals that take their nervous system structure into account (Campbell & Tobler, 1984).

As we shall see later in this chapter, most animals have a regular rest-activity cycle. It is not always possible to call the rest phase sleep, but sleep may have evolved out of such a stage (Tauber, 1984). During the rest phase, the animal is inactive and usually assumes a typical body position and may even go to a specific location to do so (Hediger, 1983). Yet, we still cannot say that animals in such a state are necessarily asleep. If, however, two additional criteria are present, then some researchers describe the state as sleep (or sleep-like). These criteria are increased arousal threshold and state reversibility (Durie, 1981).

Increased arousal threshold simply means that the animal is less responsive to stimuli. It may take a louder noise to cause the animal to flee, for example. Or you might be able to approach the animal and even touch it without any signs of it becoming defensive.

State reversibility means that when the presumably sleeping animal does respond to a stimulus, its behavior and attention level rapidly changes back to that typical of wakefulness. It may open its eyes and stand up, for example. Or its muscles may become more tense. Or it may increase the frequency of its gill movements.

Karmanova (1982) agrees that behavioral and electrophysiological criteria are useful for defining sleep in animals, but adds some vegetative signs to her list of criteria. These are things such as lowered respiratory rate and heart rate. In fact, she maintains that a lowered heart rate is the most universal and best sign of sleep in all of the animal kingdom, but that a drop in respiration rate and body muscle tone are nearly as useful.

More recently, the research group of Alex Borbély (which includes Irene Tobler) in Zurich, Switzerland has added the experimental manipulation of sleep deprivation to their list of criteria (see Borbély, 1986). They reason that if sleep (or even sleep-like rest) is of use to an animal, then being deprived of it should be of consequence and the debt repaid sometime soon in the future. This repayment may be a temporary increase in duration of sleep or sleep-like rest or a more intense manifestation of it (such as higher amplitude of delta waves following sleep deprivation).

Table 3-2 is a summary of criteria that have been useful for establishing the presence of sleep in animals. It is not necessary that each and every item on the list be present to say that sleep or sleep-like rest is occurring, but at least a significant number of these things must be observed.

With a greater reliance on behavioral signs of sleep rather than electrophysiological indicators occurs a change in the terms used to describe the stages of sleep and wakefulness by animal researchers. They prefer using quiet sleep (QS) and active sleep (AS) for NREM and REM respectively (Durie, 1981). When such states are further subdivided (especially in mammals), QS may be divided into slow wave sleep 1 (SWS1) and slow wave sleep 2 (SWS2). SWS1 (light sleep or "superficial" sleep) is typically distinguished by spindles in the EEG (Morgane, Stern, & Bronzino, 1977) and a somewhat lower heart rate than when awake (Karmanova, 1982). SWS2 ("deep" sleep or simply SWS) is distinguished by synchronized high voltage, slow waves and regular, but even lower, heart and respiration rates and somewhat lower neck muscle tension than seen in SWS1 (Karmanova, 1982). Other substates that are often identified include aroused waking versus relaxed waking (differentiated by amounts of activity and body posture) (Morgane, et al, 1977) and dozing or drowsiness.

Table 3-2 Criteria for the definition of sleep

Descriptive

1. Behavioral
   - Typical body posture
   - Specific sleeping site
   - Physical quiescence
   - Elevated threshold for arousal and reactivity
   - Rapid state reversibility

2. Electrophysiological

   EEG
   - Change from wake to sleep:
     low voltage fast waves → high voltage slow waves
     → spindles
   - Cyclic changes within sleep:
     low voltage fast waves (REM or AS [active sleep]) →
     high voltage slow waves (NREM or QS [quiet sleep])

   EOG
   - Change from wake to sleep:
     random eye movements → no eye movements (QS)
     or → rapid eye movements (AS)

   EMG
   - Progressive loss of muscle tone from W → QS → AS

3. Physiological
   - Characteristic changes in heart-rate, breathing, body temperature etc.

Functional: Regulation

Compensation of sleep deficit:
- enhancement of sleep time
- intensification of the sleep process (enhanced EEG power in the Delta range)

(Modified from Tobler I, 1984. Evolution of the sleep process: a phylogenetic approach. In A A Borbély & J L Valatx, *Sleep Mechanisms* [(pp. 207-226)]. New York: Springer-Verlag. Used with permission of Irene Tobler, Alexander Borbély, and Springer-Verlag, Inc.)

A Survey of Sleep in the Animal Kingdom

Mammals

All mammals sleep (Zepelin in Carskadon, 1993) (including humans) and they all share many of the same characteristics of sleep (Borbély, 1986; Monnier, 1983), with some notable exceptions which we shall look at shortly. Since at least one species has been studied from each of the 17 mammalian orders (Tobler, 1984), we can feel fairly confident about summarizing these similarities. They include: a) quiescence; b) typical posture; c) reduced responsiveness to stimuli; d) low voltage, fast EEG when awake accompanied by high voltage EMG; e) sleep has either high voltage slow wave EEG (QS) or lower voltage faster waves (AS); f) the low voltage waves may be accompanied at times with little or no EMG, bursts of rapid movement of the eyes and twitching of paws and whiskers (AS); g) quick reversibility to wakefulness. Also, mammals have somewhat regular cycles from wake to sleep to wake and cycles within sleep from QS to AS. Further, the percent of total sleep time occupied by AS is higher the younger the pre-adult mammal. Within this basic pattern of similarities in all mammals are species-specific differences in how it is manifested (Mukhametov, 1984). Differences may occur in total sleep time per nychthemeron, relative amounts of QS and AS, QS/AS cycle length, sleep episode length, placement of sleep relative to day/night, and arousability from sleep. For example, small mammals (who by necessity have a higher metabolic rate) generally sleep longer than larger mammals and have shorter QS/AS cycles. These smaller mammals also have a shorter life span (Borbély, 1986).

Dozing. Many mammals, but not including humans, doze (Borbély, 1986). Dozing is loosely characterized by a "sleepy" appearance, relaxation, a unique EEG pattern of a mixture of rapid and slow waves (see Figure 3-1), a small decrease in heart rate and respiration, eyes partially closed, and slightly elevated and/or low response thresholds (Borbély, 1986; Meddis 1983; Ruckebusch, 1972). Hoofed animals (pigs, horses, cows, sheep) spend a lot of time in this state. A cow, for example, will sleep for 4 hours of every 24 but doze for an additional 8. They can even chew their cud in this state. The cat (who according to one undergraduate student essay spent "most of its waking hours asleep" [Durie, 1981, p. 2]) actually is dozing a lot of the time. High

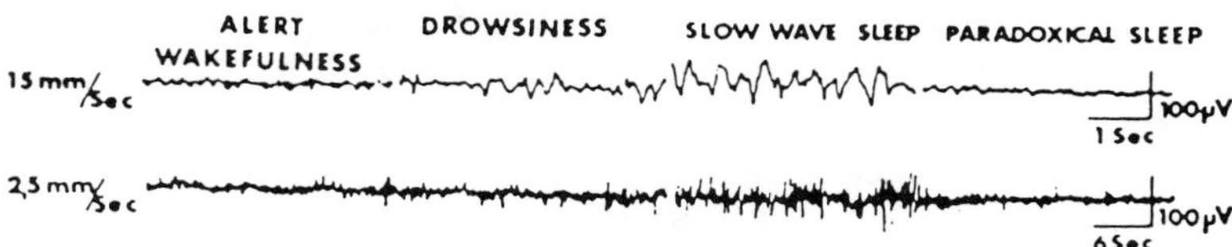

Figure 3-1. EEG for dozing compared to other states of sleep. (From Ruckebusch, 1972, The relevance of drowsiness in the circadian cycle of farm animals. *Animal Behavior, 20*, 637-643. With permission of the publisher, Builliere Tindull.)

levels of dozing have also been documented in dogs, hedgehogs, and foxes (Meddis, 1983), are dozing undoubtedly occurs in numerous other mammals.

Echidna. The notable exceptions to the general mammalian pattern of sleep are found in the Australian Spiny Anteater (Echidna) and some sea mammals. Since much importance is placed on these exceptions, we will examine their sleep in some detail.

In the early 70's, Allison and associates reported their very influential studies on the Echidna (Allison, et al, 1972). This unusual mammal hatches its young from eggs, but is a mammal since it maintains a warm body temperature. It is one of two remaining representatives of a line of mammals called non-therians (the other is the as-of-yet unstudied platypus) that branched off from the therian line about 175 million years ago. Allison and associates reported that the Echidna sleeps 12 hours of every nychthemeron cycling between QS and wake but, importantly, has never been observed to be in AS (although infant Echidna twitch during sleep as if in AS - Medis, 1989). It is not the niche or life style that results in the absence of AS, because other mammals with similar life styles that share the same niche, namely armadillos (Tauber, 1974) and moles (Monnier, 1983), do show AS. Allison and associates maintain that the non-therians never developed AS during their evolution. Not all scientists agree.

Some scientists have questioned the interpretation of the data by Allison and associates maintaining that it is equally plausible that the ancestors of the Echidna had AS but that it disappeared in Echidna over the eons (Tauber, 1974; Walker & Berger, 1980). Other scientists question the data of Allison and associates rather than its interpretation. The room temperature used for their experiment may have been so cold for the Echidna that it prevented AS from occurring (Horne, 1983b). The electrode placement used by Allison and associates is not thought to be adequate to detect important signs of AS (Meddis, 1975). The animals were in burrows most of the time when studied and thus could not be observed directly for signs of AS (Tobler, 1983).

Unfortunately, the study by Allison and associates is the only one available on Echidna or any non-therian animal. What is needed is replication of their study and extension to other kinds of Echidna (there are four in addition to the type used by Allison and associates) and the other non-therian, the platypus.

Sea mammals. For obvious reasons, sleep research on mammals that live in the sea has not been abundant. A Russian scientist, L. M. Mukhametov, and associates have managed to intensively study 11 such types of mammals, representating all 3 orders of aquatic mammals, using behavioral observations and electrophysiological monitoring (Mukhametov, 1984; 1992; Oleksenko, Mukhametov, Polyakova, Supin, & Kovalzon, 1992).

Sea mammals have a unique problem with sleep - they must breath surface air. Thus, they need to either remain on the surface of the water which, especially in wavy seas, means near constant movement or must rise to the surface to take a breath, which also requires movement. Neither of these situations is conducive to the universal component of muscle relaxation or paralysis that we see in sleeping land-based mammals. On the other hand, sea-based mammals are in a buoyant environment, so they do not have to expend much effort to counter the pull of gravity. What sorts of adaptations do these circumstances cause in the sleep of sea mammals?

The sleep in dolphins is perhaps the most surprising and instructive. Mukhametov has studied bottlenose dolphins and porpoises under a variety of experimental situations (some very long term) and has never once seen any evidence of AS! QS consisting of 50% or more delta waves is prevalent and a stage 2-like sleep, consisting of theta and delta waves with sleep spindles, does occur a small percent of the time. Wakefulness with desychronized EEG is the most prevalent state.

Another surprise is that one half of the dolphin brain may be asleep while the other half is awake! While both sides of dolphin brains may simultaneously show stage 2-like sleep (with the animal surfacing to breathe without awakening), such a situation has never been observed in SWS. That is, if one side of the brain is in SWS the other side is awake by EEG criteria. Such unihemispheric sleep can last for over 2 hours at a time. The hemispheres alternate sleeping in this way, with one hemisphere sleeping for about an hour, followed by wakefulness in both hemispheres, then the other hemisphere sleeping for an hour. Recordings from other brain areas show that this pattern is controlled from somewhere in the brain stem of the dolphin rather than being the direct influence of one hemisphere on the other. That this SWS sleep is comparable to land mammals SWS is shown by the simultaneous drop in brain temperature during SWS only on the sleeping side. Interestingly, the total amount of SWS obtained by each side of the brain is seldom equal. In some animals the left side gets more, while in others the right side gets more.

Thus, the dolphin may have both sides of the brain awake, one or both sides in stage 2 sleep, but only one side at a time in SWS. During unilateral SWS and bilateral stage 2 sleep the swimming movements are stereotypical and in circles, with regular surfacing for breathing without any change in state. In any state - asleep or awake - both eyes or only one may be open and, presumably, performing a "sentinel function."

Experimental manipulation of dolphin sleep yielded further insights. Total sleep deprivation results in increasing sleep pressure and rebound just as in land mammals. But, during the rebound sleep there was no disruption of the alternation of SWS in the hemispheres. If only one hemisphere was deprived of SWS, there was no compensation by the other hemisphere; only an increase in sleep pressure and rebound in the deprived hemisphere. Finally, if bilateral SWS was artificially induced with drugs, the animals were unable to surface to breath.

Apparently, the animal is unable to have all of its brain sleep deeply and breathe at the same time, so it sleeps deeply with only half of the brain at a time. It probably does not have any AS for the same reason; the body muscle paralysis that would occur with even unilateral AS would make it unable to breathe while in this state. For this reason, Mukhametov believes that the dolphins have lost AS in order to adapt to aquatic life.

Mukhametov also studied two kinds of seals and the porpoise. Seals can exist under water (needing, of course, to rise to the surface periodically to breathe), at the surface of the water, and on land. Both kinds of seals are immobile during sleep without maintaining any specific posture, but differ in other aspects of their sleep. Caspean seals show clear cut AS as well as other states of sleep seen in land mammals, but no unilateral sleep. When sleeping under water, Caspean seals can hold their breath for up to half an hour (Horne, 1988) then awaken to surface and breathe. (Compare this to human sleep disorder called sleep apnea discussed in Chapter 8.) There is no indication if this disrupted sleep is of good quality or not. Northern fur seals sleep on land and sea. They sleep on their side on the surface of the water with their nostrils in the air and with one flipper moving underwater to keep the animal stable, with the opposite side of the brain awake. These seals also show clear cut AS and other sleep states on land, but almost no AS in water. However, they do show occasional unilateral stage 2 and SWS as well as bilateral stage 2 and SWS. AS is always bilateral. Porpoises also have unihemispheric sleep.

Unlike research on the Echidna, some of these results have been replicated and extended by other investigators. The gray seal is reported to show QS on land, when floating, and when under the sea, but AS never occurs under water. Further, AS, when it occurs on land or the surface of the sea always precedes rather than follows QS (Tobler, 1984). States of sleep/wake have been observed to differ on the two sides of the brain in the pilot whale (Tobler, 1984). The sea cow does not appear to have AS (Tobler, 1984).

Horne (1988) cites a report on the sleep of the blind Indus dolphin. This animal lives in muddy, turbid waters of estuaries with varying currents. It must, however, be constantly on the move in order to avoid injuring itself on rocks and other debris while using its sonar. Studies (using behavioral measures only) show that it sleeps for only 4 to 60 seconds at a time (with slowed swimming) but obtains a total of 7 hours of sleep per day in this way.

Birds

Sleep in birds has been studied in 21 species of 9 of the 28 orders and was found comparable to that of mammals (Carskadon, 1993; Kryger, Roth, & Dement, 1989) but to have evolved independently. However, not enough study has occurred in birds to provide a lot of confidence about these conclusions (Tobler, 1984). Birds have desplayed rebound sleep following sleep deprivation (Tobler & Borbély, 1985). Birds show QS with high voltage slow waves accompanied by slight decrease in neck muscle tension, a decrease in heart rate to minimal values, and a low, but regular respiration rate. AS is characterized by low voltage, fast frequency EEG, irregular, but somewhat lower heart rate and respiration rate, an increase in response thresholds, some rapid eye movement (except in birds, such as owls, that are unable to move their eyes), lower neck muscle tension and/or behavioral observation of head droop). AS always follows QS but never follows wake.

The AS of birds is not entirely identical to that of mammals, however (Borbély, 1984; Karmanova, 1982; Meddis, 1983). The episodes of AS are very short - seldom longer than 30 seconds, more typically 5-6 seconds in duration - and occupy 2-10% of the total sleep time. Sound stimulation during AS does not awaken birds, but only causes them to shift to QS. They resume AS when the sound ceases.

QS differs in birds compared to mammals, too. No sleep spindles have been observed. Occasional small rapid eye movements have been observed during QS and slow waves during wake (Tauber, 1984). In mammals, delta waves progressively diminish in total amplitude as sleep continues, but not so in birds, nor is there any great difference in the amount of delta waves between sleep and wake, and there is no recovery of delta waves after sleep deprivation in birds (Tobler, 1987). Similarly, the episode length of substages of sleep does not vary over the main nocturnal sleep period in birds (Ball, Shaffery, Opp, Schmidt, & Amlaner 1987), but AS may become more frequent later in sleep.

There are some additional types of sleep observed in birds that are not present in mammals. **Vigilant sleep** is a type of sleep intermediate between QS and AS. **Unihemispheric sleep** (only one side of the brain asleep at a time) appears to be widespread in birds. One hemisphere can be unilaterally deprived of sleep by placing a patch over 1 eye and maintaining 24 hours of light to the other. The recovery from sleep deprivation in birds differs from mammals too. **Gaze-wakefulness** is characterized by a low voltage, fast EEG, reduced neck muscle tone, opening of the eyes, and slow "nontypical" movements of the eyes.

Finally, there are some additional unique facets of the sleep in birds that have been noted. Birds have been reported to be able to sleep while flying. The amount of sleep that birds get every nychthemeron depends on the amount of daylight. As the amount of daylight increases, the amount of sleep decreases, but only up to a limit (Ball et al, 1987). Pigeons (and other birds) have been observed to "peep" in their sleep. A peep is a brief opening of the eyes, something like a reverse blink. Since the frequency of peeps by a individual bird during sleep is (Lendrum, 1983):

1. increased by the presence of predators,
2. decreased by the presence of other birds, and
3. decreased by sleep deprivation,

it is thought that the peeps are a way of looking for predators.

Reptiles

Do reptiles sleep and, if so, what kind of sleep do they get? Although there is no strong agreement among researchers, the answer to the first question appears to be yes (Carskadon, 1993) in 13 out of 16 species (representing 4 of the five reptillian orders) studied (Campbell & Tobler, 1984; Tobler, 1982), especially if behavioral criteria are heavily weighted (Monnier, 1983; Tobler, 1984), but their brain waves are quite different from those seen in mammals and birds (Walker & Berger, 1980). Signs of sleep observed in reptiles include shutting of the eyes, assuming a particular body position, sometimes a specific place for sleeping, behavioral inactivity, an increase in arousal threshold, and rapid return to waking. In addition, a tonic deceleration of heart rate and a decrease in body muscle tone can be observed. Rebound of sleep following sleep deprivation has been observed in reptiles (Tobler & Borbély, 1985).

The brain waves or reptiles during sleep may differ from those of birds and mammals because they have a less advanced brain. Reptile brain waves may be less, rather than more, synchronized (regular) during sleep compared to active wakefulness and while the dominant waves may be of low frequency, they are also of low amplitude. Spike-like waves of high amplitude may occur on this background activity, beginning with the transition from wake to sleep. They become more abundant following sleep deprivation. These spikes have been called precursors of PGO spikes (Walker & Berger, 1980), similar to limbic system spikes seen in cats (Tobler, 1984), or precursors of slow waves (Tauber, 1974). Spikes during sleep were not observed in young crocodilians housed together at warm temperatures; only slow waves (some of high voltage) (Warner & Huggins, 1978). These brain waves are more like those of mammalian subcortical structures during sleep.

Assuming they do sleep, what kind of sleep do reptiles have? Opinions differ ranging from a "primordial" QS with even AS in some reptiles (Monnier, 1983) to no "recognizable" QS or AS at all (Walker & Berger, 1980). Karmanova (1982) labels reptilian sleep as "intermediate" sleep which progressed into both QS and AS during evolution of more advanced animals (see below). The evidence for AS is particularly controversial relying heavily on the presence or absence of eye movement (Tobler, 1974). Some researchers conclude AS is absent in reptiles (Flanigan, 1973a,b; Hartse in Carskadon, 1993; Horne, 1983c), while others conclude that AS can be seen in some lizards and maybe turtles (Tauber, 1974).

Amphibia

Only 9 species of the over 2500 living varieties of amphibia have been studied to date (Campbell & Tobler, 1984; McGinty in Carskadon, 1993), and the results of these studies are mixed. While all show periods of behavioral rest, only some seem to show signs of genuine sleep, while others do not. Even among those that show such signs, the sleep is not as well organized as it is in more advanced animals. Behavioral signs include resting posture and inactivity, eyes closed, and an increase in arousal threshold (except in bullfrogs). Physiological signs of sleep include reduction of respiration rate (tree frogs) and heart rate. The western toad shows a decrease in EMG, but the tree frog does not. Eye movements during sleep have never been reported in amphibia.

The brain waves of amphibia during sleep-like states do differ from that seen in alert animals. In some representatives, EEG synchrony when awake changes to low voltage, fast waves when at rest (such as in tree frogs and western toads), or no change (tiger salamander), or an increase in low voltage slow waves with on episodic kind of spiking not seen when the animal is alert (brown frog) (Karmanova, 1982 ; Tauber, 1974; Tobler, 1984).

Based on these scanty data, it is possible only to conclude that sleep-like phenomena do occur in some amphibia (ranging from ultradian activity cycles in the absence of significant EEG changes [salamander] to a slowing of the frequency and a decrease of the amplitude of the EEG in resting frogs, but not in all representatives [no sleep/rest signs in the bull frog]) (Tobler, 1982). Perhaps it is best to state that the rudiments of sleep can be seen among amphibia. Karmanova (1982) calls such sleep-like states "primary sleep" (see below). She further posits that the spike-like intrusions in the EEG that occur in primary sleep (which are accompanied by phasic motor and vegetative arousal) are the precursors of AS. In contrast to this, most other investigators have noted a low voltage, fast activity accompanying sleep-like rest states in amphibia, which resembles AS without any QS.

Fish

Most studies of sleep in fish have used behavioral criteria (Durie, 1981; Hediger, 1983; Karmanova, 1982; Tauber, 1974; Tobler, 1984; Tobler in Carskadon, 1993) with only two notable studies that have used EEG techniques. As in amphibia, fish show a great deal of variability from one species to another in sleep-like signs. Sleep has been observed in salt-water fish (Tobler, 1982). Some have very obvious sleep-like behaviors including sleeping places, body postures, lower arousal thresholds, and rebound sleep following sleep deprivation (Tobler & Borbély, 1985). Parrot fish secrete a mucous bag to sleep in. The slippery dick burrows completely under sand. Many fish flatten their fins against their bodies while others extend them away. Some seek out an overhanging ledge. Some even change color when resting. A reduction in the number of gill-beats has often been observed and used to indicate the "transition to rest." Sheat fish move their eyes 1-3 times per minute in sleep; parrot fish also move their eyes during sleep. Other fish show none of these things, especially fresh water fish. Some fish seem to be in constant motion without showing any behavioral signs of sleep. Changes in response thresholds and state reversibility have been observed in some fish, as has rebound following deprivation of rest.

Electrophysiological recordings during sleep in fish were first done on tench fish using implanted electrodes to measure "neck" EMG, EOG, respiration, heart rate, motor activity, and EEG (Peyrethon, 1968: cited in Karmanova, 1982). Three distinct phases were noted. 1) Motor activity which was much more prevalent during the night than day. 2) Complete rest; the fish was lying on the bottom of the tank without any motor activity and arousal threshold was elevated. However, there were no changes in the EMG or EEG, nor any eye-movements. 3) Intermediate phase activity was intermittent with 2 to 3 oscillating movements of the tail per minute; EMG was reduced but there was no change in brain waves. It was concluded that the rest states were nothing like sleep in mammals. (Tauber, 1974, points out, however, that these studies were done when the tench were in their yearly inactive phase and, thus, may not yield much information about sleep.)

In her own studies of physiological changes in fish during rest, Karmanova (1982) found signs similar to those seen in amphibia. Unique to the sleep-like state were single or grouped spike-like potentials rather than well formed spindles. She also observed signs of "spontaneously arising activation" during sleep-like states that included motor automatisms, eye movements, changes in heart rate, and sometimes an increase in the EMG.

Invertebrates

For years, invertebrates have almost been ignored as subjects for sleep research. Their nervous systems are so different from that of vertebrates that scientists were reluctant to describe anything in invertebrates as sleep. The little bit of research that has been done is instructive, however. Circadian rest-activity cycles have been observed in many invertebrates (Tobler, 1982; Tobler in Carskadon, 1993).

Strumwasser (1971) in a major section of a more general report on sea slugs (aplysia) described their sleep-like behavior. Although very active during the day, the sea slugs go to a specific location and assume a characteristic body position, then remain there until daylight. Interestingly, they do periodically wave their tentacles in this state, which Sturmwasser suggested may be an AS analog. He also noted that some individual sea slugs consistently sleep later than others; some are up at the crack of dawn while others only arise a considerable time after the start of the day. (How remarkably like humans!)

Observations of some flying insects suggest the occurrence of sleep. Mediterranean flour moths have increased arousal thresholds and assume specific postures (5 possible) during their daily inactive phase (Meddis, 1979). During what appears to be their deepest stage of sleep, they fold their antennae back and cover them with their wings. When this occurs, they do not react even if their wings are lifted with a small brush (Borbély, 1986). Every night, the solitary wasp digs a hole in the sand and stays there until daybreak (Durie, 1981). Flies have been noted to gather on the ceiling and remain motionless and less sensitive to stimuli (Meddis, 1975). The reaction of mosquitoes during rest varies with their body posture.

Cockroaches show distinct active/inactive circadian rhythms with specific body postures and higher arousal thresholds during rest. If forced to be active during the rest portion of the cycle, they were less active during the subsequent active time, as if tired or rebounding. This suggests that rest in the cockroach is regulated and has a function beyond immobilization or non-responsiveness (Tobler, 1984).

Activity in the nerve cells of the visual system of the bee is high when the animal is in the active (day) portion of its circadian activity cycle. The visual system can also be more easily activated by light stimuli during this time. During the nighttime (or daytime rest periods in forager bees when they crawl into empty comb cells to rest), the visual system is both less active and less reactive. They also show characteristic body postures, decreased body temperature, lower neck muscle tension, and higher arousal threshold. However, this state is rapidly reversed by an arousing stimulus (such as a puff of air) in a manner analogous to arousal from sleep (Kaiser & Steiner-Kaiser, 1983).

Scorpions have three states - active, alert, and rest - based on behavioral descriptions of activity and body position (Tobler & Stalder, 1987). They are active at night, thus showing a circadian rhythm. During the alert state, and even more so during the rest state, they have an increased threshold of arousal and a decreased heart rate. Following deprivation of alertness and rest states, the amount of rest increases, indicating that these states are necessary and regulated. Thus, the scorpion exhibits a "sleep-like" state.

Conclusions

Sleep does not appear to be a behavior exclusive to mammals. However, it appears to be best developed and most complex in them. Most mammals show very similar stages of sleep (although a select few have either lost AS [dolphins] or failed to develop it during evolution [Echidna]). Birds also show sleep stages that are similar, but not identical (significantly less AS and no change in amount of delta through sleep), to those in humans. Reptiles sleep, but a sharp difference occurs in the EEG of their sleep. Rather than an increase in amplitude and a decrease in voltage as characteristic of sleep, the opposite seems to be more common in reptiles (and in other non-mammal, non-bird species). EEG is not adequate to characterize sleep in amphibia, fish, and non-vertebrates. Therefore, more reliance must be placed on other (especially behavioral) criteria. Using such criteria, sleep-like states can be found in many, but possibly not all, representatives of lower animals.

Overall, much more data needs to be collected,with more emphasis on ascertaining arousal thresholds, reversibility of state, heart rate and respiration changes, and effects of sleep (rest) deprivation (Karmanova, 1982; Tobler, 1984). Nevertheless, efforts to find meaning in the data available have produced some interesting results. We will now review these results.

The Evolution of Sleep

Reptiles, amphibia, and fish sleep. However, unlike birds and mammals, their sleep is of only one kind. This leads to an important question. Is this one kind of sleep comparable to AS, QS, or neither? Whatever the answer to this question might be, another logically follows: what are the evolutionary steps between this unified primitive sleep in lower vertebrates and the multiple types of sleep with their cycles of higher vertebrates?

QS as the Most Ancient Sleep

One view, probably more widely held, is that QS is present in lower vertebrates, with AS having evolved in the higher vertebrates. (The most widely cited proponent of this view is Allison and associates [see for example, Allison & Van Twyver, 1970]). Several facts are used to support this view. First, QS almost always precedes AS in the sleep cycles of adult higher vertebrates. Second, reptilian sleep is thought to resemble QS of birds and mammals. The reptile shows few signs of activation during its sleep; there are few eye movements, little limb twitching, and relatively stable heart and respiration rates. However, the EEG signs of NREM sleep found in the mammalian brainstem below the cortex (see chapter 4) can also be found in sleeping reptiles and can be blocked by the same drug that blocks them is mammals (Horne, 1988).

One apparent difficulty with this theory was the discovery by Allison and associates (1972) that the Echidna does not have AS. To see why this is a difficulty we have to take a closer look at the evolution of mammals and birds. Figure 3-2 is a simplified diagram of the sequence of evolution of mammals, birds, and reptiles. The monotremes (e.g., Spiny anteater) line branches off from what becomes the Marsupials and placental mammals about 175 million year ago (at the branch labeled 1 in Figure 3-2). It is possible that the ancestor of all of them had only QS which the monotremes continued, but that the common ancestor of the marsupials and placental mammals developed AS. However, birds also have AS, and you have to trace back even further to find an ancestor common to birds and all of the mammals (point 2 in Figure 3-2). This ancestor, however, is common to many other species that do not show both QS and AS. Thus, it is no simple matter to determine when and why AS developed in animals if indeed QS is older. A partial resolution to this conundrum is to posit that birds and non-therian mammals developed AS separately in parallel with one another. That is, AS is a result of convergent evolution[1] in these 2 lines. If AS is a result of parallel evolution, then its absence in Echidna is explainable as a failure of development, although the reasons for its development in most other mammals remains unexplained.

Likewise, recent discoveries of the absence of AS in some sea mammals (such as dolphins and sea cows) requires additional explanation that complicates this theory even more. In short, it is possible that dolphins lost the AS that a common ancestor had. But this explanation itself causes its own questions about why this occurred and why other mammals have not also lost AS. The law of parsimony suggests choosing the simplest reasonable explanation; some scientists maintain that the theory that QS is the oldest type of sleep is not the simplest explanation.

AS as the Most Ancient Sleep

An alternative view starts by reexamining some of the data. The statement that the sleep of reptiles is QS has been seriously questioned

---

[1]Convergent evolution is not uncommon. The eye evolved at least 40 times independently in the animal Kingdom. Convergent evolution occurs when the environment makes strong demands on animals for which there is one best solution. For example, the ear ossicles of the monotremes and the therians are essentially the same, yet fossil evidence shows that they evolved independently in parallel (Tauber, 1974).

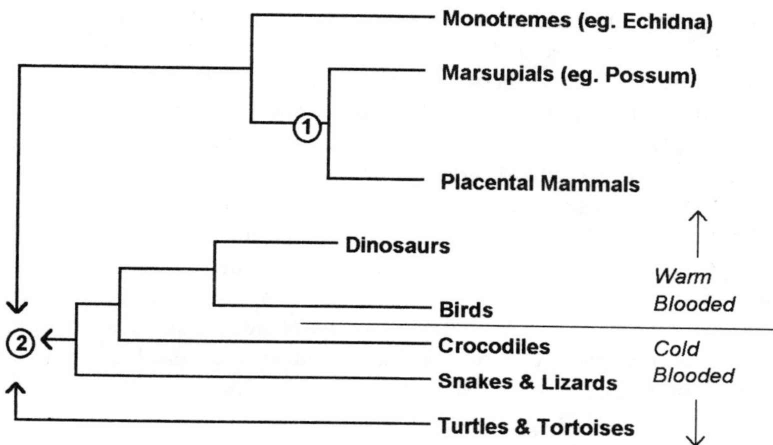

Figure 3-2. Phylogenetic tree for selected species.

(Meddis, 1979). The EEG typically found in sleeping reptiles does not resemble high voltage, slow waves of mammalian QS as much as it resembles low voltage fast waves of AS in mammals. One exception is the work of Warner and Huggins (1978) reviewed earlier in this chapter. They reported high voltage slow waves in sleeping crocodiles. However, their interpretation of other EEG waves that they collected as high voltage, fast waves has been questioned, since only 20% of the record at the best had such waves and, thus, can hardly be considered the dominant wave form of sleep.

The low levels of phasic signs during sleep in reptiles may not support the argument of the absence of AS since these animals have a low metabolic rate that gets even lower during sleep and they may not be able to produce an abundance of such signs. The fact that some reptiles and fish do show such phasic activity (although not as frequently in higher animals) is not consistent with the interpretation that their sleep is only QS. Furthermore, brain metabolic activity increases in reptilian sleep, which is more typical of AS than QS (see chapter 4) (Kilduff, Bennington, Bickler, Bartholomew, & Heller, 1989).

Meddis (1979; 1983), Walker and Berger (1980), and, more recently, Borbély (1986) have been spokespersons for the theory that AS is phylogenetically older than QS. They maintain that most descriptions of reptilian EEG more closely resemble the EEG of mammalian AS. Also, sleeping reptiles loose muscle tone, have a high arousal threshold, and show some phasic phenomena.

This theory maintains that AS is older and more primitive. It goes on to suggest that QS was a necessary development of warm-blooded animals since it is found only in them. During AS, thermoregulatory mechanisms are severely compromised (see Chapter 2), thus warmed blooded animals cannot afford too much continuous AS. During QS, temperature is regulated yet sleep is maintained. Supporting this notion is the fact that smaller animals who lose heat faster have shorter durations of AS. Also, as infant temperature regulation improves, the amount of AS declines. Some animals, such as echidna and dolphins, may have taken this to the extreme and completely replaced AS with QS.

Additional details of the changes that occur in sleep of infant mammals has been offered as support of this theory. (Karmanova, 1982). The first sleep is almost total AS with QS emerging later (see Chapter 1) and as the amount of QS increases (with coincident decreases in AS) sow waves appear, increasing in amplitude and number (Davenne, Dugovic, Franc, & Adrien, 1989). AS is tolerated in the uterus because the body temperature of the fetus is regulated for it by the mother. Birth dramatically changes this situation and, thus, QS begins to occupy more and more of sleep as the infant develops greater need and ability to regulate its own body temperature. If ontogeny recapitulates phylogeny,[2] this is an important argument.

Meddis (1979) reports additional evidence that is consistent with these arguments. Not only does AS precede QS in infant development, but spindles precede the differentiation of light QS from deep QS which, in turn, precedes K-complexes during development. The same sequence is paralleled in a ranking of species - AS seen in reptiles, slow wave sleep first in birds, spindles first seen in insectivores, differentiation between light and deep quiet sleep in carnivores, and K-complexes in primates. Finally, study of the brain mechanisms that produce sleep seem to support the theory that AS is evolutionarily older than QS. As described in Chapter 2, the areas of the brain that

---

[2]The theory that ontogeny recapitulates phylogeny maintains that the sequence of growth and development of an individual is a replay of the sequence of evolution of its species. Most biologists do not consider this theory to be generally valid.

produce AS are entirely located in the brain stem (lowest part of the brain). This part of the brain is relatively unchanged from that found in reptiles. In contrast, QS is produced by a network of structures located throughout all levels of the brain including higher structures found only in mammals. It is simpler, and more consistent, to maintain that QS emerged as the brain structures known to produce it evolved during evolution.

AS and QS Evolved Out of More Ancient Sleep-like States

A third view, developed by Karmanova, holds that neither AS nor QS is oldest but that both emerged together out of older sleep-like states. Ida Gavrilovna Karmanova is professor of Physiology and Head of the Laboratory of Comparative Physiology of Sleep at the Sechenov Institute of Evolutionary Physiology and Biochemistry in Leningrad, USSR.. She adds her laboratory observations and those of other Russians to the work of Western scientists in her book, translated from Russian, *Evolution of Sleep; Stages of the Formation of the 'Wakefulness-Sleep' Cycle in Vertebrates* (Karmanova, 1982), then relates it all to her fascinating and unique theory of the development of sleep.

In her studies, Karmanova uses a wide variety of measures to assess sleep. They include:

1) **motor activity** - present or absent; posture of the subject; tone of the somatic (including oculomotor) muscles; position of the eyes;

2) **heart rate**, characteristics of **respiration**, type of **eye movements** and other **"phasic motor automatisms"**;

3) visual and computer analysis of brain **EEGs**;

4) **Behavioral arousal** - threshold and changes of EEG and heart rate during sensory stimulation;

5) **Latencies** from wake to sleep and vice versa;

6) Effects of **experimental brain damage** and **drugs** on sleep and wakefulness;

7) **motor automatisms**; automatic, sequential movement patterns characteristic of the species such as S-shaped tail movements of fish and lizard;

8) **Brain biochemistry** during sleep and wakefulness.

Karmanova states that neither AS nor QS is the oldest. Rather both evolved somewhat simultaneously out of more primitive rest states or "sleep-like states" (SLS). She sees three major periods in this evolution of sleep in vertebrates: first Primary Sleep, then Intermediate Sleep, and finally, True Sleep.

Primary sleep. Primary sleep can be seen in fish and amphibians. It actually consists of three forms of rest. The first of these, occurring during daylight, she calls **SLS-1**. In this state, animals are immobile with a waxy flexibility. That is, their appendages or body orientation can be passively moved and the animal will remain in the new position. (This is somewhat like moving the arms or legs of a "Barbie" or "Ken" doll.) During this state, the EEG has a low amplitude with most activity in the delta and alpha or theta ranges. Intruding on this EEG pattern are "activated fragments" of spike-like activity that are usually accompanied by "motor automations" such as S-shaped movements of the tail. Heart rate diminishes, as does respiration rate, and the arousal threshold increases. The animal's eyes may be open. SLS-1 is probably the same as "resting state", drowsiness, or "quiet waking" defined by Western scientists.

The second form of primary sleep she calls **SLS-2** and it occurs during nighttime. Again the body is immobilized, but now in a rigid way. Attempts to passively move the body or its parts are resisted and if moved, they return to original state upon release (somewhat like an old-fashioned baby doll). The brain waves are of low amplitude with activated fragments of single or grouped spike-like tracings. The activated fragments are accompanied by motor automatisms similar to those seen in SLS-1.

The third type, **SLS-3**, also occurs in the dark. In this type, the immobility is one of body relaxation caused by a general drop in muscle tone. Arousal threshold is high. The brain waves are dominated by delta-like activity of low amplitude with intrusions of activated spike-like activity and very synchronized frequencies typical of wakefulness. These activated fragments are often accompanied by motor automatisms. Deceleration of the heart (to 1/2 of waking values) and respiration rates occur but with phasic accelerations of heart rate and more intense eye movements. These phasic events, however, tend to occur, independently of each other. In fish, the orientation of the body with respect to gravity may be quite altered. SLS-3 appears to involve active brain mechanisms for its production in contrast to SLS-1 and SLS-2 which involve passive brain mechanisms.

Compared to sleep in birds and mammals, primary sleep in fish and amphibians is loosely organized and not well consolidated. All three types seem to provide equal biological utility of passive rest and defense to the animal - a time of rest and energy conservation. Of these three, only SLS-3 progresses during evolution to become true sleep.

Intermediate sleep. Intermediate sleep was observed in reptiles. It is a further development of SLS-3 accompanied by a distinction between nonactivated and activated phases. During the nonactivated phase, there is a tonic deceleration of the heart and respiration rates and a reduction of body muscle tone. Also, the arousal threshold drops, yet the eyes remain open. The EEG is of low amplitude with delta rhythms dominating. The activated phase consists of a significant increase of "arrhythmic spikes" in the forebrain, together with EEG waves resembling those of wakefulness.

Absent, however, is a reduction of spinal motor reflexes during the activated stage of sleep. During intermediate sleep, phasic movements of the head and forelimbs occur together with an increase in the amplitude of the activity of the neck muscles. Also, movements of the eyes occur and the heart rate decreases. SLS-1 and SLS-2 begin to diminish in importance, although SLS-1 accounts for 45% of the sleep of every nychthemeron. The number of shifts to and from wakefulness decreases.

True sleep. True sleep is found in birds and mammals. It developed out of SLS-3 and can be divided into QS and AS. The active portions of SLS-3 and AS of homeotherms are very much similar, according to Karmanova. The ancient aspects of activated sleep include phasic heart rate increases, decreases in respiratory rate, motor automatisms, and eye movements.

Evolution of sleep. Karmanova believes she can trace the evolutionary development of sleep from primary sleep in fish and amphibians through intermediate sleep in reptiles to true sleep in birds and mammals (see Figure 3-3), because some forms of these stages are present in now living animals.

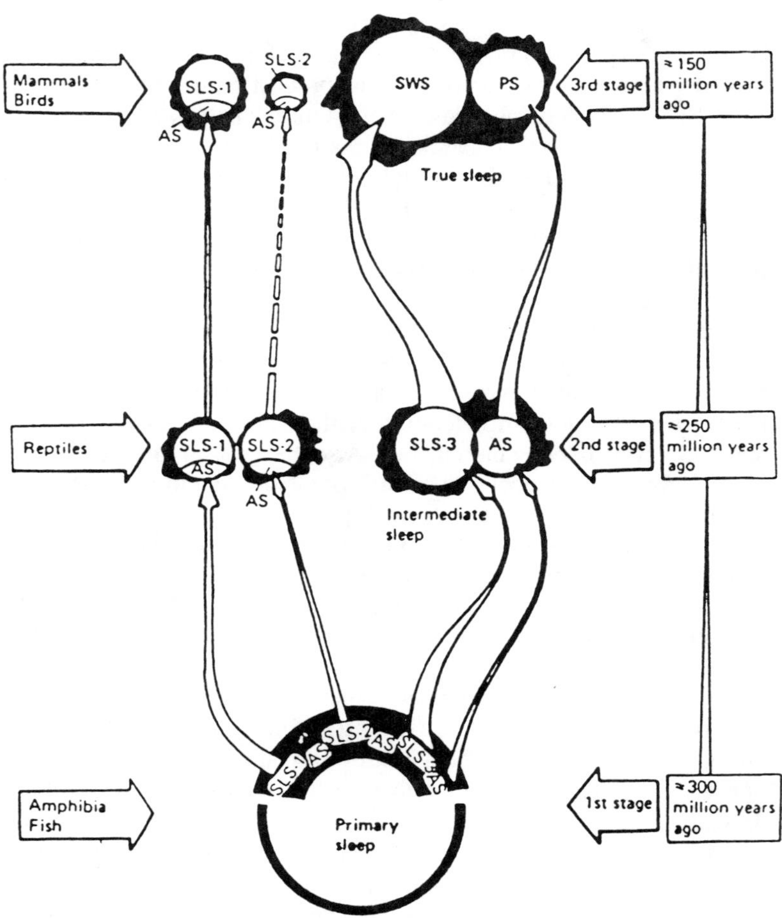

Figure 3-3. Scheme of the evolution of sleep in vertebrates. AS in this figure = activation, spontaneously arising against the background of all forms of rest and sleep. See text for details. (From Karmanova I G, 1982. *Evoultion of sleep: Stages of the formulation of the 'wakefulness-sleep' cycle in vertebrates.* New York: Karger. Used with permission of S. Karger AG, Basel, Switzerland.)

About 300 million years ago there was a circadian organization of wake and rest that occurred in fish and amphibians with SLS-1 occurring predominantly in daylight, but SLS-2 and SLS-3 happening in darkness. None of these three types of primary sleep appear to be more important than the others in these early animals. Then, about 250 million years ago, during the evolution of reptiles from amphibians, SLS-3 became more important and developed into intermediate sleep. This form continued in its development because only it contained relaxation of body muscles, which would be much more restful to land dwelling reptiles who are always opposing the pull of gravity. Rudiments of SLS-1 and SLS-2 remained, however, with little change from that seen in amphibians and fish. SLS-2 became a short transitional state between wake and intermediate sleep and seemed to have diminished in importance sooner than SLS-1. The sleep of monotremes (represented by echidna) is a later development of intermediate sleep into QS without AS.

About 150 million years ago, the third stage of sleep development could be noted and is present today in most mammals and birds. At this time, there was a progressive development of intermediate sleep into slow wave sleep with the activation occurring during intermediate sleep becoming AS (REM sleep). SLS-1 is present in birds 18-25% of every nychthemeron but in only 5% of mammals as a "transitory state between wakefulness and sleep which is often practically impossible to identify" (page 107).

This theory does not appear to be consistent with the fact that AS appears first during ontogenetic development. Karmanova points out, however, that AS in young infants manifests two "peculiarities": First, sleep onset AS is frequent, and, second, low amplitude EEG activity periods with bursts of rapid eye movements are the dominant pattern in the sleep of infants. These "peculiarities" are more like the primary sleep seen in cold-blooded animals than REM/NREM seen in adults. Also, the movements of infants during sleep are very similar to the automatic movements during states of rest in fish and amphibians. Further, the gradual development of the SWS stages in babies is similar to SWS development during evolution in vertebrates. Thus, the AS of infants that has been thought of as REM when tracing the ontogeny of human sleep (see Chapter 1), is really more akin to the evolutionary sequence of primary sleep into intermediate sleep and finally into true sleep. Thus, there are parallels in the ontogenetic development of sleep in higher mammals and the phylogenetic evolution of sleep in vertebrates.

McGinty (1979) has stated a similar conclusion. Sleep/wake states gradually emerge during development from a primitive undifferentiated state, but AS most closely resembles this primitive state. It becomes recognized as sleep as it gradually acquires its characteristic aspects.

Functions of Sleep in Animals

Examining the evolution of sleep helps provide some insight, on a broad scale, into the differences in sleep in animals. But environment plays a role in shaping the characteristics of sleep on a finer scale (Karmanova, 1982). Evolution can show us why mammal's sleep is different from amphibians sleep, but not why some mammals sleep longer than others. Evolution provides explanations for qualitative differences and environment provides explanations for quantitative differences.

First, we will list some of the environmental and individual factors thought to be important in determining characteristics of sleep in mammals and then see how they apply to sleep. Finally, we will return to the examples of animal sleep presented at the beginning of this chapter to show how these environmental and individual factors explain the sleep differences in these species. Our discussion here is limited to mammals because most research and theorizing has focused on them.

The factors shown (or at least thought) to be important in contributing to sleep differences between species or mammals are:

1) *Predator/prey proportion.* Is the animal a predator of other animals that has the weapons and skills to not only hunt other animals for food but also to protect itself? Or is the animal a plant eater who is relatively vulnerable to being attacked by other animals? Or does the animal lie somewhere between those extremes?

2) *Relative abundance of food source***.** Is the animal's source of food abundant and nutritious? Or is the food scarce and/or not very nutritious?

3) *Characteristics of the sleeping habitat.* Does the animal sleep in a relatively safe place such as a burrow or tree? Or does it sleep in an unsafe, exposed place such as the open plain?

4) Is the animal warm-blooded (*homeothermic*) or cold-blooded (*poikilothermic*)?

5) *Brain function and the degree of neotony.* Neotony means that fetal and infantile characteristics remain longer and persist into adulthood. Neotony of brain development is especially relevant to sleep differences among mammals.

6) *Body size.* Larger homeothermic animals have lower metabolic rates than smaller animals. Also, small animals are almost constantly active while awake, whereas larger animals frequently rest quietly when awake (Horne, 1988).

7) *Events and Activities* Things like hibernation, age, brooding, weather conditions, injury, mating, and feeding are included in this category.

These factors are briefly listed in Table 3-3.

How the Factors Apply

Bioadaptive. Sleep, like most other behaviors, is bioadaptive (relates to all 6 factors). According to the theory of evolution, those animals will be able to reproduce, and thus perpetuate themselves, that can adapt and survive in their particular niche. Different niches may require different survival strategies. Sleep, like other behaviors, plays an important role in the survival strategy. This is an overall explanation of variations in sleep seen in animals. Keep this in mind as we continue to explore more specific causes.

Adaptive Non-Responding. Sleep is "adaptive non-responding" at times when an animal may be vulnerable (relates to factors 1, 3, and somewhat 2). There are times in the nychthemeron that an animal may not be safe. Night time is a typical example; some animals that see well during the day and can easily perceive and avoid dangers may not be able to do so nearly as well at night. For them, it is much safer to be inactive at night. Sleep insures this. An awake animal is built to respond and be active. Sleep actively inhibits these tendencies by causing immobility and increasing response threshold. But, this is true only if the animal has a safe place to sleep. Without such a safe sleeping habitat, the animal may be even more vulnerable when asleep and unresponsive and, thus, may sleep very little and with only minimal AS (Meddis, 1983).

Vigilance Against Predators. Arousal thresholds are elevated during sleep (relative to factors 1 and 3). Some animals, especially those who are prey for many predators, need to maintain a constant vigilance against predators. If such animals do not have a safe habitat in which to sleep, then sleep, especially AS, is a dangerous situation. Such animals tend to sleep less, distribute their sleep throughout the nychthemeron rather than have one or a few consolidated sleep times, and have minimal AS (Karmanova, 1982).

Sleeping Habitat. AS is a time of muscular paralysis (relative to factor 3). If the animal is in a precarious sleeping spot or a position that requires body effort, then AS tends to be minimal.

Feeding Habits. Some animals need to feed during much of every nychthemeron (relative to number 2). If food is hard to come by (as it might be for some predators and foragers) or if it is abundant but low in readily available nutrition (as it is for some grazers) then there may not be time for sleep. In such cases, the predators and foragers need to spend a lot of time looking for food and the grazers a lot of time consuming and chewing enough to meet their nutritional needs (Horne, 1988). Furthermore, grazers may not need much sleep to

Table 3-3 Factors contributing to sleep differences between species

1. predator/prey proportion
2. relative abundance of food source
3. characteristics of sleeping habitat
4. homeothermic or poikilothermic
5. degree of neotony (of brain)
6. body size
7. events and activities

conserve energy, since grazing is relatively sedentary. Indeed, low total sleep time is consistently seen in grazing animals (Meddis, 1983).

Brain Development and Maintenance. Sleep (especially AS) aids brain development and maintenance (relates to factor 5). The infant brain begins with too many connections between brain cells. Growth and development is a process of strengthening and preserving the useful connections while weakening and loosening the less useful connections. Generally, the more a connection is used the more useful it is. AS seems, to many scientists, to be a way of using and revising useful connections, thereby actively strengthening them, while the unused ones simply passively fade away from disuse (Moruzzi, 1966; Roffwarg, Muzio, & Dement, 1966). While the growing and developing brain has a great need for this process, hence a very high amount of AS occurs during infancy, the mature brain also needs some to maintain itself, hence the continuation of AS throughout life but at lower levels. (However, Crick and Mitcheson [1983] maintain that the opposite occurs, at least in adult brains. The connections activated during AS are weakened. See Chapter 7 for more about this theory.)

Horne (1983c, 1988) carries this theory one step further. Herbivores have relatively simple brains (it does not require a complex brain to chew grass all day) that do not need much of the maintenance done during sleep and, thus, have little AS. Carnivores depend much on their brains for the flexible and adaptable behaviors that are required to hunt, stalk, and capture prey and, thus, require more AS to maintain them.

Body Temperature Regulation. Thermoregulation is inadequate during AS (relates to factors 4 and 6) but QS is a time of *regulated* fall of body temperature (Horne, 1983c). During AS, the mechanisms that enable homeothermic animals to regulate their body temperatures become inadequate, if not inactive (see Chapter 2 for details). Animals tend to lose heat during AS without any control. During QS, body temperature is allowed to fall to a lower, but regulated setting. The fall of body temperature that occurs during sleep conserves energy in warm-blooded animals, but the reduction in temperature cannot be allowed to get out of hand. QS prevents this, since body temperature falls but in a regulated manner.

A positive correlation between body size and length of AS periods has been observed. For large animals, inadequate thermoregulation during AS is not a problem because their great bulk passively stores much heat. Also, large animals have a smaller proportion of body surface to body mass meaning that relatively less of them is exposed to the environmental temperature. In contrast, smaller animals lose body temperature fairly quickly during AS and, therefore, can tolerate only brief periods of it (Meddis, 1983). But, in order to have adequate total amounts of AS, these short AS periods must occur frequently, thus a shorter QS/AS cycle occurs in smaller animals. Furthermore, independently of body size, animals living in colder climates have shorter periods of AS (Elgar, Pagel, & Harvey, 1988).

The evidence cited to support this hypothesis includes 1) the high correlation between metabolic rate and the amount of QS sleep, 2) the parallel development of QS and temperature regulation in growing warm-blooded animals, and 3) the (controversial) conclusion that poikilothermic animals do not have QS sleep.

Behavioral Temperature Regulation. For some animals, sleeping during the day is advantageous since the environment is warmer when they are inactive and, thus, they lose less precious body heat (relative to factor 4). Or conversely,sleep prevents overheating during the heat of the day. Dozing may have evolved to satisfy some of the needs of sleep, such as this one, in higher mammals without a dramatic reduction in vigilance. Higher mammals have a brain complex enough to allow such a state (Horne, 1983c).

Energy Conservation. Both QS and, especially, AS conserve energy (relative to factor 6). During sleep, and especially AS, the body is immobile, thus using up less energy resources. Further, metabolic rate drops during sleep (see Chapter 2 for details). Small animals have considerably higher metabolic rates, nearly constant activity when awake, but less stores of energy in their body. Because sleep insures immobilization, lower metabolic rate, and allows huddling in a warm nest, it is more important to small animals as a means of conserving energy. However, higher metabolic rates correlate with less sleep time independently of body size (Elgar et al, 1988).

Compare the sleep of the bat (much) to the shrew (little) in this regard. Both are about the same size and both have high waking metabolic rates. Bats have adapted by sleeping a lot, thus conserving energy, while shrews have adapted by remaining awake most of the time to feed, which burns more energy but also replaces it more rapidly (acquiring energy) (Meddis, 1975).

Walker and Berger (1980) find a high correlation between metabolic rate and amount of QS. They reason that QS (in distinction to AS) is a time of *regulated* fall in body temperature and, thus, most important for energy conservation. Other researchers find only a weak relationship between body size and amount of QS (Zepelin & Rechschaffen, 1974) or none at all if ungulates are eliminated from consideration (Meddis, 1983).

Restoration of the body. Larger animals (factor 6) spend a good deal of awake time in a relaxed, restful state that allows the body to repair and maintain itself (Horne, 1988). Small animals are almost continuously active while awake, leaving little awake time for bodily repair. Sleep serves as a time of forced immobilization in smaller animals, thus ensuring the opportunity for bodily restoration.

Sleep length. The total amount of sleep in the nychthemeron could also be affected inversely by body size (Zepelin, 1989) (factor 6) and sleeping arrangements (factor 3). Small animals that huddle during sleep and/or have a nest to sleep in may not lose as much body heat as single, exposed small animals and, thus, conserve considerable energy by sleeping (Horne, 1983c).

Events and activities Events and activities (factor 7) also affect sleep length. Time spent asleep increases prior to and following hibernation, during infancy, when brooding, during very hot or very cold weather, and following injury, feeding, and copulation (Meddis, 1975). What is eaten may also be important. The research of Danquir (1988) shows that sugars increase SWS while amino acids increase AS. Thus, he posits there is more AS in carnivores because of their high protein (amino acid) diet, but little AS in herbivors, since their diet is low in protein. He experimentally verified this by shifting sheep to a high protein diet, which resulted in high AS.

Remaining Issues

In spite of the length and complexity of this discussion, there are still several aspects of animal sleep differences that are as yet unexplained or have not been addressed (Meddis, 1983).

Why does QS have sub-stages such as SWS-1 and SWS-2 or NREM stages 1, 2, and delta? And why does it vary with species? For example, the rat has only simple QS while the cat has light QS and deep QS with slow waves.

Why do spindles and K-complexes occur in some animals but not others? Spindles can be seen in QS of mammals and echidna but K-complexes only in higher primates.

Why does dozing occur in some animals in great amounts but little, if at all, in others? Ungulates, carnivores, and some insectivores are in this state for hours out of each 24 but humans never are (except for a few college students - or so it seems).

Conclusion

Let us finish this chapter by returning to the wide variety of sleep characteristics of selected animals presented in the very beginning of this chapter to see how well they can be explained. Grazing animals have little total sleep time and get it only in brief bursts scattered throughout the nychthemeron. They may spend more time dozing than sleeping. They need to spend a lot of time feeding and chewing their relatively non-nutritious food and are vulnerable to predation, but have no safe place to sleep. Elephants also sleep little but in one single night period. They are not in danger of being preyed upon, but must spend an enormous amount of time foraging in order to get enough to eat. The tiny, short-haired shrew sleeps very little. Although it has a safe sleeping environment (its burrow) and, thus, could sleep at length safely, it must eat the equivalent of its own body weight daily in order to survive, which requires a lot of its waking time.

An old joke is, "How long does a gorilla sleep?" Answer, "as long as it wants to." There is a great deal of truth in this joke since a gorilla is not in danger of being preyed upon, so it is not unsafe for it to sleep. It also has an abundant, nutritious food source, so it does not need to spend a lot of time seeking and eating food. As a result, the gorilla sleeps 14 hours per nychthemeron.

Ground squirrels sleep 14 hours per nychthemeron, also. They too have abundant and nutritious food supplies and, even though they are preyed upon, they have a burrow in which they sleep in relative safety.

Cats and mice sleep about the same amount each nychthemeron. Cats are hunters with few natural enemies; mice are prey but have a safe nest in which to sleep (Meddis, 1975).

Bats sleep for 19-20 hours of the nychthemeron. They generally sleep in safe places but have to expend enormous amounts of energy in order to fly. They can conserve energy by sleeping, yet obtain enough nutritious food during their brief awake periods.

Baboons sleep in their safe nests, high in trees, from dusk to dawn when they are most vulnerable. They can obtain ample food by foraging alertly and diligently during daylight hours. They have a low amount of AS because of the danger of falling out of their sleeping nests during this time.

Possums get 19-20 hours of sleep. They have abundant food but are vulnerable to predation and, thus, sleep is relatively safe for them.

Some fish may not sleep. In order to breathe and remain safe from harm they may not be able to afford to sleep.

Non-mammals and non-birds have not evolved the advanced mechanisms of sleep. But even they show variations because of environmental circumstance. For example, bullfrogs show no sleep-like states, yet tree frogs do. Bullfrogs are always out in the open in danger of predation while tree frogs are safer in trees and, thus, can afford to sleep.

One criticism of such explanations is that they can explain anything but can never be scientifically tested (Zepelin, 1989). If one explanation does not suffice, simply substitute another. Prehaps this criticism is just at the present time. Yet, sleep just might serve more of one combination of functions for one species and more of another combination for another species. Sleep may just be that complex, and attempts to logically simplify its functions may be appealing but not accurate. Hopefully, more research and further analysis will lead to less speculative explanations of why there is such a great divergence of sleep patterns in animals.

Sleep, Dreaming, & Sleep Disorders

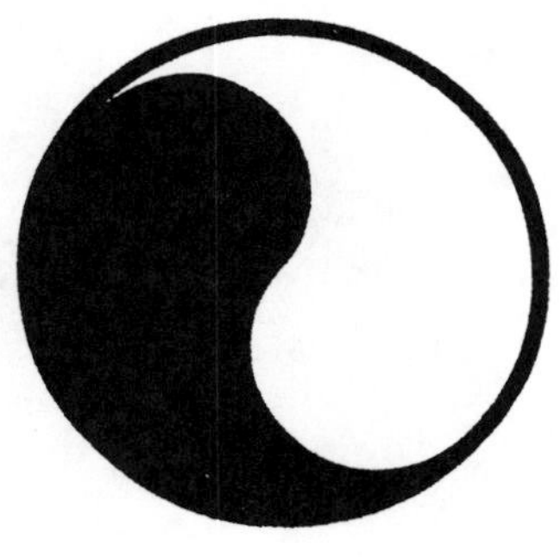

Section 2 *Dreaming*

Chapter 6

The Phenomena Of Dreams

(with Krista Hennager)

"Dreams have only been studied for about 40 years!"

A seemingly preposterous statement since there are reports of dreams in ancient literature and from all over the world: on Egyptian papyruses, in the Bible, in Freud's writings, and so on. Yet, the statement is true. Only for the last 40 years or so (since the original observation by Aserinsky and Kleitman in 1953 that REM awakenings result in dream reports) has science been able to tell when a person is dreaming in order to awaken that person for an immediate report of the dream. Prior to this, people would report their dreams after spontaneously awakening from sleep or later (often a considerable time later). These delayed accounts were not exact copies of the dream itself, but a report, often considerably altered, based on the dream. They were changed in many ways: rough edges smoothed, made more logical, some things emphasized, others ignored, and details lost.

Consider the following experiment. One night you are awakened during each REM period and asked to report on your dream. The next morning you again are asked to recall the dreams. Finally, a week later, you are again asked to report on those same dreams. In comparing the reports, several things can be seen. First, you would use the most words overall for the reports following REM awakening and the fewest a week later. Second, you would report on fewer dreams the next morning than during the night, and fewer still one week later.

Finally, the basic themes of the dream reports from the different reporting times would be the same, but details would be missing from the later reports (Faraday, 1972). Still other things would be modified or inserted to make the stories more sensible and flow smoother in the later reports.

So, until the technique of gathering dream reports by REM awakening was developed and used, the "dreams" people studied were not the dreams themselves. Rather, they were stories people told based on their dreams (Faraday, 1972). This is an important difference since the stories are changed versions of the dream, and any conclusions derived from them cannot be unambiguously related to the dreaming process.

There is another essential and related point to keep in mind. This concerns the kinds of dreams people talk about and their impression of the dominant themes of dreams. Again consider your own behavior.

Which of the following dreams are you more likely to share with others?

Dream 1:

I am fishing on a lake. It is a very calm lake - like a mirror. The sun is warm but not hot. There are a few fluffy white clouds in the sky being pushed by a gentle breeze. I haven't caught any fish, but I don't really care, even though I have been out there for hours. Its lunch time, so I get out my twinkie and root beer. They taste better than ever. Jack is now in the boat, too, and he starts rowing back to shore. I watch the ripples that the boat makes on the water and...

Dream 2:

The woods are kind of dark. You know, like at sunset. It is so quiet; I can hear myself breathe. I have this feeling that there are people or animals behind the trees. Suddenly, I realize that I am naked. I begin to run, but I know that they are running after me. I'm lost. I don't know which way to go. The creatures - oh, they're so awful: bloody, half human, half animal. I fall down. I try to scream, but nothing comes out. Now one of the creatures comes up to me, reaches out, and...

Which one would you be more likely to remember and share? The latter of course (Borbély, 1986) - the one full of sex, monsters, and violence. It's more fun, more interesting, and more people would pay attention to you. It is not unlike editing a newspaper, putting the exciting news in the headlines on page 1. This is true of everybody. We talk about our sexy, violent, creaturous dreams with a great deal of emotional concern. We may even consciously enhance them for effect. We don't speak much about the rest. Thus, it only seems that most dreams contain either sex, violence, or monsters, or combinations of them. In fact, as we shall see, most dreams are down right dull when told to other people (Borbély, 1986; Broughton, 1982), although they are important to the dreamer.

Before going on, let's talk briefly about Freud. More will be said about him in Chapter 6, but the point to be made here is that Freud was both wrong and right in his theories about dreams! He was wrong because he was not working with dreams at all, but rather with the stories his patients told (often weeks or months later) about their dreams. These stories were full of distortions and probably only resembled the original dreams. He was right, however, because these dream stories did provide information (insights) about the dreamer. The distortions were made by the dreamer by emphasizing what was important or meaningful or significant for them. Likewise, the dreamer would ignore parts of the original dream that were not important or meaningful or significant to them. In psychological terms, we say that the dream reteller is projecting their self (personality) into the story. Freud correctly used this idea to gain insight into the dreamer's personality, especially their problems, but Freud really was wrong in thinking he was working with dreams. Thus, he was incorrect when using this source of information to formulate a general theory of all dreams.

The Dream from the Laboratory

To many scientists, the study of dreams is not real science (Fiss, 1983). I was of this opinion at one time. The study of brain cells, neurotransmitters, and hormones during sleep and dreaming is real science, but not the study of dreams themselves. We have direct access to brain cells, neurotransmitters, and hormones, but we have only indirect access to dreams since we need to ask dreamers to tell us their dreams. We have no way of knowing if the subjective dream report is accurate and valid. Real science requires hard, verifiable facts not unreliable subjective data.

While it is true that access to the data is less direct and more subjective when studying dreams, it is also true that the essence of science is its methods not its subject matter. Also, just because the source of dreams has a physiological basis does not mean that we cannot also study the results - the dreams themselves.

On the other hand, the science of studying dreams is better when the dream reports are more accurate and faithful to the actual dream. Any methods that improve the reporting of dreams will improve the scientific study of dreams and dreaming.

Casually recalled dreams yield a limited, biased, and distorted sample of dreams. Scientific technology has provided us with a better tool for collecting dreams, and thus for developing theories about dreams and dream function. The dreamer in the lab can be awakened during REM and asked to immediately recount the dream into a tape recorder. This provides a report whose content is closer to the actual dream than other methods. (Much dream material has also been collected out of the lab by having a person regularly dictate dream content into a tape recorder following nighttime or morning awakenings. A person may use alarm-clock awakenings periodically through the night for this purpose.)

Reports collected following awakenings in the lab are probably closer to the content of the actual dreams. Undoubtedly, distortions of retelling still occur, but they tend to be lessened since the dreamer is less conscious (having just awakened), the time between the dream and the telling is minimal (which results in less memory loss), and conditions are better for "honest" telling. Additionally, more dreams are available for scrutinizing since more dream recall occurs when awakened during REM than following other awakenings, and experiments aimed at manipulating dream content are easier to accomplish. Thus, these dream reports get us closer to the actual dream content and, therefore, can be used to determine more about the process of dreaming. As such, they are a better research tool with which to explore the process of dreaming.

Nevertheless, there are problems associated with dreams collected during REM wake-ups in the lab. The lab setting sometimes influences the dream content, especially the electrodes, recording equipment, and the constant vigilance of technicians and researchers (Cohen, 1979).

Furthermore, the recording of dreams may make the dreamer more self-conscious.

Hall and VandeCastle reported a comparison of casually recalled home and laboratory collected dreams obtained from the same subjects in 1966. They found fewer characters in the lab dreams and fewer social interactions of physical aggression, friendliness, and sex. In contrast, lab dreams contained more misfortune but with less drama and less vividness. And, as expected, many references to the lab situation were given.

The problem with comparing casually recalled home dreams with laboratory dreams is that they are collected differently. Casually collected home dreams tend to be selectively remembered, while dreams in the lab are sampled (Cartwright, 1989). That is, we typically choose certain dreams that we have at home to remember if they are unusual in some way. Lab dreams are recorded regardless of content. Lab awakening dreams are more like being asked to report your waking experiences whenever a beeper you are carrying goes off. Home dreams are more like having you recall what happened to you recently. But what if lab dreams were collected in the same way as home dreams? Would the content still differ?

Lloyd (1987) did just that. Subjects were trained to activate a simple switch attached to their hand (prior research indicated that it is possible to learn to do so). When the switch is activated, an alarm rings, waking the dreamer, and a tape recorder is started. The awakened dreamer then dictates the dream. Half of the sleepers were at home and the other half in the lab. The sufjects in the lab also had their sleep monitored in the typical way. When the dreams that were collected were compared on several bases, no difference could be discerned.

While the lab dreams are probably more useful for understanding what dreams themselves are like and how they are produced, casually recalled home dreams yield more insight into the psychology and personality of the individual dreamer. Since the latter are also generally more available (they do not require special laboratories or equipment) and are more frequently discussed, especially in therapy, they will always be of interest. We must keep in mind, though, that casually recalled home dreams are useful mainly to gain insight about the dreamer but not the dream process. In Chapter 7, we will show how home dreams can be properly utilized by anyone for dream analysis. Meanwhile, our focus in this chapter will primarily be on laboratory dreams and the process of dreaming.

What is a dream?

Should any mentation (that is, any knid of mental activity) that occurs during sleep be attributed to dreaming? Consider the dreams reported by John in the prologue. One was vague and consisted of a single image much like a photograph or slide. The other was vivid and consisted of a sequence of images that resembled a movie or TV program. Other than the fact that they both occurred during sleep, these two mentations are considerably different. The conclusions and theories about dreams could vary considerably depending on whether one or both types of mentation are included in the definition of a dream.

Most researchers would not include both as dreams, and neither will we. A dream, for us, is a succession of images or scenes that contains action and interaction between "characters" that seems real and vivid with time going by (Cartwright, 1978; Dement, 1978; Faraday, 1972). Dreams also are internal, usually seemingly out of our control, and often contain impossible actions that are not critically evaluated while the dream is in progress. Other mentation may occur during sleep but will not be considered dreaming. Typically, this other mentation is characterized as being shorter, less vivid, less visual, less dramatic, less elaborated, less emotional, containing less action, and being more plausible and more thought-like (Cartwright, 1978; Dement, 1978; Faraday, 1972).

This non-dream mentation may not occur during sleep at all, but rather be quickly generated when turning on the wake portions of our brains. It is rather like what happens when I turn on our old Commodore PET computer - the display screen briefly is filled with a lot of random symbols. This occurs when the computer display mechanism is suddenly activated resulting in apparently random, meaningless images. These images are quickly replaced by logical information as the rest of the computer's components become activated and assume control. However, the illogical images last long enough to be observed by us. Perhaps a similar thing occurs when we awaken from sleep and "turn on" our conscious brain parts - there is a brief production of randon images.

Orlinsky (see Dement, 1978) has devised an 8 point scale for differentiation of sleep mentation:

0. Subject cannot remember dreaming; no dream is reported upon awakening.

1. Subject remembers having dreamed, or thinks he or she may have dreamed, but cannot remember any specific contents.

2. Subject remembers a specific topic, but in isolation; for example, a fragmentary action, scene, object, word or idea unrelated to anything else.

3. Subject remembers several disconnected thoughts, scenes or actions.

4. Subject remembers a short but coherent dream, the parts of which seem unrelated to each other; for example, a conversation rather than a word, a problem worked through rather than an idea, a purposeful, rather than a fragmentary, action.

5. Subject remembers a detailed dream sequence in which something happens followed by some consequence, or in which one scene, mood, or main interacting character is replaced by another .

6. Subject remembers a long, detailed dream sequence involving three or four discernible stages of development.

7. Subject remembers an extremely long and detailed dream sequence of five or more stages; or more than one dream (at least one of which is rated 5) for a single awakening.

For our purposes, we shall include as dreaming any content rated 4 or higher. A rating of 2 is not dreaming but other mentation. Content rated 3 is borderline - maybe a vague dream or the start of a dream. Other researchers have accepted only 6 or 7 as true dreaming.

REM vs. NREM Dreaming

There is general agreement that people dream during REM. Eighty to ninety percent of REM awakenings result in a dream report (Faraday, 1972). What about the other 10 to 20%? One interpretation is that dreaming occurs 100% of the time in REM but 10 to 20% of the time memory of this dreaming is "lost" during the process of awakening. We all know how hard it is to remember our dreams any-way. You wake up in the morning with the images of a recent dream still very fresh and vivid in your mind. A few minutes later you have difficulty describing even a very few vague details of the dream. In the lab, if we wait more than 3 minutes after REM has ended, the percent of dream recalled drops severely. The stuff of dreams is very ephemeral. It is possible that during 10 to 20% of REM awakenings, memory of the dream evaporates during the awakening process.

The occurrence of dreaming during NREM is more controversial (Cartwright, 1977; Dement, 1978; Faraday, 1972; VandeCastle, 1971). Using strict criteria (6 and 7 on the scale) only 7% of NREM awa-kenings yield dreaming (and this small percent may not have occurred in NREM at all, but be left in memory from a recent REM period). Almost 60% of NREM awakenings yield ratings of 1 through 7 and have been counted as dreams by some investigators. Including only categories 2 through 7 resulted in less than 50% dream reports from NREM awakenings.

One way to interpret these data is to say that dreaming occurs during NREM, but is easily lost during the transition to wakefulness (Spiegel, 1981). Or perhaps REM provides better conditions in which to remember dreaming than NREM (Faraday, 1972) since REM has been linked to memory processes (see chapter 11). However, lacking evidence to support either of these possibilities, we will assume in the rest of this book that:

1) we dream 100% of the time during REM;

2) we seldom dream, if at all, during NREM but may carry memories of dreams over from REM;

3) NREM mentation, although not dreaming, may, nevertheless, be important and should not be as ignored as it has tended to be in the past.

Analysis of sleep states using the mathematical procedure of Chaos supports the notion that dreaming only occurs in REM (or at least only complex dreams occur in REM (Röschke & Aldenhoff, 1992)

There are several bits of evidence that are not entirely consistent with the view that REM dreams differ from NREM mentation. If you are awakened from NREM toward the end of the night you will produce more dream reports than if awakened from NREM earlier in the night (Foulkes, 1966), and all reports following any awakening become more dream-like as the night goes on (Cartwright, 1978). Light sleepers give dream reports in nearly equal frequency during NREM awakenings and REM awakenings (Koukkou & Lehmann, 1983). Dream reports can be obtained by awakening a person prior to the first REM period of the night (Cartwright, 1989). Dreams typical of REM have been collected during NREM awakenings (Fiss, 1979). However, judges given only dream reports are reliably able to distinguish REM dreams from NREM mentation (Fiss, 1979). Foulkes (1985) concludes that there is but one kind of dream generator for both REM and NREM, but other cognitive processes are responsible for the difference in the reports from these two states.

One possibility is that NREM mentation is produced by the left half of our brain, while REM dreaming comes from the right half (Cartwright, 1977). In recent years, it has become obvious to brain researchers that the two halves of the brain "think" differently. The left side thinking is characterized by logical, linear thinking involving facts and numbers. The right brain, in contrast, thinking is more intuitive, global, aesthetic, and creative. The left brain relies on verbal processes, the right brain on imagery. If this is true, dreams are from the right brain during REM, and other mentations (for which we have no convenient word) are from the left brain during NREM. Early research suggested the possibility of right hemisphere control of dreaming by showing that in a small number of reports that subjects with right hemisphere brain damage lost their ability to dream. Therefore, showing that dreaming, which is an imagery process that is dominated by the right hemisphere, is also controlled by the right hemisphere. Recent evidence, however, has failed to support this view (Armitage, Bell, Campbell, & Stelmack, 1990; Herman, Rampy, Hirshkowitz, Thorpe, Bliss, & Roffwarg, 1987; Hirshkowitz & Howell, 1988). Cohen (1979) found that REM state was right hemisphere predominant, with a progressive shift over the night toward left hemisphere activation, so that the longest and last REM state of the night was most like the normal asymmetry of wakefulness, favoring the left or dominant hemisphere. This shows the complexity of the relationship between the two hemispheres (Hunt, 1989).

There is also a third kind of mentation that deserves mention (Ullman & Zimmerman, 1979). Sometimes when going to sleep (or when awakening) a person may experience a short dreamlike image: a conversation, sensation, or hallucination. These hypnagogic (when going to sleep) or hypnapompic (when awakening) hallucinations are very short and are not as dramatic as REM dreams. They occur during the transition between wakefulness and sleep, perhaps due to the shifting of brain dominance not occurring in the proper and synchronous order.

One implication of all of these factors is that it is important to ask the right questions when doing dream research (Webb, 1975). Recall how the questions were asked of John in the prologue. Not "were you dreaming" but "what was going through your mind." The former might cause people not to report other kinds of mentations which by their own definition are not dreams. Asking the latter type of question may also help prevent fabrication or elaboration of the dreams.

LUCID DREAMING

> *I am dreaming that I am running a track event. I approach the finish line and come in third place, but this is not how I want the race to end. So, I and the other competitors run backward to the start line and run the race again. This time I win!*

This is an example of a lucid dream. During a lucid dream, the dreamer is aware that they are dreaming and that it is not reality. Subjectively, the dreamer perceives themselves to be remarkably wakeful (LaBerge, 1981), although polysomnographic monitoring shows that they are clearly physiologically asleep and dreaming (Gackenbach and Bosveld, 1989). During a lucid dream, the dreamer may take an active role in resolving the dream's conflict, as shown by the example above, but not all lucid dreamers have this control over the action in their dreams. Others are only aware that they are dreaming, but do not do anything about the content of their dream. During a dream, the realization that you are lucid dreaming may be sudden or it could gradually become apparent to you.

Although spontaneous lucid dreaming occurs in only about 10% of the population (Colligan, 1982), it can be learned by many others. There are different techniques that can be used to teach a person how to lucid dream. Psychologist Patricia Garfield simply tells herself before going to sleep, "Tonight I <u>will</u> have a lucid dream"

(LaBerge,1981). A much more detailed method was created by Stephen LaBerge (1981) called mnemonic induction of lucid dreams (MILD). Briefly, the procedure entails:

1.) During the early morning hours, awaken spontaneously from a dream.

2.) After memorizing the dream, engage in 10 to 15 minutes of reading or any activity that demands full wakefulness.

3.) While lying in bed and returning to sleep, tell yourself that the next time you are dreaming, you want to realize that you are dreaming.

4.) Visualize your body lying asleep in bed, with rapid eye movements indicating that you are dreaming. At the same time, see yourself as being in the dream and realize that you are in fact dreaming.

5.) Repeat steps 3 and 4 until you feel that your intention is clearly fixed.

More recently, LaBerge has used dream incorporation of sensory stimuli (see later in this chapter) as a vehicle to learn lucid dreaming. For example, when lights are flashed into the sleepers eyes, they may be incorporated into the dream. The dreamer recognizes the lights as a prearranged cue that they are having a dream (LaBerge in Carskadon, 1993).

By learning how to control your dreams, you can stop nightmares or fly off to a tropical island for a vacation. Even children as young as 5 can learn how to lucid dream in order to fight off the characters of their nightmares. Truly skilled lucid dreamers can make people, places, and things dissolve into thin air and replace them with whatever they find interesting (Colligan, 1982).

It is believed that lucid dreaming can be used by the dreamer to help themselves. For example, it may be used as a treatment for depression. Dreamers can restructure their sense of identity and their self-image by editing the events of their dreams (Lyon, 1990). Telling people to seize control of their dreams helps them with taking control in their waking world. Sometimes though, lucid dreaming can become a problem, such as when the person realizes they are dreaming and uses this to escape the dream and thereby avoid resolving the conflict (LaBerge, 1981). Sometimes the conscious realization that they are dreaming causes the dreamer to use the attitudes and coping strategies that are used when the person is awake. This can become a problem when the dreamer wakes up as a way to avoid the unpleasant dream and, therefore, resists coming to terms with the conflict. Other dream experts believe that lucidity should be used to explore the dream rather that to manipulate it. At times it is better to see the dream through, instead of changing it or sugarcoating, it in order to confront the conflict that arises in the dream world.

Everyone Dreams but Only Some Recall

Everyone has REM sleep. One hundred percent of REM contains dreaming. Thus, everyone dreams. But not everyone recalls dreaming. In fact, no one remembers all of their dreams. Consider that each REM period may contain several different dreams (Cohen, 1979) (body movements often separate the individual dreams [Webb, 1975]), especially the longer ones during the end of the night, and that everyone has typically 4-5 REM periods per night. Thus everyone has 10 to 20 different (but often related) dreams each and every night. No one has ever recalled all of their dreams from a single night and, in fact, most people recall only a few per week. The average number of dreams that one can recall is one dream for every two nights. This is a low percentage of the total number of dreams we have (Koulack, 1991).Thus, all of us are at best poor recallers, but some are better than others. Some people never recall their dreams at all. I recently had the experience of recalling five in a single night, which is rare and unusual.

Why do people remember so few of their dreams and why do some remember more than others? The factors are many and interrelated (Cartwright, 1977; 1978; Cohen, 1979; Faraday, 1972; Fiss, 1979). We shall explore some of them.

Obviously, from what I have just said, our dreams are difficult to catch and remember. Essentially, we must awaken during a dream or within a few minutes after it has stopped in order to be aware of it. It must then be recorded or at least rehearsed quickly or it will fade forever.

Another factor that effects the amount of dream recall is presleep intention to recall dreams. Individuals and societies that place importance on dreams and/or want to recall them have more success in doing so.

Rapid awakening yields better recall. Delays in getting the conscious mind going add time between the dream and its attempted recall. However, a very sudden unpleasant awakening accompanied by a lot of physiological arousal (pounding heart, muscle tension, etc.) also seems to make dream recall more difficult.

Similarly, light sleepers recall more. These are people who awaken more often each night than typical and generally awaken quickly and easily.

Personality factors also seem to play a role, although not all sleep researchers agree on this point. Non-recallers as a group tend to be people who avoid or deny unpleasant experiences and anxieties in waking life. They also tend to be more inhibited, more conformist, and like mental things neat and orderly. Generally, they are more self-controlled. Recallers, on the other hand, tend to be more overtly anxious, more willing to admit emotional disturbances, and more self aware. They also tend to have what is called "high tolerance for ambiguity" (Hartmann, 1989).

Long sleepers (see Chapter 3) recall more dreams. The same is true of variable length sleepers during their long sleeping times. Both spend much more time in REM and thus dream more. Yet, it is equally possible that the personality factors that contribute to longer sleep also facilitate dream recall.

The nature of the dream itself may be important in recall. Long, vivid, very emotional dreams tend to be more easily remembered.

Finally, Freud was probably right when he said that people repress their dreams. Some dreams (or dream themes) are too awful for the conscious mind to handle, thus they are prevented from reaching the conscious mind.

Popular Myths About Dreams

Most dreams are black and white.

False (Carskadon, 1993). Most, if not all, are in color. We often simply do not remember the detail of color, just as we often forget other dream details. However, when people are awakened in the lab during REM and immediately asked about color in their dreams, over 2/3 report color being present. The other 1/3 may have lost that detail in the process of waking up.

Eating cheese and pickles (or sauerkraut or cold pizza or whatever) causes us to dream or dream more.

False (Carskadon, 1993). These foods, which may give us indigestion, may cause us to not sleep as well, and thus awaken more often. Lighter sleep with more awakenings may cause us to *recall* more dreams but does not cause us to have more.

Sounds or other things that occur while we are sleeping cause us to have dreams if they do not awaken us.

False (Dement, 1978). Our dreams will occur regardless, or even in spite of, any external trigger. However, such stimuli may become a part of an already ongoing dream. Many people have slept through a ringing alarm or phone because the sound became a part of their dream. This has been termed **incorporation**. Since the stimulus is interpreted to be a part of the dream and not from the real external world, the person does not awaken. Other kinds of sensations may also be incorporated, such as smells and feeling things on the skin.

I recently had such an experience. I dreamt I was eating crow wing. It was the most awful tasting thing. Yet I was at a dinner party, and everyone was watching me so I had to keep on chewing on that foul fowl. I soon awakened, however, with the worst morning-mouth I can remember. Not only was my breath awful, but I could even taste it!

Dreams occur in a flash.

False (Faraday, 1972). When the activity in your dream takes five minutes, it almost always takes five real minutes to dream it. The myth that dreams are instantaneous may have been fostered by things like a widely publicized dream by Andre Maury in the mid 1800's. He dreamt he was in Paris and amid all of the executions that followed the French Revolution. He ascended the scaffold and positioned himself on the guillotine. Then the awful blade fell. He could feel his head being severed from his body. At this point he awakened in extreme fright to find that the top of his bed had fallen across his neck just where a guillotine blade would have fallen! Later, Maury interpreted this (being hit by a part of his bed) as causing the dream - all of it - instantaneously while he was awakening.

Laboratory experiments have shown otherwise. Researchers have used incorporation to mark time in dreams. For example, water sprayed on the face of a sleeper in REM will often cause rain to become a part of the dream. When the water is sprayed and the person is immediately awakened the rain occurs at the end of the dream story. However, if the spraying is done five minutes before the awakening then about five minutes of time goes by in the dream story following the rain. Studies with lucid dreamers also lead to this conclusion (LaBerge in Carskadon, 1993). It thus appears that dreams do take time to unfold.

The eye movements of REM are following the activity of the dream.

Maybe (Antrobus, 1990). Not all sleep and dream researchers agree on this, but some research seems to support it (Herman, Erman, Boys, Peiser, Taylor, & Roffwarg, 1984). In one such experiment, extra electrodes were placed above and below the eyes so that the direction of the eye movements could be discerned. When the subjects dreamed about vertical things or activities such as climbing stairs, their eye movements went up and down. When they dreamed about horizontal things such as a big, flat lake, the eye movements tended to be right and left. Also, the intensity of the eye movements tends to correspond with the intensity of the activity of the dream. Dreams with a lot of fast action produce much more eye movement.

This evidence is not conclusive however. Maybe the eye movements determine what is being dreamed about (see discussion of the Hobson-McCarley model in Chapter 6). This might be just another example of incorporation.

Negative evidence (Tedlock, 1987) includes the fact that rapid eye movements occur during REM in fetuses, neonates, congenitally blind, and cats without a cortex. Since none of these have had visual experience, it is unlikely that they are scanning an imaginary visual field. Also, rapid eye movements differ from waking eye movements in several ways (Bridgeman, 1988; Tedlock, 1987)

Blind people don't dream.

False (Carskadon, 1993). A person who has been blind from birth will dream - but not with visual images. Their dreams will be in the other senses - especially auditory - but will otherwise contain settings, characters, and storyline. If they became blind after a period of seeing, then they will continue to dream visually but gradually replace vision with other senses in their dreams.

Other Dream Characteristics

One of the most noticeable characteristics about our dreaming is how uncritical we are of their content (Cartwright, 1978). When we are dreaming we seem to lose all of our critical, logical judgment. We take everything as real and plausible. People fly. Cars have teeth and threaten to bite us. Streets turn into carpets. We are famous movie stars. We will believe anything!

In spite of this, some people seem to dream more clearly than others (Faraday, 1972). Or at least they are able to recall their dreams more clearly. We are not able to tell which. Some people report that their dreams are very real and vivid - just like being awake. Others say their dreams tend to be fuzzy - like a poor quality TV picture.

Our emotions seem to have a greater effect on our dreams than logical, cognitive processes. While cognitive processes do influence our dreams, they are usually less important than our emotions.

Many of our dreams are quite intense with emotion-rousing occurrences. Yet strangely, we rarely really feel the pain in our dreams (Webb, 1975). We may be excited by sexual encounters during dreams, yet the actual sexual feelings are usually not there. Overall, our dreams tend to be more negative than positive (Borbély, 1986).

Our memories do, however, play a very important role in our dreaming. We very often dream about things that happened to us during the day (a process Freud named "daytime residue"; see chapter 7.) For example, a research subject broke her arm during a bicycle accident on the day that she was to sleep in the lab for an experiment on "dreaming recall following wake-ups during REM." One of her long dreams that night involved a bicycle and many problems with it.

We also tend to dream about things familiar and important to us (Hall & VandeCastle, 1966; Webb, 1975). Abstract dreams or dreams having nothing to do with the dreamer do not seem to occur. Instead we dream about our problems, our past experiences, and familiar places in our dreams. By and large, we can recognize much more as familiar than unfamiliar.

Sometimes we are an active character in our dreams and we see things through our own eyes (Hall & VandeCastle, 1966; Webb, 1975). At other times, we are observing ourselves as if we are watching a movie. Sometimes we do not appear in our own dreams or at least not directly and obviously. (Some dream theorists say that we are always in our own dreams but perhaps disguised as another character or even object; see chapters 7 and 8.)

We may repeat the same dream, perhaps several times (Cartwright, 1979). Or we may repeat some aspect of a dream, such as the same character, object, or scene. When asked about a dream, 64% of women and 54.5% of man report having had a recurrent dream. Of the people reporting they have had recurrent dreams, 77% of the females and 48% of the males reported that the dreams were unpleasant. However, the content of recurrent dreams varies with age. During the first decade of life, recurrent dreams tend to contain threats to life or safety by outside forces. For example, as a child, I, a city kid born and raised in Detroit, dreamed that I was in a barn encircled by trucks, tractors, and other farm vehicles. Their headlights looked like eyes and their grills like hugh teeth in wide open mouths.

During the second decade of life, recurrent dreams contain various themes of concern about competence, involving things like shame and failure, where we disappoint ourselves. Beyond the second decade, recurrent dreams concern still fewer outside forces causing unpleasant consequences and more dreams of self-caused problems.

Cultural/Historical Views About Dreams

What are dreams? What do they do? Throughout recorded history (and probably even earlier) people have asked these questions. The kinds of answers that have been given can be grouped into four categories (after Webb, 1992):

1. a different reality/co-reality
2. omens
3. reflections of waking life
4. artifacts of brain activity.

Lets explore each of these in turn.

Different Reality

GANAKA VAIDEHA SAID: "Who is that Self?"

Yagnavalkya replied: "He who is within the heart, surrounded by the Pranas (senses), the person of light consisting of knowledge. He, remaining the same, wanders along the two worlds, as if thinking, as if moving. During sleep (in dreams) he transcends this world and all the forms of death (all that falls under the sway of death; all that is perishable).

"On being born, that person, assuming his body, becomes united with all evils; when he departs and dies, he leaves all evil behind.

"And there are two states for that person, the one here in this world, the other in the other world, and, as a third, an intermediate state, the state of sleep. When in that intermediate state, he sees both these states together, the one here in this world, and the other in the other world. Now whatever his admission to the other world may be, having gained that admission, he sees both the evils and the blessings.

"And when he falls asleep, then after having taken away with him the material from the whole world, destroying and building it up again, he sleeps (dreams) by his own light. In that state the person is self-illuminated.

"There are no (real) chariots in that state, no horses, no roads. There are no blessings there, no happiness, no joys, but he himself sends forth (creates) blessings, happiness and joys. There are no tanks there, no lakes, no rivers, but he himself sends forth (creates) tanks, lakes and rivers. He indeed is the maker.

"On this there are two verses:

"After having subdued by sleep all that belongs to the body, he, not asleep himself, looks down upon the sleeping (senses).

Having assumed light, he goes again to his place, the golden person, the lovely bird.

"Guarding with the breath (prana, life) the lower nest, the immortal moves away from the nest; the immortal one goes wherever he likes, the golden person, the lovely bird.

"Going up and down in his dreams, the god makes manifold shapes for himself, either rejoicing together with women, or laughing (with his friends), or seeing terrible sights.

"People may see his playground, but he himself no one ever sees. Therefore they say, `Let no one wake a man suddenly, for it is not easy to remedy if he does not get back (rightly to his body).'

"Here some people (object and) say:

"'No, this (sleep) is the same as the place of waking, for what he sees while awake, that only he sees when asleep.' No, here (in sleep) the person is self-illuminated (as we explained before)....

"That (person) having enjoyed himself in that sleep (dream), having moved about and seen both good and evil, hastens back again as he came, to the place from which he started to awake. And whatever he may have seen there, he is not followed (affected) by it, for that person is not attached to anything....

"As a large fish moves along the two bakds of a river, the right and left, so does that person move along these two states, the state of sleeping and the state of waking.

"And as a falcon, or any other (swift) bird, after he has roamed about here in the air, becomes tired, and folding his wings he is carried to his nest, so does that person hasten to that state where, when asleep, he desires no more desires, and dreams no more dreams.

"There are in his body the veins called Hita, which are as small as a hair divided a thousandfold, full of white, blue, yellow, green and red. Now when, as it were, they kill him, when, as it were, they overcome him, when, as it were, he falls into a well, he fancies, through ignorance, that danger which he (commonly) sees in waking. But when he fancies that he is, as it were, a god, or that he is, as it were, a king, or 'I am this altogether,' that is his highest world."

That excerpt was taken from the Brihadarmyaka-Upanishad from India (as translated by F. Max Muller, 1974. Dreaming an intermediate state. In R L Woods & H B Greenhouse [Eds.], *The new world of Dreams* (pp. 125-126). New York: MacMillan.) Its origin has been traced back to about 1000 B.C. In it we see a clear example of an attempt to explain dreaming as an existence by the dreamer in another world. Also contained in this excerpt is the warning not to awaken the sleeper (dreamer) lest she does not get back to her real waking-world body.

This is but one example. Throughout the world and history there have been many variations of this notion. One such notion is that the dreamer's spirit travels suddenly to, and exists in, a different place totally unrelated to the place of his waking existence. A variation of this notion is that the different place is related to the place of waking existence. Also included in this category are complex philosophical theories in which dreams play an important part.

Examples of a totally separate existence include the Eskimos of Hudson Bay and the distant, unrelated Pantani Malay people. Both have a similar explanation of dreaming; the sleeper leaves his body during sleep and enters another world. The Tajal of Luzon will severely punish a person who awakens a sleeper because of the danger that the person will be lost forever from his body.

The beliefs of many of the ancient Greeks fit in this category (Coxhead & Hiller, 1976). To them, Hypnos was the god of sleep and his son Morpheus the god of dreams. Yet the stuff in dreams - the people, objects, the places - are older than the gods and very close to primeval origins. While the dreamer rules his individual dreams and Morpheus rules the world of dreams, their existence is beyond both the dreamer and Morpheus. Greeks did not have dreams; they were visited by them. The Pythagoreans felt that the soul was freed from the body during sleep and was able to go upward to interact with higher beings. This notion has its roots in the Egyptians who believed that Id (the spiritual double) exited the body during sleep.

Hippocrates, the Greek founder of modern medicine, saw the soul as able to perceive the causes of illness in dreams by judging the balance of the body's functions. The body is well when dreams are good representations of the waking world. If something is not as it should be - for example, a black sun - there is something wrong with the organ of the body that corresponds to the sun. Hippocrates also felt that at night, when the mind was free from its conscious duties, it was then able to express in dream imagery the physical condition of the body. Therefore, the dream was capable of giving early warning to illness, and would thus make it easier for diagnosis and treatment.

Plato held that spirits came near the dreamer to impart ideas and relay orders of gods through the dream. This idea was further developed by the Neo-Platonists, later adopted by the Gnostics, continued by the Occultists of the Renaissance, and continues with the Theospophists and the Mystics of our century.

Co-reality

Other people see dreams as a co-reality with our waking life (Coxhead and Hiller, 1976). The most famous example is that of the Senoi of Malaysia at the beginning of this century. They feel that if a dreamer wins a dream battle with the spirit of an enemy, then that enemy becomes a friend who will be able to help him in future dreams or in waking life. The Senoi gather each morning in family groups to discuss and analyze their recent dreams. Attempts are made to bring back something from the dream that can be shared with the group, such as a song or dance. The ultimate goal of a Senoi is for his various souls to leave the body during dreaming and interact with distant people and objects.

Many other widely diverse cultures such as Kurdish, Kamchatka, Borneo, or Zulu see actions during dreams as having the same reality as actions during waking. To dream of adultery is to be an adulterer. An offense in one is an offense in the other. A gift received during a dream requires the dreamer to return the favor in waking life. An insult given while dreaming requires an apology the next waking day. (Try to imagine what your life would be like if you had to do this with your dreams!)

A vivid example of dreams having a co-reality with waking life is dramatically seen in the following report entitled "Sex Dreams of the African Ashantis" by R.S. Rattray (1974).

> *I have heard of a case of a sexual dream where the disclosure of the dream cost the owner his life. It would not be easy to obtain a better example of how real events are held to be which pass before the sleeper. Such dreams mean that "your soul desires that woman's soul," stated my informant. "If you dream that you have had intercourse with a woman with whom*

you have never had sexual relations, it means that you will never in all your life have sexual intercourse with that woman, because your soul has already devoured her."

If you dream that you have had sexual intercourse with another man's wife and any one hears of it, and tells her husband, then you will be fined the usual adultery fee, for your soul and hers have had sexual intercourse. If you ever dream such a dream you should not tell anyone, but very early next morning you should go to the midden heap, which is also the a women's latrine, and whisper to it and say "Suminna ma so dae bone emma no nye sa". (O midden heap, I have dreamed an evil dream, grant that it may never happen like that.) Any bad dream you must carry away to the refuse heap, where everything bad is put.

If you dream that you have sexual intercourse with someone who is now dead and with whom you have had sexual relations during her life, then your penis will surely die; but this does not happen if the dream is about some woman now dead, but with whom you have never had sexual relations during her life.

Some notions of dreams are even more complexly intermingled with philosophical notions, as in the following myth from the Uttoto Indians of Colombia (from Coxhead & Hiller, 1976). They use dreams to explain the creation of the world.

In the beginning, the Word gave origin to the Father.

A phantasm, nothing else existed in the beginning; the Father touched an illusion, he grasped something mysterious. Nothing existed. Through the agency of a dream our Father Nai-mu-ena (he who is, or has, a dream) kept the mirage of his body, and he pondered long and thought deeply.

Nothing existed, not even a stick to support the vision: our Father attached the illusion to the thread of a dream and kept it by the aid of his breath. He sounded to reach the bottom of the appearance, but there was nothing. Nothing existed.

Then the Father again investigated the bottom of the mystery. He tied the empty illusion to the dream thread and pressed the magical substance upon it. Then by the aid of his dream he held it like a wisp of raw cotton.

Then he seized the mirage bottom and stamped upon it repeatedly, sitting down at last on his dreamed earth."

A third century B.C. Chinese philosopher asked, "Am I a man dreaming of being a butterfly or a butterfly dreaming of being a man?" (Ullman & Zimmerman, 1979) Bertrand Russell has said, "I do not believe that I am now dreaming, but I cannot prove that I am not" (Ullman & Zimmerman, 1979). Heraclitus maintained that as consciousness is fire, hence life, knowledge, and reason. Sleep (as is death) is when the soul escapes from the fire of life but only founders in moisture. Dreams are located near OKEANOS ("damp mists of time where consciousness is swamped by vague unknown") (Coxhead & Hiller, 1976, p 6).

Omens

The attitude that dreams have prophetic functions has a long history. Dreams in The Odyssey play a frequent role in predicting and giving guidance for the future. There is an Egyptian Papyrus of 1350 B.C. that is a dream book giving help in interpreting dreams. This tradition continues even today, for you can buy books claiming to help you analyze your dreams in such a way as to foretell the future.

Various cultures have had special people designated to interpret dreams such as priests, elders, and so on. In many cultures, these people were very powerful and influential. The Greeks had over 600 temples where people would sleep in an attempt to have dreams of guidance. Often, the priests at these temples interpreted the meaning of these special dreams for the dreamer.

Perhaps the most familiar prophetic dreams are found in the Bible. "If there is a prophet among you, I the Lord will make myself known to him in a vision; I will speak with him in a dream," (Numbers 12:6). When God spoke to the Israelites he did so directly such as to Jacob who "dreamed that there was a ladder set upon the earth...and behold the Lord stood above it, and said: I am the Lord, the God of Abraham your father and the God of Isaac; the land on which you lie I will give to you and your descendants," (Genesis 28:12). At other times, the dreams sent directly to the Israelites were less direct in meaning, but nevertheless obvious. One example is the dream of Joseph: "Hear this dream that I have dreamed: behold, we were binding sheaves in the field, and lo, my sheaf arose and stood upright; and behold, your sheaves gathered around it, and bowed down to my sheaf. His brothers said to him, 'are you indeed to reign over us?'" (Genesis 37:5).

The dreams of Gentiles, however, were more cryptic and always required interpretation by a Hebrew (with God's help). The following story from Genesis chapter 41 is a familiar example.

> *After two whole years, Pharaoh dreamed that he was standing by the Nile, and behold, there came up out of the Nile seven cows sleek and fat, and they fed in the reed grass. And behold, seven other cows, gaunt and thin, came up out of the Nile after them, and stood by the other cows on the bank of the Nile. And the gaunt and thin cows ate up the seven sleek and fat cows. And Pharaoh awoke. And he fell asleep and dreamed a second time; and behold, seven ears of grain, plump and good, were growing on one stalk. And behold, after them sprouted seven ears, thin and blighted by the east wind. And the thin ears swallowed up the seven plump and full ears. And Pharaoh awoke, and behold, it was a dream. So in the morning his spirit was troubled; and he sent and called for all the magicians of Egypt and all its wise men; and Pharaoh told them his dream, but there was none who could interpret it to Pharaoh.*
>
> *...Then Pharaoh sent and called Joseph, and they brought him hastily out of the dungeon; and when he had shaved himself and changed his clothes, he came in before Pharaoh. And Pharaoh said to Joseph, "I have had a dream, and there is no one who can interpret it; and I have heard it said of you that when you hear a dream you can interpret it." Joseph answered Pharaoh, "It is not in me; God will give Pharaoh a favorable answer."*
>
> *... Then Joseph said to Pharaoh, "The dream of Pharaoh is one; God has revealed to Pharaoh what he is about to do. The seven good cows are seven years, and the seven good ears are seven years; the dream is one. The seven lean and gaunt cows that came up after them are seven years, and the seven empty ears blighted by the east wind are also seven years of famine. It is as I told Pharaoh, God has shown to Pharaoh what he is about to do. There will come seven years of great plenty throughout all the land of Egypt, but after them there will arise seven years of famine, and all the plenty will be forgotten in*

the land of Egypt; the famine will consume the land, and the plenty will be unknown in the land by reason of that famine which will follow, for it will be very grievous. And the doubling of Pharaoh's dream means that the thing is fixed by God, and God will shortly bring it to pass..."

In the New Testament, too, dreams play an important prophetic role.

... an angel of the Lord appeared to him in a dream, "Joseph, son of David, do not fear to take Mary as your wife, for that which is conceived in her is of the Holy Spirit; she will bear a son, and you shall call him Jesus, for he will save his people from their sins" (Matt 1:20-21).

Why does the Bible portray the dream as omen so frequently? One of the main purposes of the Bible is to show the relationship of God and human beings in ways that are easily understood. One way to do this is to tell stories using common, contemporary examples. At the time that the Bible was written, the common understanding was that the dream often served to foretell the future. This prevailing attitude was used in some of the stories. If the Bible were written today, many of the stories would be different in details - perhaps with stories and parables involving computers and space travel rather than fishing nets and tall towers. If dreams were used in the modern stories, they would probably not be used as omens, for that is no longer the prevailing attitude toward them. Nevertheless, the way dreams are used in the Bible reflects the serious regard people then had for dreams.

Although no longer the prevailing attitude, the notion that dreams can have predictive value is still somewhat popular in the Western world. Many people buy the dictionary-like books that claim to interpret the meanings of objects, people, or events occurring in dreams. Many of the meanings are purportedly predictive of the future. There is, however, little basis in fact for such books, and they are held to be of limited, if any, value by dream researchers. At best, they should be considered as entertainment rather than as having practical value.

Psychic Dreams. More serious is the current research which is going on to explore the psychic value of dreams (Moorcroft in Carskadon, 1993). Telepathic, precognitive (seeing the future), and clairvoyant (thought transfer or perception of current but distant events) dreams are being investigated. In all psychic dreams, awareness seems to bypass normal senses. Spearheading these endeavors for over the last 20 years has been Montague Ullman, a psychoanalyst.

His interest started in 1950 when a woman told him two dreams which he thought were very similar to a film he had been watching during the night when the woman's dreams occurred (Demming, 1972). Since the woman had been in analysis with him for a long time, he felt good "rapport" with her. He wondered if this was not an example of clairvoyance through dreaming. This notion has intrigued him so much that in 1962 he formed the Wm. G. Menninger Dream Lab at Maimonides Hospital in Brooklyn. He continued there until 1974 when he resigned to give himself more time to devote to teaching and working on dreaming.

Imagine now that you and a friend were a subject in his research (Ullman, Krippner, & Vaughan, 1989). After being shown around and the procedure explained, your friend is prepared for a typical sleep study and goes to bed. At this time, in an isolated room you blindly select one of 12 reproductions of famous paintings and then spend the rest of the night concentrating on it. You comment on it, redraw it, color over parts of it, etc. You were probably also able to manipulate actual items that were shown in the painting.

Throughout the night, your friend was awakened ten minutes after the start of each REM period and asked to report on what he or she was dreaming. The next morning the sleeper also commented about their dreams. Any similarity between the dream report and the painting upon which you had been concentrating is considered evidence of telepathy.

But there is more. Your friend is then shown the 12 reproductions and asked to pick out the one that most resembles her dreams, then the one that next most resembles her dreams, and so on until all 12 have been ranked. If the reproduction you had been focusing upon was among the top 6 choices, Ullman considered it evidence of telepathy. In one experiment, 10 of 12 subjects ranked the chosen painting among the top 6. Over many experiments, the percent of time the chosen painting was among the top 6 was greater than chance. (To be sure that there was no inadvertent signals given by the experimenter, Ullman had a colleague who was unaware of your choice show your friend the twelve pictures and had other naive judges evaluate the dream reports for content.)

On occasion, the research produced a "Bull's Eye". This occurred when the dream was obviously like the picture. Perhaps you had picked out Van Gogh's "Fishing Boats at Saint-Maries-de-la-Mer" (see Figure 5-1) and your friend dreamed of a beach or boardwalk on some kind of seacoast. The boardwalk was somewhat raised up. In fact, the dream reminded your friend of Van Gogh.

In spite of the occasional Bull's Eyes and somewhat better than chance dream reports, the evidence remains unconvincing (Hansel, 1980). The success rate is not very strong and the degree of the similarities depends greatly on interpretation. More importantly, appropriate controls were apparently not done. One such control might have been to have you pick one of the twelve pictures but not look at it at all. In all other ways, the experiment would be conducted as above.

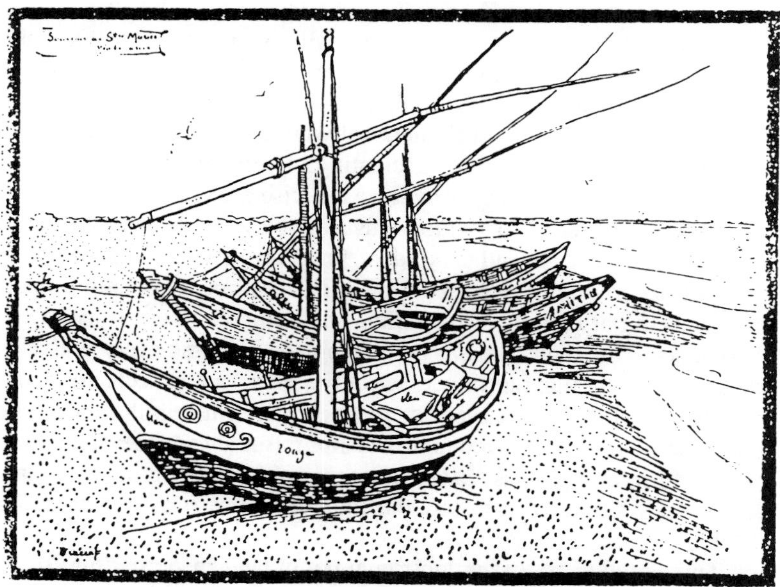

Figure 5-1. Van Gogh's Fishing Boats at Saint-Maries-de-la-Mer. From a private collection. Used with permission.

Would the results consistently differ from those reported when you had concentrated on the picture? We simply do not know. Until such control experiments have been faithfully done, we must not place too much credence in these experiments and regard their conclusions as tentative at best.

Another famous example of psychic dream research was done in the 1930s just after the baby of the world famous flier Charles Lindberg was kidnapped (Murray & Wheeler, 1937). The researchers used newspapers to appeal to people to submit their dreams about the fate of the baby. Thirteen hundred reports were submitted before the fate of the baby was actually known. Of these, only 7 contained content that resembled in some way the characteristics of the burial scene and even they were considerably more wrong than right. In most of the dream reports the baby was still alive. Other incorrect aspects of these reports contained aspects of false speculations widely reported in newspapers.

As Reflections of Waking Life

Each and every night you do something seemingly extraordinary. You create, produce, and view the equivalent of several TV programs. True, there really is no TV equipment nor live characters or actual scenes; these things are all figments of your creative imagination. But that makes it all the more fascinating. Every one of us has this tremendous creative ability, which we exercise each and every night.

These self-created TV programs can be said to resemble soap operas more than any other kind of program. They contain a lot of emotion-laden drama. We dream of things that are personally important to us in our current waking life - important on an emotional level. Like a good TV show, dreams do not contain each and every mundane detail of waking life, but rather, select the important aspects and focus on them. Often these aspects are distorted for emphasis or are symbolic in order to convey more meaning. But always they are things that have meaning to us in our current, waking life on an emotional level. Always, these dreams are our total creations. (Cartwright, 1977; 1978)

This is the view that is most commonly held in our culture today about dreams. They are creations of our mind that echo our waking world. They are reflections of our current concerns, our selves, and our current situation. They are not exact replicas - that would be boring and not very helpful. Rather, attention is focused on the important elements in ways that are useful and meaningful.

Although this approach is the most popular and prevalent now, it is not new. Aristotle maintained that just as we perceive when awake, we perceive in sleep (Borbély, 1986). While awake, perceptions may outlast the stimulus. We can look directly at a tree then turn away from it and still know it is there by visualizing it in our minds. So too, we perceive things in our dreams even though the physical stimulus is not present. According to Aristotle, the sources of these perceptions may be internal or external. Yet they are exaggerated since the "intellect" is not working with the "senses." He states that they are distorted just as "eddies in a great river...(are often) broken into other forms by collisions with other objects." Also, our emotions have a great deal to do with these exaggerations and distortions.

Thomas Hobbs in the 1650's maintained that dreams are reflections of imaginations in sleep that were the results of earlier sense events which were remembered (VandeCastle, 1971). Specific dreams, he asserted, may result from stimulations to the sleeper. Anger results in heat in parts of the body when awake; in sleep, heating of these body parts causes anger to raise up in the brain and then to produce dream images.

It probably was Freud who is most responsible for popularizing the attitude that dreams are a reflection of waking life (Freud, 1900). Dreams, he stressed, are creations of the dreamer's mind - a kind of wish-fulfillment. Most often these wishes are disguised in symbols but, nevertheless, are basically and truly based on what is important to us and what has happened to us. Furthermore, according to Freud, these dreams are of great benefit to us, for they allow us to be rid of the pressure of unfulfilled, yet unacceptable desires. We will elaborate more on Freud's dream theory, as well as the theories of those who followed him, in Chapter 7. Important for us at this point is the fact that Freud made the idea that the dream is a reflection of our waking state prevalent and popular in our culture.

As Functional States

Not all contemporary scientists accept the notion that Freud and his followers are correct. Nor do they believe that dreams are foretellers of the future or involve other psychic phenomena. They also reject the notion of dreaming as existence in another reality. In fact, they maintain that dreams are secondary accompaniments of brain activity. Most of the details of this attitude are based on recent research into brain anatomy and physiology, states of sleep, sleep in animals, and even modern computer technology. Yet it is not an entirely new notion. In his book *On Dreams* (1901) Freud states that he is not in agreement with the idea espoused by many of his contemporaries in the medical community that dreams are naught but accidental, meaningless "disconnected activity of separate organs or groups of cells in an otherwise sleeping brain..." (page 14).

The modern versions of this approach range from the idea that REM sleep is necessary to exercise the eyes so that they coordinate properly to analogies of reprogramming computers. It is a complex task for the brain to coordinate the functioning of the two eyeballs and the separate images that come from them. Thus, according to one theory (Snyder, 1966), the brain moves the eyes and makes necessary adjustments during sleep to enable proper waking functioning. In the process, the stimulated parts of the brain that are involved with vision, generate the images we call dreams. These images are, however, totally meaningless since they are a secondary result of the efforts of the brain to maintain visual coordination.

Just as computer hardware needs up to date software instructions to function properly, the brain, according to another theory (see Faraday, 1972), needs to regularly accommodate and assimilate its functioning in order to be able to the process new experiences and information which are constantly being acquired during waking life. This reprogramming is done during sleep when many parts of the brain do not have to be fully functioning. However, in the process of reprogramming, parts of the brain are artificially activated giving rise to random images which we call dreams.

Nobel prize winner Frances Crick, together with Graeme Mitchison, has proposed that dreams are the result of the brain's way of ridding itself of unwanted, unnecessary memories (Crick & Mitchison, 1983; 1986). They begin with the finding that the brain has the capacity for too much learning. Some of the things that are accidentally learned may, in fact, be detrimental. Or some of the interactions among brain cells that spontaneously occur during growth may resemble memories but are really quite useless. In order to get rid of these superfluous and harmful memories, the brainstem, during sleep, randomly stimulates the forebrain. Any assemblies of brain cells (i.e., memories) that are stimulated in this way may be meaningless and are greatly weakened in the process. Thus, for Crick and Mitchison, the function of dreaming is to forget. Any conscious remembering of the content of the dream is quite accidental and may even be counterproductive since it may serve to restrengthen the memory. (Dreams as functional states are further discussed in Chapter 6.)

Critical Comments

Of the four cultural/historical viewpoints about dreaming, the third, reflections of waking life, is the most widely held in our part of the world. That we leave our body and exist in a parallel reality while sleeping does not fit well with our understanding and beliefs of bodily and mental processes. Nor do many people believe that dreams in some way can predict the future. It is difficult to explain, given what we know and believe, how this could happen. True, there are some people who believe that either, or both, of these can and do happen. Often this belief is quite strong, but these people are few. Such individuals are especially rare among scientists and others who have carefully studied dreaming.

Why, then, do these ideas persist? Some people have dreams in which these things seem to occur. They seem very real. Since some people have no other immediate explanation, they are led to believe in out of body or psychic occurrences as being real. There are, however, alternative explanations that are more consistent with modern psychological knowledge.

Our knowledge and impressions of the world and all that is in it depend on processes occurring in the brain (Kalat, 1992). For example, our eyes send electrical impulses to special parts of our brain which interpret them as varying degrees of light and dark, often with color. Further interpretation of these signals results in the perception of trees and people and other things we recognize. We know this from scientific study of the brain. But these brain areas - as wonderful and efficient as they are - can be tricked into producing false perceptions. Visual illusions are one example. We can "see" things that are impossible to build out of real materials. Movies provide another example. Although we "see" continuous movement, what is projected on the screen is only a sequence of still images; but they occur so fast in sequence that our brain perceives continuous movement. In other words, our brain creates an impression of reality as best it can. It does this when we are asleep too. Sometimes, in some people, the reality that is created is of being out of one's body. This may seem very real and very vivid, but it is a creation of the brain, nevertheless.

Likewise, the impression that our dreams sometimes come true can also be explained. Our memory ability is really quite poor - especially for details (Myers, 1992). Numerous experiments have shown that we probably forget more than we remember. This is especially true of dreams, as already discussed in the beginning of this chapter. If we do not remember our dreams well - especially the details - then it is not really possible to tell that they "come true."

Perhaps it would be like this report from one of my students:

The event:

We were at grandpa's farm. I went for a walk by myself toward the hill that was part of the pasture. I had new white nail polish on. It was a beautiful spring day. Suddenly, gramp's new white puppy ran over the hill toward me and wanted to play.

The dream report:

It was just like the dream I had the week before. In the dream, I was in my backyard putting white polish on my nails. I was sitting on the ground on a bright, warm, sunny day. I looked up and there was a hill covered with wild flowers extending from our backyard, and there was a white puppy running down the hill toward me. It came up to me and playfully kissed me.

The event - and the report of the dream - occurred several days after the dream. Since our memories of dreams are poor, it is likely that the event influenced the dream report, especially the details. This, too, is backed up by much scientific research showing that memories of events of all kinds, not just of dreams, are influenced by later events and by the process of describing them. One example comes from research by psychologist Elizabeth Loftus on eyewitness reports (1979). Subjects were shown movies or slides of events. At various times later they were asked to describe what they had seen. They were sure that they saw things they had not. Errorless reports were rare! As few as 25 to 40% of the details were accurate. Even asking them if something was in the movie or slides (when in fact it was not) often led to subjects saying it was present and they were absolutely sure of it. Thus, it may seem like the dream predicted the event, but a better explanation is that the memory of the dream was unintentionally altered in such a way that it resembled the event.

Another psychological dynamic is important here, too. We tend to notice, and think about, and talk about those few dreams that do seem to come true while the thousands of other dreams that did not appear to come true are ignored. Thus, even the occurrences of these seem-to-come-true dreams are in reality rare.

Ann Faraday provides another explanation which she calls "detective work" (Faraday, 1972). Our waking experiences include much more than we can consciously pay attention to. Usually, we attend to the important things. But sometimes we may fail to consciously pay attention to something important such as a weak rung on a ladder. Our unconscious mind is aware of it though, and in dreaming may focus on this ignored but important thing. Thus, we might dream of falling off of a broken ladder. The next time we use the ladder it does indeed break. What might appear at first to be a precognitive dream was really the result of an unconscious perception manifesting itself in our dream. The emphasis here is that the dreaming mind has power not to clairvoyantly predict but to use clues unconsciously perceived when awake as the basis for logical predictions of consequences.

And yet... In spite of the scientific knowledge that is the basis of the above conclusions, we cannot completely deny the possibility that out of body or predictive dreaming can occur. To deny such possibility would be to dogmatically adhere to a mistakenly narrow understanding of science. In fact, science can never prove the non-existence of anything, so we must maintain that such things are possible. However, science can and does assert the likelihood of the existence of things, and in this case the likelihood is small. Thus, until their existence is shown, we should proceed with the assumption that they do not really exist.

What would constitute good evidence of their existence? For out-of-body experiences, I am not sure. However, it is possible, but difficult, to produce and examine evidence for predictive dreams. The dreams would have to be recorded and stored immediately after their occurrence and then correlated with later events. In this way, the event could not influence the dream content. Such an experiment would be difficult because of the sheer volume of dreams and events which would have to be recorded and correlated, but is possible in theory.

What evidence supports the idea that dreams are a reflection of waking life? There is not a lot of scientific evidence, but other kinds of support are overwhelming. Examination of thousands of dream reports by hundreds of investigators almost always has led them to support the idea that people create their own dreams about their own lives and concerns. This impression is overwhelming. It becomes especially strong when modern dream analysis is done. Analysis works too easily and too well for it to be anything else. (See Chapter 8 for three contemporary methods of dream analysis.)

The fourth approach - that dreams are artifacts of brain activity - is based on scientifically gained knowledge. Why is a version of this theory not more widely accepted? Probably because relatively few people are knowledgeable enough about the brain mechanisms that underlie these theories to even understand them. (Count yourself lucky for you are now among those people who do.) It takes time for specialized scientific ideas to become widely accepted.

Perhaps, ultimately, more important are the questions of the validity of these kinds of brain mechanism theories and the question of their incompatibility with the most widely held attitude that dreams are reflections of waking life. Each of these brain mechanism theories is based on some or even quite a lot of knowledge of the workings of the brain and mind. Yet they also contain many assumptions and speculations. So much so that much more research needs to be done with the aim of testing these assumptions and speculations before they can be considered valid enough to displace the idea that dreams are indeed significant. Even so, these theories are not entirely incompatible with dreams as being meaningful as the Hobson-McCarley activation-synthesis model shows (see Chapter 7).

Common Elements of Dreams

What kinds of things do people dream about? Common folklore and Freud's writings leave the impression that dreams are full of sex and violence. But as you found out at the beginning of this chapter, this is not really true. It only appears to be true because people remember and tell others more of these types of dreams than of others. If not always sex and violence, what then do people typically dream about?

Calvin Hall and associates have collected and carefully assessed thousands of dream reports from hundreds of people (Hall, 1953; Hall & VandeCastle, 1966). In 1953, Hall reported on the home dreams of 10,000 ordinary people using a method he developed called "content analysis." He categorized and counted the frequency of the occurrences of events, characters, scenes, and so on. He made no attempt to analyze the meanings of these dreams; he simply tabulated their contents by the characteristics of the dreamer. He then summarized the characteristics of their content noninterpretively with a great deal of precision. This method allowed him to be very objective and quantitative. His work gave a more accurate impression of what people dream about than anything that had preceded it.

For example, he found that younger people remember more dreams than older people, and females more then males. The higher one's IQ., the greater the number of dream reports. Color was reported in 1/3 of the dreams, but more in the dreams of women and young people. The most common emotion was hostility, with 63% of dreamers directing an unfriendly or violent act toward another person. Only 2% of these acts were murder. Two thirds were of apprehension, anger, or sadness. Only 1 of 5 were exciting or happy. Thus, healthy people tend to have "bad" dreams.

In 1966, Hall teamed with Robert VandeCastle to do content analysis of 500 home dreams from one hundred male college students and 500 home dreams from one hundred female college students. Most of these dreams were rather dull and boring, but all were at least somewhat personal. There were great differences between the dream reports of females and males. (In fact, experts can tell if a dreamer is male or female simply by reading the dream report.)

The dreams of the females contained more indoor scenes, while the male's dreams were set out-of-doors more often. The females more often reported the setting of the dream to be familiar and people were in them more frequently. These people tended to be familiar rather than strangers. There was less sexual content in the dreams of females, but when it did occur it was with a familiar person. Females noted clothing more often than men and were more color conscious overall. They also placed greater emphasis on emotionality.

Dreams by males tended to be more action oriented. There was more aggression which was also more physical than that found in the dreams of females, but it was less frequent against an unfamiliar male. Males in male dreams tended to be identified by their vocation and job or males in male dreams tended to be less friendly,but if friendly they tended to be in a protective or helping relationship. Sex was more frequent in male dreams and usually with a stranger as a partner even though, generally, other females appearing in the dreams of males tended to be known.

Are these differences between the dreams of males and females due mainly to biological differences or acquired through the influence of culture? Krammer, Kinney, and Scharf (1983) cite evidence in support of the cultural transmission hypothesis. The differences between the dreams of men and women vary from culture to culture. Within each culture the pattern is consistent with the amount of contact between the sexes and their social experiences. Since the role of women in our culture has changed since the original Hall and VandeCastle studies, Krammer and associates reasoned that there should be parallel changes in the differences between the dreams of men and women. The results were in support of this reasoning when examining the REM awakening dreams of 11 males and 11 females. They found some traditional differences to have changed. Things previously different but now equal include 1) the percent of dream recall (about 72%), 2) the dreams of misfortune (about 10%), 3) the amount of social interactions (close to 50%), and 4) the level of aggression (12%).

Other changes from past studies included 1) more interactions with single males in the dreams of males (which the authors interpreted as reflecting more openness with regard to homosexuality in our culture), and 2) more thinking in the dreams of females. Finally, other differences were still present, but the degree of difference had changed:

1) women's dreams are still more intense;

2) men's dreams still contain more;

   a) strangers;

   b) sounds;

   c) lack of color;

d) references to old age;

e) fullness;

f) large sizes;

g) crookedness.

Other surveys have shown some themes to be very prevalent among college students. Some of these are presented in Table 5-1.

Table 5-1 Percentage of College Students Who Have Experienced the Following Dream Themes:

	Percent
1. Falling	83
2. Being attached or pursued	77
3. Trying repeatedly to do something	71
4. Schools, teachers, studying	71
5. Sexual experiences	66
6. Arriving too late	
7. Eating	62
8. Being frozen with fright	58
9. A loved person dying	57
10. Being locked up	56
11. Finding money	56
12. Swimming	51
13. Snakes	49
14. Being inappropriately dressed	46
15. Being smothered, unable to breathe	44
16. Being nude	43
17. Fire	41
18. Failing an examination	39
19. Seeing oneself dead	33
20. Killing someone	26

(From R.M. Giffith, O. Miyago, & A. Tago, 1958. The universality of typical dreams: Japanese vs. Americans. *American Anthropoligist, 60,* 1173-1179.)

Things that Change Dreams

Dream themes do not remain stationary. They often reflect changes in the dreamer's physiology and emotional states. (This is good evidence that dreams are meaningful and not just random, meaningless activity). Examples of this include how dream content varies with culture, can be modified by suggestion, and changes during therapy (Hunt, 1989). Also, survivors of sexual abuse have more frequent and more intense nightmares (Penn, Wood, & Bootzin, 1991). Research examples include stimuli (stressful movies, hard IQ tests, events discussed in psychotherapy (Koulack, 1991)). (While reading Koulack's book, I took a mid-afternoon nap and dreamed about reading accounts of experiments involving influencing the content of dreams!)

Pregnancy

One of the best examples of how emotion and physiology change dreams is the changes that occur in dreams during a women's first pregnancy (Maybruck, 1986; Stukane, 1985). Pregnancy involves both changes in physiology and psychological/emotional state - either or both of which may greatly change the content of dreams.

Early in pregnancy (sometimes even before the woman knows she is pregnant) her dreams turn introspective. She dreams much more about what is happening to her than before. Certain things are typically dreamed about that subtly relate to the pregnancy. Dreams of fertility and the ability to reproduce, dreams of small animals (thought to represent the small fetus), and dreams of miscarriage (stemming from the fear of having a miscarriage). In some dreams, the fetus may be depicted as dangerous or intrusive.

Some of these dreams may reflect the woman's ambivalency about being pregnant. On one hand, she may have positive feelings about creating a human being and of having a baby of her own to care for. Yet, this same event probably also means significant changes in her body for the next several months and changes in her lifestyle for several or more years. Is she ready for such changes? Does she really want them? Is this the wrong time? All of these things, plus many others, seem to manifest themselves in her dreams early in pregnancy.

By the second trimester, many pregnant women begin to judge themselves and their significant others and, at the same time, the subtly of the dreams disappears. One common theme is whether she will be an adequate mother. She dreams of being a bad mother and of all sorts of things that can go wrong. These reflect common, mixed emotions about readiness for parenthood.

She also focuses on her relationships with others. Dreams of her relationship with the father of the baby (whether her husband or not) occur especially if there is a problem in the relationship. Dreams of her relationship with her own mother and comparisons between herself and her mother are also frequently reported.

Other dreams focus on the pregnancy itself. Dreams of babies replace dreams of small animals. In not a few of these dreams the baby is abnormal (reflecting a concern that probably all mothers have about having a "normal" baby). The baby-as-intruder type dreams may also continue from the first trimester.

By the end of the second trimester, many women report dreams containing more appealing fetal symbols. But they report dreaming about also a wide range of disasters in various settings depicting unresolved issues such as labor and delivery, careers, money concerns, and marital relationships.

During the third trimester, women report remembering more - often many more - dreams. Sleep is more disturbed during this trimester (see chapter 4) and lighter sleep with more wake-ups causes more dreams to be remembered (see earlier in this chapter). In the dreams themselves, some earlier issues continue, but new ones also emerge.

The woman may continue to dream about her relationship with and comparison to her own mother. Also continuing may be dreams of abnormal or unusual babies.

New themes emerge that focus on herself. Especially prevalent are dreams about the now obvious change in her own body. But she may also dream about being the very special focus of attention by others.

Toward the end of pregnancy,dreams of the birthing process emerge. Dreams of what labor is like are often reported. In one experiment, women who reported several dreams of labor - usually difficult and/or long labor - actually subsequently had an easier or shorter labor in reality. Additionally, many women report dreams about their OB-GYN at this time.

These are typical dream themes reported by women during their first pregnancy. Subsequent pregnancies bring some changes in themes. Especially notable are concerns about adequacy of being a mother and her relationship with her own mother being replaced by concerns of how the new child will relate to the others in the family and even her own ongoing relationship with her existing children.

The dreams of expectant fathers are also different from non-expectant males (Siegel, 1983; Stukane, 1985). Unlike the dreams of pregnant women which may be either caused by physiological or psychological changes or a combination of both, these differences in the expectant fathers must be psychological.

Early in the pregnancy, the expectant father has dreams that center on sex and nurturance versus machismo. Much concern with sexual identity and masculinity emerge in the dramatic increase of dreams with overt sex in them. Yet, the newly expectant male also has dreams of being very nurturant and caretaking. At the same time, he also may have dreams of macho roles and behavior as if in reaction to his feelings and thoughts of nurturance.

By the second trimester, the dreams of nurturance continue, but the dreams of sex are replaced by an increase in dreams about his identity. He dreams about his comparison to his father and his childhood family. His dreams reflect his concerns about his role in the pregnancy process, specifically about being left out! Sometimes he may dream about being pregnant himself. He may also dream about his relationship with his wife.

During the third trimester, the dreams of the expectant father are less about his childhood family and more about his current family, especially his wife. Dreams occur about her body, what the child will be like (a high percent are dreams about sons), and, as the due date approaches, the birthing process.

Comparison of the dreams of expectant women and men is interesting. Early on both are focusing internally on themselves and the changes the pregnancy implies for them. By the end of pregnancy the dreams of both the mothers and the fathers are more oriented toward the baby, the process of birth, and each other.

Menstrual cycle

Pregnancy is not the only psychobiological factor that has been shown to have an effect on dream content. It may be affected by a woman's menstrual cycle (Carskadon, 1993; Cartwright, 1977; VandeCastle, 1971), with more friendliness toward other characters and more awareness of uterine functioning during menstruation, but more friendliness between the dreamer and males during the preovulatory phase, and heightened narcissism after ovulation. Yet, even these factors were shown to be influenced by the personality of the dreamer. For example, girls who desired to be a housewife reported more friendly interactions with males and with familiar characters in general. Girls from one parent homes reported dreams with fewer familiar settings, fewer familiar characters, more aggressiveness directed toward them from others, and more adversity.

Major life changes

Divorce

Rosalind Cartwright and associates (Cartwright & Lamberg, 1992; Cartwright, Lloyd, Knight, & Trenholme, 1984) have studied dream changes in 200 recently divorced men and women. Divorce typically generates much stress and it may be accompanied by depression. For example, in a study by Trenholme, et al (1984), 19 women going through divorce or separation and nine nondepressed married women who had never considered divorce were studied. The stably married women dreamt of the laboratory and experiment during the study, while the other group of women had dreams with themes involving threat. Those divorcing women who were also depressed had fewer positive motives in their dreams than the women who were coping well with their divorce. The dreams of all those seeking divorce contained more harm-avoidance,while the stable, married women had more affiliation motives. The dreams of happily married people typically have many themes throughout one night; in contrast,divorcing but not depressed women had dreams resembling the patterns of people who are under stress.

The dreams of the divorcing and depressed women seem to be stuck in the rut of a past event (Lamburg, 1988),and are reflections of low self-esteem, feelings of failure, and fears of the future. Furthermore, their dreams are in chaos instead of being a sequence of images that tellsa story. There is no clear focus to them. The dreams were only of the past,with little present or future focus to them. Divorced women never dreamed of themselves as wives. As the depression abated,the mood of the dreams became less negative, and they began to dream of being separated or about being ex-wives and began to dream of the future.

Depression in divorcing women is expressed in dreams as having more anxiety and threat directed at themselves rather than at others. There are often feelings of inadequacy that are attributed to themselves and not to others. Motives in their dreams are more negative and tend to dominate the end of the night, which probably accounts for why these are most easily remembered in the subjects.

In addition to dreaming, the sleep of depressed, divorced women also differs in another way - REM latency. REM latency is shorter in women who get depressed after they have divorced and they have more REM-type dreams filled with strong emotions. Interestingly, it is these women who show a moderately good adjustment one year after the divorce, although not as good as women who divorce but are not depressed. Those divorced women who show normal REM latency and are depressed have fewer REM-type dreams and have poorer adjustment one year later. Therefore, according to Cartwright and associates (Cartwright et al, 1991), a short REM latency may not be a sleep "abnormality" and may be used as an indicator of which divorced, depressed women will have a shorter course of depression.

Cartwright has taken the negativity of the dreams of divorcing women and has used it to help her patients with their depression. She believes that dreams "mirror emotional problems, and that 'bad' dreams can be turned around to a positive outcome" (Cartwright, 1989). Cartwright uses "dream reshaping" to help depressed women. This is similar to lucid dreaming, but with specific emphasis for her patients to take control of their dreams and, in essence, their lives (Lyon, 1990). So, by using their dreams, these depressed women can work through the negative feelings and come to terms with their divorce and start sleeping and dreaming better.

Age

The age of the dreamer also has an effect on dreaming and the content of dreams (Cartwright, 1978); of adult men and women, ages 17 to 70 years, the group who had the greatest quantity of dreaming were people in their college years. It was found that as we age, dreaming and interest in dreams decline. Also, visual imagery (Fein et al., 1981) and bizarreness of REM dreams decline with age. Thus, upon awakening, dreams may be less memorable. Dream themes that relate to family decline with age and that there are slight decreases in dream aggression with age.

The dreams of children differ from those of adults in many interesting ways. As with adults, however, different insights about dreaming are gained when working with home dreams versus those gathered in the lab during REM wake-ups. Both kinds of studies agree that the length of dreams increases as the child gets older and that animals are more prevalent in the dreams of children than adults.

In other ways, lab versus home dream reports by children provide divergent information. First, let us examine the spontaneously recalled dreams of children sleeping in their own beds at home. As with adults, boys report less about clothing but more about various kinds of implements. Girls dreams also tend to be longer and contain more people. The adult pattern of an equal number of males and females occurs in the dreams of females, but the two times as many male characters in the dreams of males does not appear until sometime between 6 to 9 years of age. Common characters that appear in children's dreams are family members, known persons, strangers acting like other people, and animals. The settings that were most common were the home and recreation areas. The dreams were relatively realistic without fantastic characters and bizarre activities.

The percent of home dreams containing physical aggression is higher in children than in adults, and much of this aggression is directed toward the dreamer. Apprehension is the most common emotion in the dreams of children and is about twice as frequent as it is in the dreams of adults.

The high frequency of animals in the dreams of children is a fascinating and interesting phenomenon. As Figure 5-2 indicates, over 60% of the dreams of four year olds contain animal characters, but this percentage drops with age reaching a steady level of only 7.5% by age eighteen. Dogs and horses are the most frequent animal characters in the home dreams of children and adults, but children's dreams also are populated with more frightening animals such as spiders, lions, tigers, and alligators. Such creatures constitute over one fourth of the animals in children's dreams but less than 10% of the animals in the dreams of adults. The dreams of males contain fewer mammals than the dreams of females.

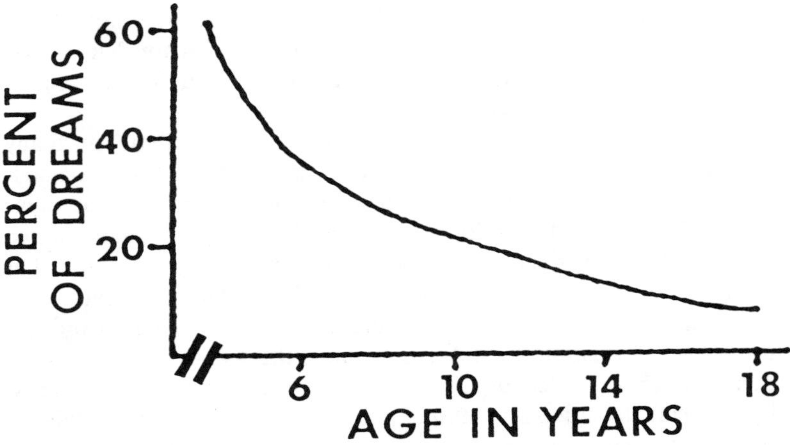

Figure 5-2. The percent of the dreams of children that contain animals (after Foulkes, 1982).

Why is there an emphasis on animals in the home dreams of younger children? Carl Jung would say they are archetypes - universal themes present in the minds of each and every human being (see Chapter 7). He also would state that the reduction of animals that occurs with age recapitulates the evolutionary development of human beings with the archetypes sinking deeper and deeper into the unconsciousness. To Freud, dreams about animals are the inherited remains of primitive "Totemistic Thought" of human ancestors.

Robert L. VandeCastle (1971) tested these notions by comparing the home dreams of children in our culture to those of adults in contemporary but primitive cultures. He found striking parallels. One fourth to one half of the dreams of primitive people contain dreams of animals and, like children, the dreams of such people show a fusion of waking and dreaming realities. In another study, he compared the dreams of adults in our culture that contained animals with those of children. The more animals (and the fewer humans) there were in the dream the more the dream, contained other aspects characteristic of children's dreams. They were shorter, and the dreamer was more often the victim of physical aggression. All of this together suggests that the dreams of children are more primitive.

More recently, the dreams of children have been studied using REM awakenings in the lab (Foulkes, 1982). Three and four year olds reported dreams on only one-fourth of such awakenings. This increased to two thirds by ages nine and ten and remained at about that level thereafter. At no age was the typical dream frightening, nor was there any evidence of a dominance of primitive impulses or fantasies, nor of complex archetypical, primitive mythical dreams. Rather, just as in adults, these dreams were reflections of the concerns, events, and emphases of the waking life of the dreamer. The major difference was in the cognitive complexity of these dreams. At each age, the dreams show the level of thinking ability of the child that parallels the thinking ability demonstrated by the child when awake. As thinking ability progresses with age, so does the complexity of the dreams. When dreaming, then, children are able to conceptualize their world and their feelings no better nor no differently than when awake.

The dream reports of three to four year olds are typically short - 1 or 2 sentences - and lack much emotion or interaction. The settings are usually unspecified, such as in the dreamer's home, or out-of-doors. Typical characters include the dreamer and their family members, but seldom strangers. Animals are frequent characters in their dreams. These animals tend to be familiar to the dreamer; usually they are domesticated species rather than mythical or exotic. Furthermore, these animals are in human, home-like situations such as in fairy tales or cartoons.

Five and six year olds report dreams that are twice as long as those of three and four year olds. These dreams usually have a story line, although often quite simple, that contains interactions. These stories are more like vignettes that are not totally filled in. Characters most often are nuclear family members and animals. The settings are most often the home or places of recreation. Play activities are most often portrayed and these activities are most often initiated by the dreamer. Overall, the dreamer as a character begins to become more active - a trend that continues into other ages.

Subplots begin to appear in the dreams of seven and eight year olds. The themes are things that are meaningful to the dreamer with an especial emphasis on becoming an adequate adult male or female. These dreams, rather than being primitive, are rather cognitively advanced.

The dreams of the late preadolescent are rather well organized. They are as full of purpose and as real as any dream of an adult.

Differences between males and females are obvious. Other characters more often initiated aggression than did the dreamer, and the overall level of this aggression was higher in the dreams produced by boys. Seldom, however, was the aggression directed toward the dreamer. By this age there are fewer family characters and settings; this is especially true of boys' dreams.

Early adolescence (age 13 to 14) ushers in more complex and more obscure dream metaphors, coupled with less literal content. Whereas action and activities had previously been the almost sole means of carrying out the plot, speech now acquires more of this role. Overall, the dreams of girls are more pleasant than those of boys at this age, yet the dreams of both boys and girls reflect the turbulence of adolescence. Characters approach each other much less on a social basis than before, but such interactions are still more prevalent than hostile approaches. Some of the dreams of this age are without context.

In comparison, the dreams of children gathered at home show some similarities but also some important differences to the dreams collected in the lab. Both show developmental trends in frequency, length, complexity, and high percentage of animal characters at younger ages that diminishes with development. As with adults, the dreams collected in the lab are different in that they appear to be more bland with less primitive, archetypical content. We must, then, again conclude that the dreams from the lab show us more about the process of dreaming, but that the home dreams are more psychologically insightful into the personality and concerns of the individual dreamer.

Dream themes continue to change with age in adults. Generally, the young dream more about morality and guilt, the middle aged about aggression and sexuality, and the elderly about illness and death (Cartwright, 1979).

Creativity in Dreams

Dreams may provide creative solutions to problems (Cartwright, 1977; Broughton, 1982). For most of us, our thinking tends to be very rational while we are awake. But when asleep, our thinking changes to fanciful, and we thus look at things in a different way. Sometimes these fanciful dreams provide clues to solutions to problems of all sorts.

There are several famous examples. Ellias Howe had been trying for years to invent the sewing machine. He was unsuccessful until he had a dream in which he was a captive of an African tribe that gave him 48 hours to perfect the machine. When he failed, they threw spears at him. There were two things that were different about these spears. First, they had a hole just behind the sharp tip. Second, whenever these spears hit the ground, they bounced up again,then dove back into the ground, only to bounce up again, and so on. Upon awakening, he realized what the dream was telling him: move the hole from the dull end (as it is in a hand sewing needle) to the sharp end, then have the needle penetrate the cloth repeatedly without going completely through it. These two clues provided the help he needed to be successful in inventing the sewing machine.

There are some things we should notice in this example. Howe had been working hard on the problem during his waking life. In this case, he had been doing so for a long time. He also had a lot of emotional involvement in the problem and experienced a lot of frustration because of being unable to solve it. All of these elements - being familiar with the problem, having worked on it a lot while awake, and emotional involvement with it - seem to be necessary for dreams to provide creative solutions to problems.

Another example is provided by a dream of James Watt which led to an improved way to make lead shot. He had been involved with making lead shot the old way - a block of lead was cut into pieces and formed into spheres as best as possible. However, this method produced a lot of irregular shot which performed somewhat less than optimally.

In his dream he was caught in a rain storm. But this was no ordinary rain storm for it was raining molten lead! Watt must not have been attuned to his dreams for he did not realize that this dream was offering him the idea for an improved shot-making method. He had the same dream a second time. Again, to no avail. Finally, after another repeat of the dream, he realized what it was telling him. The result led to the development of the shot-tower. This is a tall, narrow structure from which molten lead is splattered down the center. During their fall, the drops of lead assume a spherical shape, cool and harden thus landing as near-perfect lead shot.

Other examples include Kekule's discovery of the benzine ring following a dream of snakes biting their own tails. Also, Bohr has been reported to have had a dream of our sun and its planets during which the sun solidified and the planets crashed on it. This led to his discoveries of atomic theory. (Bohr later denied this, however.)

Creative dreaming is not limited to science. The arts also give us many famous examples of creative dreaming. For example, when Robert Lewis Stevenson was badly in need of money and had been struggling to write a story, he had a dream that led to the idea of his famous, "Dr. Jeckel and Mr. Hyde". "The Rhyme of the Ancient Mariner" by Colleridge was a result of a dream. While writing down another dream, Colleridge was interrupted, and when he was able to return to the task he could not remember the end, thus "The Kubla Kahn" is unfinished. Tartini, the Italian violinist and composer, dreamed that he had sold his soul to the devil and then he handed the devil his violin. Thereupon, the devil played the most enrapturing sonata. Upon awakening, Tartini grabbed his violin and attempted to reproduce the sounds from the dream. Although he felt his efforts were much less than what he had heard in his dream, it did result in his best work, "Devil's Sonata".

Dreams may not always provide answers and solutions. And even when they do, the dreamer has to be alert and knowledgeable enough to recognize that the dream is providing solutions. Nor is this type of dreaming a substitute for hard work. In all cases, the dreamer had been working on the problem before the dream and had to do considerable work after it. The dream, however, did provide the necessary creative elements that led to successful completion of the task.

Nightmares

When discussing dreaming, it is impossible to avoid the topic of nightmares, those frightening intrusions upon our sleeping tranquillity. They actually come in three varieties which can differ greatly from one another (Association of Sleep Disorders Centers, 1979; Hartmann, 1984; Hauri, 1982).

Night Terrors

During the night terror or incubus attack (Kahn, Fisher, & Edwards, 1978; Kryger, Roth, & Dement, 1989; Mahowald &

Ettinger, 1990), the sleeper suddenly is aroused, accompanied by profuse sweating, panting for breath, and heart rapidly pounding. The sense of impending doom pervades their mind, accompanied perhaps by an image of a threatening person or monster. The dreamer may scream and move about and perhaps wet the bed. Agitated and destructive sleep walking may also occur. Attempts to console the dreamer are typically frustrating for they seem confused and disoriented - perhaps not totally awake - and have a dazed, "far away" look on their face. The person may converse, yet not seem completely present. The dreamer may soon fall back asleep (especially if young), but may have another nightmare in 15 to 30 minutes. In the morning they may remember little if anything about the whole thing.

This type of nightmare in many ways is not related to normal dreaming. Rather than occurring during REM, it comes out of SWS which, as we saw in Chapter 1, prevails during the first third of the night. Seventy percent of sleep terrors occur during the first NREM period of the night. Detailed studies have shown that such nightmares tend to occur toward the end of a SWS period. Furthermore, the longer and deeper the preceding SWS, the stronger the intensity of the night terror. It appears that the night terror does not awaken the sleeper and cause the bodily effects, but that a sudden arousal from deep SWS first causes the arousal (the EEG showing alpha waves) and bodily effects, then the mind fabricates the frightening image in response to these bodily changes. All of this is often accompanied by a simultaneous body movement. Heart rate may shoot up from normal or slightly below to over three times normal - possibly the greatest, sudden increase in heart rate achievable in humans. The heart rate decreases in the subsequent 45 to 90 seconds and is essentially normal in 2 to 4 minutes.

The night terror is not really a dream at all. Rather than a long, elaborate sequence of fright, it is a brief, often vague image. While it usually is an elaboration of the sudden changes in the body (specifically, autonomic arousal), it may also involve a return to a waking conflict. This report of Gloria's night terror is typical:

I myself don't remember the dream very well. I only remember waking when it was over and finding my roommate hovering over me with a frightened look on her face. Apparently, I woke her when I yelled "BOMB" and began hunting through my bed sheets. When I awakened, my heart was pounding and I was breathing fast and hard; I felt panicky like something awful was about to happen and I had to do something about it, but I couldn't. I don't remember much more other than I was about as scared as I have ever been.

Other typical sensations of night terrors include (Broughton, 1968):

-being crushed
-being struck by a sudden force
-things closing in
-being trapped in a small area
-being left alone or abandoned
-choking on or swallowing something

Night terrors tend to be more frequent in those susceptible to them during periods of stress and fatigue. In some sufferers, night terrors can be elicited by sounding a buzzer during SWS sleep. They are also more prevalent in males than in females. (For more on night terrors see Chapter 9).

REM Nightmares

Strong, intense REM dreams are the second type of nightmare. These are called, appropriately enough, REM anxiety dreams or true nightmares. Because they occur during REM, especially toward the end of a long REM period, they are more prevalent later in the night. The frightening content has a gradual build up during a sequence of images and events, There may be various stages of intensity. The dreamer has both immediate and morning recall of its long and detailed content. Less bodily (autonomic) arousal accompanies this kind of nightmare. Perhaps some increase in heart rate and breathing occurs prior to arousal, but it is gradual and slight and occurs only if the dream was especially frightening. However, increase in REM phasic activity is common. Overall, the dreamer displays less panic. Leslie's nightmare is a good example of this type.

The setting is my hometown. Daytime. I am in the passenger seat of my best friend's car. Jeannie, 21, is driving. Kathy (another good friend), 22, is in the back seat. We were driving to the apartments in town. There had been a big snow storm the previous evening. We had heard that the three-story apartments were covered completely with snow. We went to see them.

All scenery was vivid and colorful. I knew the area well. We were in the back parking lot looking at the snow in amazement.

We were about to leave; backing up we got stuck in the snow. I told Jeannie if she backed straight up into the elementary school parking lot we would miss the snow drifts. As she was backing up, she was turning the wheel. We were heading toward the cliff at the side of the parking lot. I told her to straighten the wheel or else we would go over the cliff. She didn't listen to me. I began screaming at her. Kathy didn't say anything.

There wasn't any snow in that parking lot. I couldn't see any anywhere. We went over the cliff. I was screaming and crying. I could feel the branches from the trees whipping my face as the window was open. I was praying to God as we were descending. We were going extremely fast. I saw a lot of blurred images like trees, bushes, mud, and rocks.

I woke up before crashing. I was crying and frightened. I remember everything in the dream perfectly.

Typically, the dreamer responds to the threat in the dream with a sudden movement - both in the dream and in reality. This movement is followed by the awakening and may even cause it.

REM anxiety dreams occur in all types of people and at all ages. They tend to be more frequent during times of emotional distress. Some people seem to be more susceptible than others to them. Severe, chronic sufferers are often treated with psychotherapy.

Posttraumatic Stress Disorder

Posttraumatic Stress Disorder (PTSD) usually follows a severe trauma such as combat experience, natural disasters (flood, earthquakes), rape, torture, being a prisoner of war, or being detained in a concentration camp. PTSD in Vietnam combat veterans has been studied intensively. Their disorder is often characterized by the reexperiencing of a traumatic event in the form of repetitive dreams, recurrent, intrusive daytime recollections, and dissociative flashback episodes (DSM-III R). PTSD nightmares are likely to occur in REM and Stage 2 sleep, but they may occur in other stages of sleep as well (Delaney, 1991). There are two forms of PTSD according to time course. The first is acute, that is, coming on right after the trauma, and the second is delayed, which comes on some six months or more after the trauma. It is possible that the sleep and dream patterns may be different in these two conditions, but it is likely that these disturbances are central to both the acute and delayed PTSD, so they will be discussed together.

There are two symptoms of PTSD that are reported more than any other: 1.) recurrent dreams and/or nightmares related to the trauma and 2.) sleep disturbances or abnormalities. Frequent nightmares have been reported in 68% of recent Vietnam combat veterans with 59% having one or more nightmares per month (Ross, Ball, Sullivan, & Caroff, 1989). PTSD veterans usually report awakening after a dream which involves the reliving of the trauma. They also experience strong emotions that are appropriate reactions to the original traumatic event such as rage, intense fear, or grief. Many of their dreams contained elements of death, dying, or a threat to self, accompanied by anxiety or fear. For the most part, the actual traumatic event is replayed over and over again in the dream. Only half of the PTSD subjects dreams were about Vietnam and the other half were related to other aspects of their lives (Kramer, 1990). This showed that they were not exclusively dreaming about their Vietnam experience, even though in their waking state they felt that to be the case.

The second symptom that was reported in dream-disturbed Vietnam combat veterans with PTSD was clear disturbances in sleep. They often showed decreased slow wave sleep, an increased wake time, decreased REM percentage, and delayed REM onset (Kramer & Kinney, 1988). Subjects with PTSD slept more poorly and arouse spontaneously in NREM sleep (across the night) more often than the control subjects who did not have PTSD. Sleep of PTSD subjects was more easily disrupted by random noise that would lead to an awakening; however, upon awakening, they were unaware of the source of the noise. This would leave them experiencing the awakening as frightening. The delayed REM onset might possibly be explained as a coping strategy to avoid the reexperiencing in the dream (Kramer & Kinney, 1988).

Treatment for all kinds of nightmares is covered in Chapter 9.

Sequence of Dreams Through the Night

Another way to see the significance of dreams is to examine their sequence through a night. This can be done by awakening a dreamer in the midst of each REM period during a single night. Rosalind Cartwright (1977) has done this many times with many different dreamers and has determined that the dreams of a night are related to one another. Each has meaning by itself, yet the series forms an interrelated whole. (A recent experiment done in Europe using very different analysis techniques resulted in evidence consistent with this hypothesis [Cipolli, Baroncini, Fagioli, Fumai, & Salzarulo, 1987].)

The first dream introduces and reviews the themes. These themes reflect the dreamer's responses to waking life, especially on an emotional level. The dreams of the next two REM periods relate the theme to the dreamer's remembered past. The dreamer uses memories that have a similar emotional theme or tone. As this series progresses, the theme becomes clearer and clearer. The final two REM periods produce dreams that blend early and recent memories and may also project the theme into the future. These are not attempts to predict the future, but rather possible outcomes or even impossible outcomes that, nevertheless, help relieve the emotional tension that initiates the dream series. In these projected outcomes, the dreamer explores their hopes and fears, which is usually beneficial emotionally. However, if the theme is very threatening, the last REM periods may contain dreams that come to the defense of the self.

It is interesting in this regard to think that the dreams that are spontaneously recalled at home most often tend to be the last ones of the night. This is a bit like reading the last chapter of a novel and trying to understand what the entire book is about.

In her book *Night Life: Exploration In Dreaming* (1977), Cartwright gives a thorough example of one such sequence of dreams through the night. Jerry, a medical student, had a first dream that was short and without a developed plot. He dreamt of the electrode leads and how they plugged in. He kept unplugging them and then trying to plug them in again correctly, but never seemed to feel that he got them quite right.

During his second REM period, he dreamt he was driving to the lab with another subject. There was some confusion about who had to stop for a stop sign - their car or the other one in the intersection.

Eventually, the other car stopped, and Jerry's car proceeded through the intersection.

The third REM period dream was about Jerry returning a book to the library (a condensation of the Chicago Public Library, The University of Illinois Library, and Cook County Hospital, which were all aspects of educational institutions in his life). All was going well until he was not able to determine where to put the book, which made him agitated. He eventually left it somewhere (although he was not sure where or how), yet still he remained in the library.

REM period four seemed to produce a dream that took him back to his childhood. He was making mud pies on a beautiful, warm summer day. He described the procedure for making the pies and what they were like in some detail. He was successful, for the pies turned out quite nice. Some girl (stranger) was helping him, but he was definitely in charge.

Finally, in the dream of REM period five, he was again young (about 4 years old), and his mother was giving him a bath while he sat on a tall stool. She was washing his ear with a white wash cloth, tugging at the ear lobe in order to get the inside clean. It did not seem to be a pleasant experience.

The overall theme of this series of dreams appears to be anxiety about his self-competence. This is the theme declared in the first dream - wanting to get the plugs in correctly but being unable to do so and feeling frustration and anxiety about it. The next two dreams directly carry on this theme in vignettes from his recent past - driving to the lab but not being sure who has the right-of-way at an intersection and trying to return a book to the library but not being confident about where to put it. Dream four appears to be complimentary. He goes back to a much earlier time in his life during which things were simpler, he was in charge and able to easily and successfully complete the job, and all was happy and bright. Dream five shows us that he both rejects the return to the past as the solution and has the awareness that even then he was often dominated by someone in authority who showed him how incompetent he was in taking care of himself. These final dreams seem to tell him that neither going back to a simpler life nor relying on external authorities is a completely satisfactory future solution to this basic problem.

This pattern of dreams through the night holds for dreams during sleep when the presleep affect level (amount of stress or upset) is moderate (Cartwright, 1979). If affect level is low (everything is going well, but not so well as to excite you) then the dreams are not ordered and may have many themes. However, if the affect is high (a really bad or really good day) then a single theme may be repeated throughout the night (and possibly successive nights) with little resolution, if the stress-producing events are not being coped with adequately during waking hours. Another variation occurs in depressed people; the sequence does not end up in the present or future, but instead stays with the past events.

Conclusion

The discovery of the phenomena of dreams leads to speculative insights about the function of dreaming. Surely something so complex and so related to the dreamer's personal life must have important functions. Yet, these functions are not so obvious as to bring unanimous agreement about them. We will explore this issue further in Chapter 11.

Chapter 7

Theories of Dreaming

(with Elaine Hoversten and Connie Foxworthy)

Our current understanding of dreams, their meaning, and how to analyze them are all intertwined. In this chapter we will review several theories that exemplify this. Each theory was chosen because it has been historically important in introducing new ideas about the nature of dreams and about dream analysis or because it has significantly modified old theories. These theories were selected from among many possibilities in order to demonstrate the wide range of such theories. It is not possible to do an adequate job of completely and adequately presenting any one of these theories in one short chapter. What follows is an introduction to these theories that attempts to emphasize their important aspects, especially the things that make each distinctive and important. The reader is directed to the references for each of the theories from which deeper and more complete understanding and appreciation of them can be gained.

A major change in the attitude and approach to dreams began with the work of Sigmund Freud, so we will first explore his theories and methods. Freud popularized a whole new way of thinking about how the mind works, with particular emphasis on the role of dreams. Prior to Freud, most people tended to view dreams as coming from a source external to themselves (see Chapter 6). (However, many scientists prior to Freud saw them as meaningless products of the sleeping brain.) Freud changed this popular notion for people in the Western world to dreams as being meaningful creations of the dreamer's mind. From this basic notion, Freud developed many new ideas, including those that became his theory of dreams.

After Freud, numerous others accepted these new ideas but were critical of some, or even many, of the working details of his theories. Carl Jung's theory, while not the first modification of Freud, has become the most popular and influential. Calvin Hall approached dreams and their analysis as a scientific psychologist rather than as a therapist, and thus offered new and important insights. More recently, several brain scientists (most notably Hobson and McCarley) have offered theories about the source of dreams that take as their starting point a knowledge of how the brain works, but each arrives at different and sometimes unique conclusions. Finally, the theory of Seligman and Yellen combines ideas from both the brain sciences, psychology, and the study of dreams themselves to formulate their theory.

Freud

> *One of the most common types of dream-formation may be described as follows: a train of thoughts has been aroused by the working of the mind in the daytime... During the night this train of thoughts succeeds in finding connections with one of the unconscious tendencies present ever since his childhood in the mind of the dreamer, but ordinarily repressed and excluded from his conscious life. By the borrowed force of this unconscious help, the thoughts, the residue of the day's work, now become active again, and emerge into consciousness in the shape of a dream." (Freud, 1958, p. 265)*

Almost everyone, whether they have taken a psychology course or not, has heard of Sigmund Freud. Freud's theories introduced a new and startling look at human-kind. In our day and age these theories, isolated from the historical context in which Freud wrote, may seem to be bizarre and overly fixated on issues of sexual conflict. Thus, in order to understand this perspective better, we need to begin by taking a brief look at what influenced Freus's theories.

Born in 1856, Freud lived and practiced medicine in Vienna, with its atmosphere of strict Victorian moral codes. (So pervasive were these codes that, for example, tablecloths extended to the floor, hiding the table legs, in order that males not be aroused by the reminder of women's legs!) Living in this Victorian society influenced Freud and his thinking, and it is not surprising to find that it also influenced his theories.

Freud did not study large numbers of average people to derive his theories. Rather, he relied on experience with his troubled patients and his own life events. In 1900, he published his theories in what many regard as his most important work, *Interpretation of Dreams*, which contains many of his own dreams and his own interpretations of them. Freud's theory of dreaming has three basic aspects (Hunt, 1989): 1) why dreaming occurs, 2) how dreams are formed, and 3) a method of dream interpretation.

Because his approach was new and unique, Freud coined many terms for the concepts and techniques that he used. His ideas were the basis for the theories of many others that followed him, and these other theories also adopted much of his terminology. Therefore, as we discuss his theories, we will also emphasize the more important terms that are part of it.

Freud's belief that all behavior, including dreaming, is motivated by powerful inner, and usually unconscious, forces is called **determinism**. The content of dreams is determined by unconscious forces so strong that they may be too disturbing to think about freely when awake. Consider this: a happily married man may unconsciously desire to have an affair with his neighbor. For him, to think about this may indeed be disturbing, so the topic remains on an unconscious level. But it continually exerts pressure for expression. This unconscious desire thus manifests itself in one of the man's dreams as a **wish fulfillment**. But since our married man may recall his dream upon waking from sleep, his mind transforms the dream content so that the dream is a **disguised** version of his true unconscious desire. The undisguised, underlying content Freud called the **latent** (or hidden) **content**; what is remembered upon awakening is the **manifest content**. In the example above, the latent content of desiring to have an affair with his neighbor may result in a dream with a manifest content of the man being a business partner with his neighbor.

Freud considered the transformation from latent to manifest content an important psychological process that he called **dream**

work. The transformation process of dream work acts as an editor to **censor** the disturbing material by covering it up with a disguise. Also, an important part of dream work is **secondary elaboration**. This occurs when thoughts and impulses are transformed into a visual format and a storyline is added through the process of **dramatization.** According to Freud, censorship also occurs upon awakening. When a person recalls their dream, the person tries to capture its essence as best as they can and attempts to discover the meaning of the dream. To illustrate, recall your own experiences of waking up and reviewing your own dreams. Perhaps you dreamed of a casual acquaintance being in your class. But you believe it was your friend and your mind changes the memory of the dream to be consistent with your belief. Now when you recall the dream, it was your friend who was in class.

When recalling a dream, we often can recall some of the events, people, or sights as having recently been a part of our waking experience. Perhaps during the day you saw someone you have not seen for a long time. That night you may dream about her. Or perhaps you ride your bicycle for the first time in months, then dream about a bicycle that night. Freud believed that often the content of our dreams is made up of these and similar occurrences of **day residue**. Events that happen during the day and memories that are called upon during that day often become a part of the dream during the process of secondary elaboration.

Two or more unconscious thoughts often merge together into a single image or event in our dreams. When this occurs, our sleeping brain has gone through the type of dream work called **condensation**. In turn, this means that many single images or events in our manifest dream may be **overdetermined**, that is, determined by the condensation of numerous latent dream thoughts. This can be done because much of the manifest content of dreams is **symbolic**, and a symbol is capable of conveying multiple meanings.

Another term Freud used to describe dream work was **displacement**. This process is a part of censorship. If an unconscious desire, emotion, or thought is too threatening to the dreamer, it is transformed into an insignificant component of the dream. Freud saw many neutral objects and events in his own and his patients' dreams as displaced sexual thoughts or desires. Hence to Freud, a dream of a box and a knife was actually about a vagina and a penis in a disguised form.

Because dreams are protective disguises of unacceptable unconscious/latent thoughts, the dreamers themselves cannot understand them fully without the help of an analyst. Freud developed and used the analytic technique of **free association** to uncover the true meaning of dreams. His patients were instructed to talk freely about whatever came to mind when thinking about their dream or elements of it. Freud then used the association to discover the patient's underlying conflicts. His therapeutic methods relied heavily on the symbolism which the dreaming mind presented (and also on the early childhood experiences his patients professed to have had). After weeks, months, or years of analysis, the conflicts would be worked through in this way and Freud would close the case.

Freudian analysis of dreams is still practiced today, but is not as popular as it once was because of its heavy emphasis on sex and childhood experience. Yet we owe a big debt of gratitude to Freud for opening up dreams to analysis and starting us on the road to understanding what dreams really are.

Jung

Dreams, I maintain, are compensatory to the conscious situation of the moment." (Jung, 1974, p. 38)

Carl Jung was a Swiss psychologist and colleague of Freud. He broke from Freud in 1913 when he realized his dream theories were taking a much different direction than those of his mentor. The following synopsis of Jung's theories is derived from his books *Dreams*, (1974) and *Man and His Symbols*, (1964). Also used was Mahoney's (1966) review of Jung's work, *The Meaning in Dreams and Dreaming: The Jungian Viewpoint*.

To Jung, humans have a built-in mechanism to stay healthy. Dreams are a part of this tendency toward health. They serve as a communicator between the unconscious and conscious in order to establish a "balance" of emotional well-being. This process begins when dreams with a specific meaning arise from our unconscious and attempt to add something to our conscious knowledge. For example, there may be certain events in your conscious life which you are not paying attention or are repressing. But this doesn't mean they cease to exist - they simply enter your unconscious. Here is a specific example: A man walks by a ladder on the side of his house. He does not consciously note that this ladder has a broken rung. But this information is taken in and enters his unconscious without him realizing it. That night he dreams that he falls off of a ladder and breaks his leg. This information was brought out in a dream by his unconscious because his conscious had not taken note of this very important bit of information. In this way, dreams can aid the dreamer in maintaining health, be it physical or emotional health.

In addition to portraying events in our lives, other aspects of ourselves appear in our dreams. What Jung called the **"shadow"** is the dark, repressed aspects of personality that press for recognition. For example, a respectable but overly puritanical young woman might have a sexually uninhibited, wild female motorcycle gang member that often appears in her dreams chasing her and causing her problems. These aspects of the shadow need to be appropriately integrated into the rest of the person, and it is up to the unconscious to insure that they are.

It is through the symbolic images of our dreams that the unconscious reveals these things, rather than through rational thought (more typical of the conscious mind). These symbolic images are not disguises. Rather, they are used by the unconscious to put back the emotional energy that has been stripped away in our every-day life. Our conscious ideas are so barren of emotional energy that we do not really respond to them anymore. We state things as accurately as possible and discard all the excess baggage. The dream language used by the unconscious puts some of that psychic energy back in, so that we are forced to pay attention to it. It uses symbolic images to bring things to our attention strongly enough to make us change our attitude or behavior. It is through this process that dreams make us whole. They tell us about parts of ourselves that we are ignoring, suppressing, or not using. Dreams reveal, not conceal.

Some of these parts of ourselves make up our **personal consciousness**. These are things experienced by the individual, but not at the level of awareness. They may have been forgotten, may not have been intense enough, may have been repressed, and so on. They differ from one person to the next, because each person has unique experiences during life. Dreams enable other aspects of our unconscious to be expressed. Things which have not been a part of our personal conscious occasionally arise from the unconscious. When this happens, the **collective unconscious** is being expressed. The collective unconscious is composed of **archetypes,** which are predispositions or instincts that all people have inherited from primitive humans. They are seen in the similarities of the motives and images in the dreams, fantasies, and myths from the past and present. This is a very important part of Jung's theory. He believes that archetypes serve as a bridge for people to be connected back to nature, because we are too often dehumanized in our scientific society. Archetypes form a link between the ways in which we consciously express our thoughts and a more primitive, more colorful, and more imaginative form of expression.

Examples are the best way to understand what Jung meant by archetypes. Every child is born with a mother archetype which innately makes the child respond to her in a certain way - such as perceiving her as nurturant and by being dependent on her. One archetype already mentioned is the shadow. Two other very common archetypes described by Jung are the **animus** and the **anima**. The animus is the male element in the female unconscious and the anima is the female element in the male unconscious. For example, the anima image is innate in each male child and begins to develop from the mother's effect on her son. The anima may soften his macho character and make him sympathetic, warm, moody, and jealous. A man must come to terms with this part of his inner being in order to be a complete person. A very masculine man may appear to have nothing feminine about him. But underneath, there are very feminine aspects. These are carefully guarded and hidden in order to prevent being described as "feminine." It is because of this attempt to repress as much of this femininity as possible, that the anima accumulates in the collective unconscious and must be brought out through dreams. But just like the personal unconscious, archetypes express themselves in their own language. These symbols in our dreams are strange and difficult for us to understand, so during analysis we need to attempt to translate them back into conscious language that will make it easier for us to interpret the meaning of our dream.

Therefore, Jung believed that the main function of our dreams is to be the message carrier between the conscious and the unconscious. By using symbols, our dreams attempt to do two main things:

1. Bring the mind of our primitive ancestors back into our present conscious, and

2. Alert us to everything that is repressed or neglected or unknown by re-entering that information to our conscious to bring it to our attention.

The role of dreams, to restore our psychological balance, is referred to by Jung as **compensation**. If this balance between the conscious and unconscious does not stay healthy and active, Jung believed that psychological disturbance is very likely. Dreams aim at self healing.

In contrast to Freud, Jung did not believe that the function of dreams is essentially sleep-preservation and wish-fulfillment. He stated that dreams are compensatory to the conscious situation at the moment. They preserve sleep whenever possible, (that is, they function automatically during sleep), but they do break through whenever their function demands it - when the contents of the unconscious are so intense that they must counteract sleep in order to have a compensatory function. This is experienced when, for example, we are awakened from sleep by a nightmare that is trying to tell us something very important.

Although Jung believed that wish-fulfilling dreams did exist, he did not agree with Freud that wish-fulfillment should be the sole criterion for interpreting a dream. He stated:

> *It is certainly true that there are dreams which embody suppressed wishes and fears, but what is there which the dream cannot, on occasion, embody? Dreams may give expression to ineluctable truths, to philosophical pronouncement, illusions, wild fantasies, memories, plans, anticipations, irrational experiences, even telepathic visions, and heaven knows what besides. (Jung, 1933, p 11)*

One of Jung's biggest contributions was the introduction of the possibility of dream interpretation by and for "ordinary people." Rather than focusing on how dreams analysis can help neurotic or emotionally disturbed people, as Freud often did, Jung developed theories and techniques of dream interpretation centered around the non-neurotic or "normal" person. When interpreting dreams, according to Jung, one must remember that a dream is a product of the total psyche. By this he means not just the personal psyche, but everything that has ever been of significance in the life of humanity (through archetypes) - a "psyche of humankind." The analysis and interpretation of dreams gives us insight into the structure of both the personal psyche and the collective psyche.

Amplification is the main technique developed by Jung for use in dream interpretation. This refers to the process of elaboration, or expanding on ideas and images present in dreams in order to make the problems of the dreamer stand out more clearly. Two steps are involved. The first is **personal amplification** - asking the dreamer to explore and describe any and all possible associations (thoughts, feelings, and recollections) that they can make when recalling a dream. Each image is discussed to make possible associations to the dreamer's life. For example, *Boat*: "When I was a kid, I wanted a toy boat for Christmas, but my parents never gave me one." The second step is **objective amplification** or explanation usually by a dream analyst. In this stage of dream interpretation, associations are not at all personal, but rather very collective. They correspond to the symbolic images from the very primitive collective unconscious. For instance, *Boat*: "A means by which you can get there'." These objective associations are also discussed to determine possible explanations for dream images.

As is evident from Jung's technique of amplification, the primary aim of interpreting dreams is to make dream material serve the dreamer. Dreams are diagnostically valuable facts. But in order to interpret a dream correctly and allow it to help a person function, we need thorough knowledge of the conscious situation of the dreamer at that moment. Without this knowledge, it is impossible to interpret a dream correctly. We must know the preceding experiences from the conscious life of the dreamer in order to untangle what the unconscious has composed in the dream. A dream from the unconscious has the ability to add something to our conscious knowledge and if it does not, then it has not been interpreted correctly.

Jung suggested that dream analysis is not really a technique that can be learned and applied according to a certain set of rules. If specific rules are used, the individual psychic personality gets lost. Dream interpretation should come from the dreamer, from what exists in his or her psyche, so that it can serve the dreamer in the best way possible. He advised people to meditate on, or have **"interior dialogue"** with, the characters in the dream. For it is the dreamer who knows his or her dream better than anyone else and, therefore, can interpret it most accurately.

Jung did state, however, that some contributions from a dream interpreter or analyst are necessary to make material clearer to the dreamer. An analyst and dreamer working together with a series of dreams can provide the best interpretation. Dreams in a series can throw light on one another and possibly show progression of ideas or events. In any such situation, a comfortable and unthreatening relationship must exist between the analyst and the dreamer during the interpretation. The intuition, imagination, and intelligence of both the analyst and the dreamer are very important and must be freely shared.

Unlike Freud, Jung believed that the dream interpreter should not use free association with a patient unless absolutely necessary. One should pay more attention to the actual form and content of dreams, rather than using free association to branch off on a new train of ideas. Such associations can be a waste of time in dream interpretation. The dream itself should be its own interpretation. Jung suggested staying as close as possible to the actual dream - only the material that is clearly part of the dream should be used. For example, you should not automatically interpret a huge necktie as having sexual connotations, but rather, question why the unconscious chose a tie to get its message across. The interpreter must also decide if the symbols in a dream are related to purely personal experience, if parts of the dream are actually parts of the dreamer's own personality, or if the dream was derived from the collective unconscious (the instinctive archetypes).

Jung built upon Freud's theories of dreams, expanding and adding to them. To Jung, dreams are based on more than just infantile sex and aggression. We should not endeavor to travel back to the sources of the dream as Freud suggests, but rather endeavor to finish off the revelation process of the dream. Dreams serve as our partner, not our opposer. They exist to reveal inner resources that are necessary to our emotional well-being. They can be very positive and uplifting experiences.

Hall

In short, the images of our dreams are pictures of our conceptions. We study dreams in order to find out what people think during sleep. (Hall, 1966, p. 10)

Calvin Hall was a university professor of Psychology prior to becoming the Director of the Dream Research Institute in Santa Cruz, California. He was the first to apply the scientific method to the study of dreams in order to determine *what* people dream about (see Chapter 6). Subsequently, in 1953, he published *The Meaning of Dreams,* which developed out of both his Freudian and scientific studies of dreams. The following discussion is from a subsequent edition of that book (Hall, 1966).

Hall derived his ideas from the study of thousands of dreams collected from hundreds of normal people - people just like you - not patients or clients. He was the first to do this on any major scale. It is interesting to note that when he finished his scientific study, he concluded that Freud was essentially correct about the nature of dreams. Freud's disturbed patients dreamed in the same way as Hall's normal subjects. For example, Hall's male subjects often revealed the Oedipal complex in their dreams, as did Freud's male patients. The basic nature of dreams, Hall concludes, appears to be the same in all people, regardless of their psychological health. The details of the content and focus may differ between normals and patients, but the basic underlying processes are the same.

Hall saw the dream as "a succession of images, predominantly visual in quality, which are experienced during sleep" (Hall, 1966, pp. 2-3). These images represent the ideas or conceptions of the dreamer that are typically found below the level of consciousness. They are a projective representation of the content of the mind in pictorial form. He even called them hallucinations, since they typically occur in the absence of any immediate real-world stimulus. He did recognize that external, sensory stimuli sometimes generate dream content, but he said that they are neither responsible for the generation of the dream, nor are they typically accurately portrayed. For example, a ringing telephone may become a fire alarm in a dream. These, he said, are akin to waking illusions where a real stimulus is misperceived. Real-world stimuli may become a part of dreams in another way according to Hall. People, things, or events of our recent waking experience may show up later in our dreams. Freud called this daytime residue, although Hall did not use that term. For Hall, dreams are a projective pictorial representation of the present content of a person's mind and an embodiment of a person's thoughts.

Hall felt that people dream only of things that are of personal importance to them but not current events, even catastrophic ones. For example, none of the hundreds of dreams he collected from many US. citizens shortly after the first atomic bomb was dropped on Japan contained any reference to that event. Neither do people dream about other impersonal things. They do not dream about politics or economics. Nor do they dream about sports. They do not even dream very much about business or work. Rather, dreams are very personal - a "letter to oneself" about things that are important to the dreamer.

One thing that dreams do especially is to show what a dreamer really thinks of themself in the absence of the facades maintained by the waking self. Dreams are like a magic mirror that shows what is below the surface of the dreamer. Another thing people dream about is how they see other people and what they feel about them. This is not an objective picture of others. Rather, it is the personal subjective portrayal of others as found in the mind of the dreamer.

The dreamer may have more that one conception of themself and others. Some of these may even be contradictory, since logic is not important in dreaming. For example, the dreamer may conceive of their mother as warm, intelligent, aloof, absentminded, assertive, productive, weak-willed, and disorganized. These various conceptions may all manifest themselves within one dream or some in one dream and others in another dream. The dreamer is perfectly free to say whatever she feels in her dreams. In this regard, Hall pointed out that each aspect of the dreamer's personality is often symbolized by a different character in a dream.

Dreams also show how the dreamer views their world, the space that the dreamer lives in, or how it in some way affects them. This subjective world is never an exact replica of the "real" world, and two different people will certainly have two different views of the same "real" world. Our dreams reveal our subjective world.

Additionally, dreams show our attitudes toward our impulses. When asleep, our mind is is free of external controls and free to think of impulse gratification. We also dream about the ways we would like to satisfy our impulses and what prohibits their satisfaction. The conflict between conscience and impulse is better seen in dreams than anywhere else. For example, does the dreamer see sex as fun or evil? Would he like to have sex with his wife in a variety of exotic ways, or is he attracted to other women? Does she constrain herself sexually because of moral conscience or because of fears of inadequacy? These, or any number of other possibilities, may reveal themselves in dreams.

Nightmares are more extreme examples of this, according to Hall. "The nightmare is the price he [the dreamer] pays for doing something wrong" (Hall, 1966, p. 16). That is, nightmares picture what penalties the dreamer will incur if their conscience is ignored. For example, following yielding to temptation that result in a sexual indiscretion, a person may dream of being horribly maimed. Note here that Hall is saying that it is not the impulse (in our example, the sexual impulse) that triggers the dream, but the person's attitude toward the impulse.

Finally, and most importantly, dreams show the conflicts and problems of the dreamer. Most of the information gained from dreams comes from this source. Hall defined conflicts as the opposing conceptions that are constantly struggling and fighting with one another. In dreams the real, authentic problems surface rather than the delusions and pretensions of waking life.

Hall stated that we never dream about things that are simple, settled, and with which we are truly comfortable. Dreams do not reflect our accomplishments and joys. Quite the contrary. The source of our dreams is "unresolved tension" and life's complexities. For example, a husband does not dream about his wife if all is stable and satisfying between them. But if there is obvious or underlying tension, she may frequently appear in his dreams. Hall means several important things by this. Dreamers create their own dreams out of material present in their mind, focusing especially on material that is below, often deep below, the level of waking consciousness. This material typically has its source in things perceived, but not focused upon, when awake. Since the dreamers create their own dreams, they determine who is in them and what things become a part of them. Furthermore, everything is put into the dream for a purpose and is important. How these things are included and combined is usually very clever. The dream is a very creative product, but it comes out of our unawareness. We do not consciously create our dreams.

Symbols are an important aspect of dreams. Hall believed that they serve the same function in dreams that they do in waking life. He called symbols "pictoral metaphors", and he emphasized that they are intended not to obscure, but to clarify. They express thoughts better and they convey meaning more precisely and economically. Symbols are used in dreams not to hide something, but to express it in the best way possible. They are a form of thinking used especially in dreaming. Symbols are a concise way of presenting complex and hard to understand ideas. They can often make visible, things that are otherwise invisible (such as feelings). Hall suggested that we also might use symbols because they give an esthetic quality to dreams. In waking life, humans use symbols in poetry, figures of speech, slang, advertising, and other kinds of expression. In sleeping life, humans make use of symbols in dreams.

But the presence of symbols in dreams does make it more difficult to assess the meaning in dreams, thus the need for dream analysis or interpretation. Since dreamers are the ones who created the dreams and chose what symbols to use, the dreamers themselves should be an important part of interpretation process. If the dream does not make sense on the face of it (as some do), then the dreamer must work with it and its parts and symbols to get at its meanings. Sometimes it will be obvious to the dreamer what a symbol stands for, so the analyst first should just ask the dreamer what they feel the symbol means. If that does not work, then the analyst should try having the dreamer free associate to the symbol.

Like Freud, Hall believed it is best to free associate while comfortably lying down in a quiet location. Unlike Freud, Hall believed that you need not have a psychologist, psychiatrist, or analyst present to free associate. Anyone who is willing to let go without suppressing or controlling, or trying to edit can free associate. The dreamer can best recognize the accuracy of the symbol interpretation because the true referent is in the dreamer's mind, not in an actual object or activity. "Anyone who can look at a picture and say what it means ought to be able to look at his dream pictures and say what they mean." (Hall, 1966, p. 85). It is not necessary to have elaborate theoretical knowledge, because the meaning of the dream is in the dream itself. Hall advised not to read some theory *into* a dream; rather read the meaning *out* of the dream. The goal of dream interpretation is to convert images into verbal ideas.

Hall believed that you should not work with only a portion of a dream. A dream is "an organic whole" and should be analyzed that way. In fact, he recommended looking at a series of dreams rather than each dream separately. Each dream is like a chapter in a book. While each chapter may contain a lot of information, only by reading the whole book can you understand what the author is saying. Each dream contributes something toward the whole, but is not whole in and of itself. Similarly, Hall felt you should consider the interpretation of one dream only as a hunch until verified by the interpretation of other dreams. If it does not agree with other dreams, then consider it wrong.

In this way, interpreting dreams is like fitting together the pieces of a jigsaw puzzle. Try various combinations of dreams to see how they fit together until a meaningful whole emerges. On occasion you may have what Hall called "spotlight" or "bareface" dreams whose meanings are obvious, and thus need little interpretation. If such a dream is available, use this one first, then work with other, more complex, dreams in the series. Try to take small steps from the simple to the complex. Each dream supplements and complements the others of the series. What is not forthcoming in one dream may be revealed in another.

Hall's dream theory derives from Freud's theory and contains many similarities to it. Things like the basic assumptions about the unconscious nature of dreams and the importance of symbols are the same in both theories. But Hall, like Jung, broadened the scope of Freudian dream interpretation by emphasizing the importance of working with a series of dreams and the personal, contemporary nature of dream content. He also eliminated the need for a trained analyst to interpret dreams, believing instead that each of us is best capable of interpreting our own dreams.

The Brain Scientists

To this point, we have been reviewing dream theories that originate from the phenomenology of dreams and a psychological base. We now turn to three dream theories that use knowledge of brain functioning as their starting point. Because of this biological base, these theories are quite different from those just reviewed. Although they all start with brain functioning, the activation-synthesis model of Hobson and McCarley, an unnamed hypothesis by Crick and Mitchison, and Winson's theory each have their own unique aspects.

Hobson-McCarley

Alan Hobson and Robert McCarley are both employed at the Department of Psychiatry at Harvard Medical School. Hobson is a brain research scientist and McCarley is a psychiatrist. Their "activation-synthesis" model of dreaming (McCarley, 1978; also Hobson, 1989;1991; Hobson and McCarley, 1977; McCarley and

Hobson, 1979; McCarley, 1981; 1989) is a fascinating extension of their reciprocal interaction model for the control of NREM/REM cycling (see Chapter 2).

In that model, Hobson and McCarley describe a functional organization of the brain that is unique to sleep. REM is a result of activation of the "REM-ON" area located in the pontine reticular formation, which in turn causes the phenomena of REM to be produced, including the characteristic EEG, body muscle paralysis, bursts of eye movements, and other "phasic" phenomena. This REM-ON area also cuts off most sensory stimuli from the brain. In other words, in the absence of motor output and sensory input, the brain is virtually isolated during REM.

According to the activation-synthesis model, dreaming is also a result of the activation of the REM-ON system. The REM-ON system excites five systems of your brain in addition to those that produce REM sleep. These are 1) motor (movement control) neurons, 2) areas that produce stereotyped behaviors, 3) memory areas, 4) areas responsible for emotions, and 5) higher portions of sensory systems. Your brain then tries to make sense of the **activation** of these systems using a process called **synthesis**.

Commands are issued by your brain for body movement and behaviors during REM, but no movement actually occurs in response (except for the eyes), because the neurons that carry such information to your muscles (the alpha motor neurons) are prevented from doing so by your REM-ON system. Yet, a copy of the original movement command is sent to higher regions of your brain, just as always. When this movement command arrives at the higher regions of your brain, you may perceive a character in your dream to move or a change in the visual scene.

The parts of the brain that control your emotions or store your memories may also be activated in REM. This may occur either directly by your REM-on system or indirectly via the activation of your motor or sensory systems. In this way, the aspects of your personality become part of your dream. (This important aspect of the activation-synthesis model has frequently been ignored or missed by its critics.)

When the simultaneous **activation** of any or all of these are **synthesized**, you experience your dream. This process of synthesis is no different from what occurs when you are awake. All of us constantly synthesize the available sensory and motor information with our current affective state and then draw upon our memory banks of similar experiences and meanings in order to understand it. When awake, our sensory information is usually very much related to our motor information and seems "normal." For example, when we stroke a furry cat we see and feel our hand moving across the fur at the same time that we sense the muscles of our arm producing the stroking movements. When asleep, the activation of the various components at any time are not so well related, yet the brain synthesizes them into a single entity. The result is often the bizarreness we perceive in our dreams. For instance, the sensory part of our brain may be activated to produce the image of a wall, while the muscle command area of the brain is sending out signals to produce walking, thus we dream of walking through a wall. When awake, our perceptions usually flow smoothly because the sequence of sensory/motor activations follow one another in an orderly fashion. But when asleep, what is activated at one moment may not be related to what is activated next, thus bizarre shifts occur in our dreams. We are in a boat at one instant and in class the next. The difference between dreaming and being awake, then, is not the process of activation and synthesis, but the source of the activation: more external (and sequential) when awake, almost entirely internal (somewhat random) when in REM.

It is important to note that Hobson and McCarley are very careful in how they describe the relationship between the physiology and the psychology of dreaming. They specifically state that the activation-synthesis physiology does not **cause** the dream to be experienced. That is, dreamin,g cannot be reduced to brain cell activity. Rather, they state that the neural activity is paralleled by the experience of the dream or when a dream is experienced there is a correspondent activation of certain brain areas. Neither the physiology nor the psychology is primary to the other; rather they occur simultaneously. This is the same relationship known to occur between the physiology and psychology of our senses. For example, when something touches our body, the frequency of discharge of neurons involved in our sense of touch corresponds to the intensity of touch that we perceive. In another example, when you identify a particular sound, there is a parallel and unique pattern of neuronal impulses in the auditory system of your brain. The psychology in these examples is nothing more than a different conceptualization of the physiology. So too in dreams.

Hobson and McCarley do not maintain that dreams are meaningless. After all, motivational states, memories, emotions, even the movement patterns that are activated in your brain during REM, are products of your experiences and personality. While the synthesis of these elements may be unusual, the elements themselves are not. Furthermore, your personality characteristics determine the meaning placed on a specific stimulus regardless if its source is external (as in waking) or internal (as in dreaming). For example, if you have exaggerated concerns about your personal safety, then your descriptions of your waking and dreaming life will be filled with threats to your physical well being. Thus your dreams may contain information that is relevant to you and revealing about you. Such information can be useful in psychotherapy. But Hobson and McCarley do warn that this should not be carried too far; it does not follow that each aspect of a dream has symbolic meaning.

Crick and Mitchison

Francis Crick (a Nobel Prize winner in microbiology) and Graene Mitchison (Crick's associate) have developed a theory of REM sleep and dreams that relies in part on the activation synthesis hypothesis of Hobson and McCarley (Crick & Mitchison, 1983; 1986). Crick and Mitchison give the activation-synthesis process a function that results in a very startling conclusion: we dream in order to forget! They base this hypothesis on their review of the functional capabilities and the organization of neurons in the cerebral cortex of the nervous system.

The cortex, they surmise, functions as a network of cells that is capable of many different momentary patterns of interconnections. Our memories consist of these various patterns of interconnections. However, when such a system is modeled using computers, it develops unwanted associations which may be either malfunctional or by eventually overload the system. In the brain, such unwanted associations can occur during rapid building (growth) of the system or by learned, but meaningless, random associations of stimuli. One way of compensating for such unwanted associations is to enlarge the storage capacity of the system (brain). Another, more advantageous, way is to keep the capacity of the system (brain) small, but reduce the strength of the unwanted associations by some kind of "unlearning" process.

During REM, the normal inputs and outputs of your cortex are virtually cut off and the brainstem more or less randomly excites some cell associations in the cortex (see the Hobson-McCarley model above). Any associations excited in this way tend to be **reduced** in strength just a bit. Crick and Mitchison speculate that repetition of this process serves to weaken **any** memories, random or meaningful. However, since spurious associations tend to be weaker, initially, than legitimate memories, they are weakened more severely, leaving the legitimate memories clearer. Furthermore, it is the recently created associative nets and that are most likely to be excited in this way, and thus are most vulnerable to the weakening process. Dreams are the awareness of the mixture of whatever is activated by this process. Since the activation is more or less random, dreams have a bizarre quality.

This theory leads to an explanation and an unusual implication. Recurrent dreams, according to this theory, occur because certain things tend to awaken sleepers, such as their name being called or certain meaningful content of the dream. The awakened sleeper then attends to the content of the dream, which reinstalls it in memory (i.e., strengthen the associations that underlie it). This strengthened memory is more likely to be activated again in the future, thus repeating the whole process. Finally, this theory implies that when we remember our dreams we are defeating their function of weakening associations and therefore, any attempts to increase dream remembrance should be avoided!

Winson

Jonathan Winson, a brain scientist at Rochefeller University, has proposed a theory of dreams that comes out of his work on the neuroscience of memory, the Hobson-McCarley hypothesis, and some of what is known about the nature of dreams.

Winson's research, and that of others, shows that an area of the brain called the hippocampus (lying between the thalamus and the cortex - see chapter 2) plays a key role in memory. Without the hippocampus, new learning is not processed into long-term storage (Kalat, 1992). In awake, sub-primate animals, the hippocampus shows a distinct pattern of electrical activity called theta rhythm (very uniform brain waves of 4 to 7 hertz) when the animal is learning something necessary to survival, such as finding food sources or finding safe places to flee to when pursued by a predator. But these same hippocampal theta rhythms also occur during REM sleep. They are triggered by the same brainstem REM-ON mechanisms that Hobson and McCarley say trigger other brain areas (see Chapter 2).

Winson maintains hippocampal theta rhythms reflect the reprocessing or strengthening by the hippocampus of the newly acquired survival-important memories. In other words hippocampal theta during sleep occurs during a kind of off-line memory processing.

Although hippocampal theta rhythms have not been demonstrated in primates, Winson speculates similar processes may also occur in humans. For humans, dreaming during REM may reflect the processing of memories that are important to our psychological survival, especially involving the complex interpersonal relationships and complex personalities of humans. This survival memory processing function has no need to even reach consciousness. We are only consciously aware of the dreams that are occurring as we awaken. Dreams,therefore, have deep psychological importance and meaning that may be the very essence of the unconscious. Winson refers to Cartwright's studies of dreaming in divorcing people (see Chapter 6) as evidence of the psychological importance of dreaming although he states that the topic of the dreams of a particular night are typically not predictable.

For Winson, much of the formulation of the content of our dreams and its bizarre character depends on our personality and complex associations "culled" from our memory. It follows from this that interpretation of dreams requires the dreamer to track the dream's contents to "relevant or similar events" - usually childhood experiences. In sum, to Winson our dreams are biologically relevant because they perform important psychological functions.

A Combined Theory: Seligman and Yellen

The final scientific theory about dreaming is even more psychologically based but also adapts the biologically based Hobson-McCarley model of how dreams are generated.

In 1987, Martin E. P. Seligman and Amy Yellen developed their theory of dreaming. Martin Seligman is an experimental psychologist who has contributed much to our understanding of the process of learning. This theory is a result of an essay written while Seligman was a visiting scholar at the Max-Planck-Institute fur Bilderingsforschung, Berlin, and at a dream seminar at the University of Pennsylvania.

Seligman and Yellen describe a classroom demonstration that serves as a basis for their theory. The instructor crumples a string of sequentially blinking miniature Christmas tree lights into a loose ball. The lights now appear to blink randomly. The instructor then turns on a tape of Beatle's music. Soon most students report that the lights appear to blink in synchrony with the song. When the instructor turns the music off, the randomness of the blinking again becomes apparent to the students. This demonstration shows how a pattern is imposed on something unpatterned. It's irresistible. We cannot help but do it, because our brain does this automatically. So too with dreams.

Seligman and Yellen's main idea is that dreams consist of three elements: (1) sensory (primarily visual) bursts, (2) emotional episodes, and (3) cognitive synthesis. The visual bursts (and to a lessor extent, other sensory bursts) are essentially random during sleep. The emotional episodes are largely random, also, but much longer lasting. Cognitive synthesis puts it all together and forms a pattern which we experience as a dream.

The visual or other sensory bursts are sudden and brief. They are an irregular series of hallucinations that are unrelated to each other or the ongoing dream. They occur during rapid eye movements due to trigger mechanisms in the pons (see Hobson & McCarley's theory presented above) and are coincident with PGO waves. These sensory bursts provide "the skeleton" or "architectural elements" of the dream.

The contents of the sensory bursts are in part determined by various sources. One is daytime residue (see Freud's theory above). Another source is remote residues from memories of prior waking experiences or even memories from prior dreams. Some remote residues may occur frequently enough to trigger recurrent dreams. Sometimes genuine (i.e., not hallucinatory), concurrent sensory inputs (for example, sensations from posture or indigestion) may also be a source of sensory input during dreaming.

The emotional bursts also fluctuate like the sensory bursts, but they are much longer lasting with more gradual onsets and offsets. This is probably due to their hormonal (or similar chemical) source which, by their very nature, change more gradually and are longer lasting than brain activity. Yet, the limbic system of the brain and the autonomic nervous system are also heavily involved with emotions, both when awake and when dreaming. These emotional bursts may be weakly influenced by the other two dream elements, but are primarily randomly generated. That is, some images or products of synthesis may generate some emotion by their very nature (such as images of monsters provoking fear) just as they do when we are awake.

The contents of the emotional episodes may come from various sources. First, current concerns from the recent waking life are an important source. Especially unfinished concerns. Dreams may be useful for resolving these and broadly point to the meaning of the dream. Second, our current physiological state play an important role. This includes things like hunger and thirst, anxiety and tension, and our hormones. Third, old unconscious concerns also influence emotional episodes. Finally, the age of the dreamer is important for there are different emotional concerns at different ages.

These first two elements - visual bursts and emotional episodes - might be likened to the components of a thunderstorm. The rain, like emotions, waxes and wanes in intensity while lightening and thunder, like sensory bursts,occur suddenly, irregularly, and briefly and capture our attention.

The third element, cognitive synthesis, is the brain's attempt to combine the visual bursts and emotional episodes with the ongoing dream by constructing a reasonable plot. This process takes the sensory and emotional elements and weaves them together, adding whatever it takes to make the story as logical and coherent as possible. This process of synthesis is the same one that occurs when we are awake; the difference is the nature of the sensory and emotional elements. When we are awake, the sequence of our sensory perceptions are usually continuously related to one another and are more related to our emotions, rather than being discontinuously random, as in dreams. Still, when awake our brain creates our reality for us out of these perceptions and emotions, but it has to do less "filling in" than it does when we are asleep. This same process explains why we may incorporate real sensory stimuli, such as a ringing phone, into our dream rather than waking up.

The filling-in is primarily visual. However, these created-for-continuity visual images are not as vivid as the visual burst hallucinations. They are, rather, more like closing your eyes and trying to imagine a visual scene compared to actually looking at the scene. The difference in these two visual aspects can be noted in dream reports: visual bursts are vivid and in the center, while integration results in images that are more peripheral, smaller, with fewer details, and which cannot be scanned.

There are limits in how the cognitive synthesis process is to smoothly integrate the elements that compose a dream. Images previously created to fill-in may suddenly be bizzarrely transmogrified (changed or altered in structure, form, or appearance) when new vivid sensory bursts occur in the continuing attempt to generate a consistent story line. Also, only the most recent aspects of the on-going dream are integrated with new sensory bursts and emotional episodes. The result is like a meandering social conversation that twists and turns as the most recent topic leads to the next association and soon people are talking about things far different from what they were discussing just a few minutes ago. This is in distinction to a good lecture where remote, as well as recent, topics are very tightly related even after an hour or more. A good lecture, unlike a social conversation or dream, has a specific goal in mind from the very start.

This theory differs from others in how this third element - cognitive synthesis - has the dreamer playing a more active role in the production of the dream. Also, in this theory the images are not metaphors whose purpose is to convey emotional content.

How do dreams differ from reality? There are three ways according to Seligman and Yellen (1987). First, sensory events are usually sequentially continuous when we are awake. For example, when we watch a baseball game, we see the pitcher wind-up and throw, then the batter swings, next the ball is rocketing toward the left field bleachers, the batter is running the bases, the scoreboard changes the score, and so on. Discontinuities are more common in dreams. The pitcher winds-up, the batter swings, and starts to run, but is now running up an escalator at an airport in a frustrating effort to get to class.

Second, emotions may change rapidly when we are awake as we perceive events. For example, we are calmly watching a TV show when there is a loud bang upstairs. We are immediately tense and afraid with heart racing but calm down quickly when we realize that a friend dropped a big book on the floor. In dreams emotions may become very intense, but they change more gradually and consistently than when we are awake. For example, you become more and more fearful as the car continues out of control down the mountain road.

Third, waking cognitive integration is broad-based with multiple influences, both immediate and remote. It is something like a mosaic view from a distance - many pieces are combined to give coherence. Dream cognitive integration is more sequential, like following a sequence of clues on a treasure hunt. Each clue leads to the next but is less related to earlier clues.

According to this theory, it is in the integration of the dream ,as a result of cognitive synthesis, that the meaning of the dream should be sought. That is in the vaguer, less clear, less central images. This is the part of the dream that most reflects you as an individual. Just as different people see vastly different things in the same ink-blot because of their vastly different personalities and ways of seeing the world, so too will different people create vastly different dreams out of the same visual bursts and emotional episodes. It is this personal uniqueness of the synthesis that is most informative about the meaning of the dream for the individual.

However, Seligman and Yellen maintain that their theory says nothing about the functioning of dreaming. However, they maintain that it does allow for certain possibilities. First, it allows that dreaming gives practice in integration of sensory and emotional inputs to the brain. Second, it allows for CATHEXIS (the attachment of emotional energy upon an object) when pairing visual images with emotional states. Finally, it allows for problem solving by the way images are integrated with one another and with emotions.

Summary

In this chapter we have reviewed several important and representative theories of dreams. Some of these theories are basically psychological in their nature, while other theories are more physiological. Some see dreams as "improvisationist" (the dreamer combines whatever elements of mental activity happen to occur) versus as a "movie" (the dreamer starts with a story and brings in the elements necessary to portray that story) (Seligman & Yellen, 1987). Hobson & McCarley would be an example of improvisationist, while Freud and Jung are examples of movie. Others see dreams either as a compromise between primitive and disruptive tendencies and more advanced mental processes, or as non-language, emotional expressions on the same level as waking mental processes (Hunt, 1989). Examples of the first are Freud and Hobson & McCarley, while an example of the second is Jung. Others insist that we reject subjectivity and study dreams only in the lab (that is the method of prime importance). In contrast are those who place the dream itself first, saying the methods should follow.

Not everyone would agree that dreams are meaningful or even that a chapter such as this one should be written. Many of my colleagues in the Sleep Research Society conclude that since Hobson and McCarley have shown that dreams are a result of random activation of the cortex by the pons, dreams are a meaningless epiphenomenon. Others reach the same conclusion from a psychological perspective (see Hunt's 1989 summary of the ideas of Foulkes) - dreams are the result of the lawful integration of more or less, randomly activated recent and long term memories. Although this results in a structured storyline, there is no communicative intent. Hence, dreams do not mean anything and interpretation of them is meaningless.

Which theory or approach is correct? At this point in time, we do not have enough information to determine the answer, but I believe we can anticipate that some time in the future we will have the requisite information. At the very least, we can at least expect continuing changes in these theories about dreaming.

Each of these dream theories has been criticized. The proponents of one theory have easily found and often vocally proclaimed the weaknesses of the others. It is not necessary to detail the individual criticisms of these theories since, in the end, we would be left with a welter of confusion or with nothing. One criticism valid for them all is the low ratio of facts-to-assumptions. The reason for this low ratio is because either the theories cannot be scientifically tested using present methods or available methods have not been sufficiently applied. We included the theories in this chapter - however imperfect - for two reasons. First, they are all we have at the moment. While not perfect, some, if not all, may contain aspects of the truth about what dreams really are. In the future, more accurate theories will probably adapt the best parts of them, or at least use them as a springboard to even better theories. Second, current approaches to dreams in the scientific laboratory, in the therapists office, in the popular press, and in the minds of modern humans are heavily influenced by these theories. Until something better comes along, they cannot be ignored.

The history of science is full of many "speculative" theories - that is, theories based more on intuition than on hard data. Most of these were not well received by the existing scientific establishment of their time and were ridiculed and called names like "crack-pot." A few, however, have proven to be quite accurate. "The earth is round, not flat" and "the earth revolves around the sun, not the sun around the earth" are two such examples. At the moment, we cannot really tell which of these dream theories, if any, are valid and which are crackpot. Perhaps in time we will know. Until then, we will have to live with a variety of highly speculative theories of dreams.

Compare this situation to the history of our understanding of two issues from physics (Rechtschaffen, 1983). At one time, most humans were comfortable and secure with the notion that the physical world was made up of very solid materials which we could see, touch, and hold. The discovery of sub-atomic physics changed that notion. Still, humans saw matter and energy as interacting but, by nature, very different. Then Einstein discovered the famous equation $E=MC^2$ which forever changed our understanding of the relationship between material and energy.

Perhaps in trying to understand the relationship between dreams and the brain, we are in need of an Einstein to discover an equation showing the relationship between the two. Until such time, we must work with concepts and their distinctions that we don't fully understand.

We can assume that one of these must be correct (Rechtshaffen, 1983):

A. Dreams are the result of physiological processes of the brain;

B. Dreams are the result of mental processes of the mind;

C. Dreams are the result of both mental and physiological processes.

Currently, we cannot disprove either A or B. But that does not mean we should compromise and accept C, since if either A or B is correct, C is incorrect. So we have to live with the possibility that any of the three could be correct. Meanwhile, we recognize that a theory that strongly espouses one or another of these can be useful. Such theories help organize the available knowledge and suggest further research. They also offer opponents of one or another of the possibilities, a clear and focused target for criticism. Both the research and criticisms generated help further our knowledge and perhaps will be the basis from which a future "Sleep-Einstein" will develop an equation that more truly shows the nature of dreams.

Perhaps Cartwright (1989) is pointing us in the right direction. She sees two sources of dream theories - those that start with the dreams as their basic data, as opposed to those that are based on knowledge of the brain. The first group tends to see dreams in response to psychological needs, while the second group tends to see dreams as having little or no meaning. But these are not irreconcilable, dichotomous choices. An emerging way of looking at how the brain works is termed parallel distributed processing. That is, rather than doing linear processing (doing one thing, then another, then another, and so on) the brain/mind processes and stores information through simultaneous interaction of several simple, but interrelated, elements. Our minds are made up of various patterns of such brain activity that help us meet our biological and psychological needs. When we do or do not get these needs met, we experience emotions which are stored in *parallel* in the brain, *distributed* among various patterns in varying degrees of strength. When asleep, emotions resulting from not having a need met when awake stimulate different parts of these patterns, because the brain is functionally organized differently. This results in complex imagery that comes from stored memories and past associations related to meeting similar needs. Some of this was stored visually, others by name, and so on, in different brain locations. Dreams are the product of these parallel and distributed activations.

Chapter 8

Three Modern Methods of Analyzing Dreams

"How can I best make sense of my dreams?" "Who can I ask to tell me what my dreams mean?" These and other similar questions are often asked. In this chapter, we will explore and compare three modern methods for interpreting dreams that are based on what is known about dreaming and that seem to work reasonably well. These are the methods of Ann Faraday, Montague Ullman, and Gayle Delaney.

First, let me describe my biases about dream interpretation. In agreement with all three of these people, I believe that the dreamer is the best person to interpret his or her own dream. You cannot go to somebody (or some book) to do this for you; you have to do it yourself. What others can do for you is to show you how you can do it more easily, better, and more completely. It's similar to learning to play tennis. One way is to do it on your own; you could grab a racquet and a ball, go to a tennis court, and start playing. You could learn tennis this way, and with time, might even become pretty good. But it would be much easier and probably faster if you took lessons from a tennis pro. This is similar to what Faraday, Ullman, and Delaney can do for you. They are your dream professionals, eager to teach you what they know about dream interpretation.

In many ways, all three theories are similar. All are familiar with the theories and methods of their predecessors Freud, Jung, etc. and build on their foundations and borrow freely from their techniques. Yet, unlike the methods of Freud and Jung, none of the methods used by these three are derived from elaborate, well defined theories. Rather, these modern approaches are more pragmatic; they simply do things because they work. It is true that all three have some basic assumptions about what dreams are and what they are for. And, in fact, they share many of those assumptions. Yet, one could not call these assumptions a fully developed theory.

One important assumption about dreams that all three approaches share is that dreams are the creation of the dreamer and are very personal. Each one of us authors, often participates in, and is the sole audience of our dreams. We dream about things emotionally important to us. What we dream about is of importance to us in our present "here and now" existence. Not only the main story line, but also the minor details are personal, current, and significant. For this reason, Ullman, Faraday, and Delaney all agree that the dreamer is the best person to analyze his or her dreams for their meanings.

All three methods agree that our dreams focus on cares and concerns that are of immediate importance to us. They relate to our past only if that past is affecting us now in some way or offers some helpful information. Our dreams are trying to help us in some way. They help us deal with our emotions, our relationships with others, our problems. We often use people and things from our waking experiences of the past day or two when creating our dreams - what Freud called "day residue" - but only if we need to work on something connected with them or use them as a vehicle to deal with something else. For this reason, it is important when doing dream analysis to look at waking events that precede the dream and even at your presleep thoughts.

The three approaches agree that analysis is necessary because dreams consist of visual metaphors and symbols. Such metaphors and symbols can convey much more meaning - especially emotional meaning - than more literal ways of presentation. Each element of a dream may represent multiple, and often complex, things simultaneously. While some symbols may be generally the same for all people, most are unusually created by each individual dreamer. Dream interpretation endeavors to separate out the various meanings of symbols into a logical, verbal form. It is in the means of doing this that the three methods differ.

But, you must be careful not to place so much emphasis on the symbolic elements of the dream that you lose sight of the story line. The sequence of happenings in dreams may also have a great deal of significance.

Yet, you need not be concerned if every aspect of a dream does not make sense. For many dreams - especially the longer ones - total understanding is usually not possible. Be pleased and satisfied with the success you do have - not frustrated with those elements that stubbornly refuse to yield to analysis. If they are important enough, they will manifest themselves in other dreams and perhaps, later, you will discover their meaning. With all three methods, successful interpretation has occurred when some insight has been gained. It may be insight about oneself, a significant other, or anything of importance to you, the dreamer. The dreamer has to feel good about this insight and be able to make use of it in waking life. When this happens, the interpretation is successful.

In addition to symbols and metaphors, our dreams make use of puns and other plays on words. Not only just for the humor but because such word games can also convey much meaning. A good example is Judy's dream.

Following an evening during which she was worrying about a topic for her church youth group, Judy reported remembering a long dream. In part of it she finds a green-silver charm bracelet. Judy examines it more closely and finds a charm with a little hole "where you put money in a little bank for coins, and I looked and next to it was sort of a plastic thing that looked like a church where folding money could go in ... and it said St. Benedictine Monastery on it."

The overall theme of the dream, of which this is a segment, involved security. In this portion, money is represented directly - coins and folding money - and indirectly - the charm bracelet was green-silver, which are the colors of money. The coins (small change) go into a small but (apparently) metal bank - very secure. The paper money (of more value) went into a plastic church (a less secure structure) labeled Benedictine Monastery. Judy attends Saint Benedict's Church and monastery sounds similar to monetary, hence the pun "(Saint) Benedicts Monetary" representing a not so secure place in which many resources have been placed.

It is in the *methods* used to interpret dreams that Faraday, Ullman, and Delaney differ. As might be expected, each of them does it somewhat differently. Ullman's method requires a group of several people. Delaney's method does not but does work best with one person in addition to the dreamer. Faraday's method does not require a group, but works better with one. Ullman's and Faraday's methods are somewhat rigid in procedure - especially the order in which one must do things. Delaney's is much freer.

In my experience, it does not appear that any of the three is right and the others wrong; all three methods work. It is rather like traveling to a destination; you can walk through the woods with a group of friends, bicycle on the backroads with another person, or drive on the highway alone. Each method gets you to the destination but with different experiences along the way. But before we become familiar with these methods of dream analysis, we need to explore how to improve dream recall.

Hints On How To Remember Dreams

Some people may need help in recalling their dreams - or more of them. Research has shown that several factors affect dream recall (Cartwright, 1977; 1978; Faraday, 1972):

1. Presleep intention. Falling asleep with the intention and desire to recall your dreams improves their recall.

2. Rapid awakening. Slow, gradual awakening results in poor recall. On the other hand, a sudden, startled awakening is detrimental, also. Best is awakening as rapidly as possible without startling the mind or body.

3. Light sleepers recall more dreams. There may not be much you can do about this - it is just something that we know occurs.

4. Personality factors influence dream recall. Things such as high anxiety levels and inner orientation seem to help recall (Cartwright, 1977).

5. Length of sleep. Long sleepers recall more dreams than short sleepers. Long sleepers have more REM (see chapter 3) hence more time for vivid dreams and thus have more from which to recall.

6. Cultural and social attitudes. More individual dream recall is reported in those cultures that value dreaming and dream recall.

7. Repression. Freud may have been correct that we sometimes cannot face the reality of some of our dreams and thus repress their memory from conscious recall.

8. Awakening during REM. Little elaborate dream recall occurs when awakening from NREM stages but much more from REM awakenings.

Based on these factors and our knowledge about dreams, the following hints will improve dream recall (Delaney, 1988; Faraday, 1972):

1. Have recording materials handy. Some people have a pad of paper and a pencil at bedside or others prefer a tape recorder. Memory of dreams fades fast. The sooner the dream is permanently recorded, the better. Such preparation also indicates a presleep intention to recall.

2. Record the dream as soon as possible.

3. Quickly review or rehearse the key parts before recording.

4. Do not be overly concerned about getting everything down in correct order. (You can reorder it later.)

5. But do try to record everything including details, no matter how irrelevant. Also, especially note the mood or feelings of the dream.

6. Add any associations that EASILY occur at this time.

7. Note any events of the prior day that may be relevant.

Faraday's Method

First in *Dream Power* (Faraday, 1972) and later in *The Dream Game* (Faraday, 1974), Ann Faraday has described and illustrated her method of dream analysis. She is a British psychologist who became frustrated and disillusioned with the slowness and unsatisfactory results of traditional Freudian analysis. She then moved to Jungian analysis, which she found moved more rapidly but mystified and complicated the dreams when a more simple interpretation seemed to be better. Then, working with a group of others - both professional and non-professional - she began exploring and developing alternatives for dream analysis. By trial and error, the following three-stage method evolved.

The first level is LOOKING OUTWARD; here one simply sees if the dream is telling some facts, relatively undistorted, about the waking world which had not been fully comprehended as important. Another name for this level is OBJECTIVE TRUTH.

The second level is the LOOKING GLASS (the British word for mirror). The dream on this level is viewed as a reflection of the dreamer's conception about life, which may be distorted and very subjective. (The label came from the book *Through The Looking Glass* by C. S. Lewis. When Alice went through the looking glass, some things were much as they were in the ordinary world, but others were "as different as possible"). It can also be called SUBJECTIVE TRUTH.

The third level is LOOKING INWARD. At this level, the dream is seen as providing insight into the dreamer's own character and personality. Another name for it is PERSONAL TRUTH.

The three are to be always used in the same sequence and, even if nothing results in the earlier levels, one should go on to the subsequent ones. The feeling of the entire dream is important at all levels. For example, a heavy, sad feeling from the dream should cause us to look for a different kind of meaning at all three levels, than if the dream had a light, happy feeling.

Looking Outward (Objective Truth)

The method for this initial level is quite simple. Look at each dream in a common sense way to see if it is simply saying something that is in fact true. Do not dig too deeply; if it's not fairly obvious, it's probably not there. Such truths are presented in an open, undisguised way.

The source of such information is subconscious perceptions by the waking mind that were never consciously registered but that are significant and important. The mind subsequently calls our attention to this information by placing it quite straightforwardly in a dream.

There are a variety of types of this level of dreaming that Faraday has discovered. One is the simple reminder dream which is about some specific event which has been forgotten but requires immediate attention. An example might be dreaming about your dentist to remind you of your appointment tomorrow that you made a while back.

Another example that came out of one of my groups is the following dream by a pre-med student. "I was playing racquetball in the racquetball court at Luther College. I was playing all by myself. Rather than hitting a ball, I was hitting a molecule. Every time that it hit the "front" wall the molecule changed. Before I would hit the molecule, I had to yell out the reagent(s) that changed it from the previous molecule." She recognized that the dream was reminding her to learn the reagents for an exam coming up at the end of the week.

Another type is the warning dream in which continuing concerns of your waking life that you are ignoring are made the focus of the dream. The dream goes on to show what may happen if you continue to ignore the situation and thus "gives you a warning." (This is not a prediction of the inevitable, but one logical, possible conclusion to the situation).

In one of my dream groups, a grandmother told of a very frightening dream she had the night before her young grandchildren, whom she had not seen in over a year, were coming from out-of-town to visit for a few days. In the dream, one of the children got some matches out of a low cupboard and began lighting them. This resulted in a fire in which the grandchildren were trapped. The next morning this grandmother went through her house and "childproofed" it by placing all dangerous things such as matches, chemicals, and knives in inaccessible locations.

A similar kind of dream is one in which some "truth" seems to come out in a dream through paranormal clairvoyant means. An example of this happened to one of my students, Rona. She had recently had a couple of dreams about her steady boyfriend. They were dreams "of him with other women in intimate, compromising situations." Although she was sure that they were completely false, she began to make some inquiries and finally confronted him. Eventually, the truth came out - he had started having "one night stands" with other women.

Rather than attributing these to some psychic phenomena, Faraday says they can usually be explained by some antecedent events which logically lead to the dream content.

Looking back on it all, Rona realized that the dreams nearly forced her to become aware of little clues about her boyfriend she had been ignoring in waking life. When she asked where he had been when she had telephoned the day before, he had suddenly become evasive. About the same time he had stopped coming over to her house as much as he used to. And he seemed to be picking fights with her. Once, he slipped and called her by another name.

A similar type of dream is one that seems to predict the future. Such pseudo-precognitive dreams can better be explained by the power of our subconscious mind doing some "detective work" rather than some supernatural powers of the mind.[1] For example, Anna had the following dream episode:

> *The next scene took place with myself, my other older brother, and his wife. We were at a boathouse on a river or swamp. It was very murky water and swamp-like. All I remember is that off and on my brother was in the water and once I was also. When we were leaving the area by boat, we forgot our money on the dock. We had taken our money out of our pockets earlier. When we went back, the money was gone.*
>
> *The next day, I lost my wallet in the locker room after swimming class. When I went back to look for it, it was gone.*

When questioned, she recalled that she recently had almost forgotten her books in the locker room one time and was about to leave another time when she saw her wallet laying on the floor. What her subconscious brain was telling her might happen because of these recent events, actually did then happen.

Another example of an objective truth dream is seeing something about another person which is quite true but about which you were not consciously aware. Again, it is the subconscious mind which perceived the truth about this person and placed it into the dream.

Joe had the following dream about his new roommate of about two weeks. It followed a discussion about some noisy drunk students on

---

[1]In her more recent book, *The Dream Game*, Faraday (1974) states her belief that some ESP may in fact occur in dreams but only when an under dog (see later in this section) of the dreamer is especially threatened by top dog's threats of death or disaster. (In this case, under dog activates his normally unused paranormal abilities.)

their floor during which the roommate stated that he thought drinking was stupid and inconsiderate to other people.

I was in a bank in Minnesota, the bank was not familiar to me, but the town was. It's about 20 miles from my grandma's farm. I don't know what I was doing in there, but then my roommate walked in. He was supposed to be skiing in Wisconsin, but had to come to cash a check. He was so drunk that he could hardly stand up and the manager wanted to throw him out. He protested, saying that he wouldn't drink. I even had a hard time talking to him until we got out of the bank.

Two weeks after this dream, the roommate entered treatment for alcoholism. Something about the roommate's protest about drinking was insincere and Joe's unconscious mind detected this and produced the dream as a result.

Looking Glass (Subjective Truth)

Each of us perceives differently the people and situations that make up our lives. These subjective reactions and perceptions are exemplified in our dreams. Analysis of dreams at this level can tell us something about our current perceptions of reality, as well as something about ourselves, since how we view things partially depends on who we are. We can see this first by just looking at the content of the dream "as is," followed by seeing what associations we have to the details of the dream. This is very similar to the word-association method that Freud used. Let your mind react freely and openly. Say whatever comes to mind, no matter how ridiculous. For certain types of characters or objects, the associations are directed by questions that help get to the meaningful associations more quickly.

People

Intimates. When we dream about people who are currently a close and important part of our lives, they, in all likelihood, represent themselves. We should ask why we are dreaming of these people. Thus guide your associations with the following question: "What does the dream tell me about my present feelings or thoughts about this person?" (Faraday, 1972, p. 190). The meaning often depends on what the character is doing and what is being done to him or her, as well as the general situation. If this fails to produce results, try just associating more freely with the thought of the person.

It is possible that characters in your dreams that are currently an intimate part of your life are symbolic. If a literal interpretation of them makes no sense, then treat them as symbols for someone else entirely (but with similar characteristics) or a part of your own personality. Tom had such a dream.

> *On this night I remember a couple of things. First, I remember seeing some other people trying to climb a steep cliff. My roommate was one of them, but he only had stumps for legs and I remember seeing his artificial wooden legs hanging on a wall. Later I tried to climb up this - 45 degrees - or actually I was pulling myself up. It was a long way up, and [I] was just pulling myself up and over when I woke up. I remember some of the rocks being loose, but I still think I made it, although I didn't think I would.*

Since his roommate did not have wooden legs in real life, this could not have been a literal dream, but rather symbolic. Since by the end of the dream it was Tom who was climbing without using his legs; he quickly realized that his roommate in the dream was a symbol for himself. He came from a lower class environment and none of his family had ever attended college. He felt he had "no legs to stand on" and had to "pull himself up" by a lot of effort but often had doubts if he would "make it."

Intimates from the past. Characters from our dreams may be people we were close to earlier in our lives but with whom we are no longer in close contact. Such characters usually represent parts of ourselves which we have taken from them. Furthermore, some recent event has triggered the reminder of these persons and the parts of us that they represent. When associating to these characters, pay particular attention to the associations that are about the characteristics of the individual. A good example of this can be found in Dave's associations to his dream.

> *Me and my dad (who in reality has been dead for three years) were driving from Northfield, Minnesota to Decorah, Iowa in a van. (The van was one that our family, at one time,*

owned but has since sold. This van often broke down.) In this dream, it broke in a desolate spot of a 4 lane highway. It was a hot, dusty, summer day. We looked up at a house and saw one of my college friends dressed up in an elegant tux. He served us food and drink using silver service and silver cups. He served some kind of pastry things. My dad said, "let's take the food to the median so we will not get hit by traffic - and it's nicer."

Dave's associations to this dream included a vacation that he and his dad had taken when he was 8. They were driving on the same highway at night when they ran out of gas. Dave was scared but his dad was calm and decisive saying, "Let's pop open the hood and wait for help." He then stated that this reminded him of other times when his dad would do nothing to help himself in troublesome situations, but wait for things to get better. Recently, Dave had had a lot of "breakdowns" in the flow of his waking life but was doing nothing about them other than waiting for things to get better or to have solutions (rescues) served up to him on a silver platter, just like his dad always had. Before interpreting this dream, Dave had not realized that he was doing so.

Dreams of our childhood are of this type. They can stem from "voices" from the past that are still alive in us and are influencing us now, and probably in maladaptive ways. Then, too, it might be that something that is occurring now is reminding us of the past.

Friends and colleagues. We may dream about people that are currently a part of our lives but whom we do not consider to be close and intimate. Such characters may be in our dreams for one of several reasons.

First, the dream may simply reflect how we feel about these people. This may be obvious from the dream or may require some associating to the character. Dan's dream fragment is a good example. "All I can remember was my new boss got castrated. It seemed real and unpleasant at the time." Dan admitted that he did not like his new boss because he acted so "macho."

Second, the character may stand for another person in real life, especially if we are no longer in contact with the character in the dream. Something in common between the character out of the past and the person he or she represents caused the choice. Associations about the dream character may both trigger a realization about who is represented and our feelings about the real person.

Susie was an older, single student nurse who had been dating a drummer in a local rock band for several months, and things were beginning to get serious between them. The following is her dream report.

> *This dream seemed pretty real, but there were a lot of things that were vague. I was walking home from school carrying a backpack. I walked into this house which supposedly I lived in, (it wasn't my house in real life) and this guy named Mark was sitting there waiting for me. I've only talked to this guy once in real life, so I really don't even know him. He used to be our neighbor back home before I started college. He wanted me to give him a kiss, but I said I had to brush my teeth first. Then we were just sitting around, talking away, like we'd known each other for years. I remember telling him I really liked him and that I was having fun.*
>
> *The next thing I knew, we were going to a movie. I had never been to this particular theater before, and didn't know what movie was showing. Pretty soon I noticed we had someone else along with us, a little boy about 4 or 5. It ended up that he was Mark's son. The theater was really crowded so we all couldn't sit together. I sat with the little boy and Mark sat somewhere else. After the movie was over, we went somewhere else, although I don't remember where. It seems like it was an apartment or something. Anyway, we were sitting there talking and Mark said he had been married and divorced 3 times. He was laughing and making a big joke out of it. I thought it was pretty funny too. All I remember saying was, "You're a pretty high risk," and that was the end of the dream. I felt pretty confused during the whole dream.*

When associating to Mark in the dream, she realized that he stood for her boyfriend and she was confused about liking him. She admitted that she knew that he was a little unstable and had had troubled relationships with women in the past, but she had been ignoring these things. She concluded that the dream was telling her that "something was off the mark" with her boyfriend. Not long afterward, she broke up with him.

Third, the character may be a part of the dreamer's personality. Again, the results of association to the character may yield insight, but this time about the dreamer's own self.

Finally, the character may be a symbol of something else entirely. That is, neither the actual person characterized in the dream, nor a different person symbolized by the character, nor a part of ourselves. Free, honest, and open association can show us what the character means.

People with whom the dreamer is not personally acquainted. Often the characters in our dreams are public figures, historical characters, or fictional persons. Since dreams are always personally relevant to the dreamer, such characters must be symbolic. They may stand for someone else, something else, or a part of our personality. The key questions with which to guide our associations here are: Why this particular symbolic character rather than another? What aspects of the character make him or her the character of choice in this dream?

Steve had a dream about Tommy Smothers of the Smother's Brothers. Since Steve had never met Tommy Smothers, he must have been symbolic. In the dream, Tommy was lecturing on music with the song "Heat of the Moment" by the group ASIA playing in the background. The only thing Steve remembered that Tommy said was what a "liberal form" of music this was. At this point Steve woke up and the song was actually playing on the radio.

Since the song and the group singing it was an incorporation from an actual stimulus at the time, it was unlikely that there was much symbolism there. However, associations to Tommy Smothers quickly produced the following.

> *Why did your dream mind choose Tommy Smothers?*
>
> *Tommy Smothers . . . that's like my Prof. Tom Caruthers who we jokingly call Tommy. I had him in class today. Tommy is also like Tommy Gun.*
>
> *What about Smothers?*
>
> *Well (chuckles), Prof. Caruthers kind of looks like Tommy Smothers and, I just realized it, he has a machine gun style of lecturing that sometimes smothers us. Just yesterday I was wondering why I didn't want to go to class even though I like it.*

Strangers. We are not always able to clearly identify the characters in our dreams. Yet, they may have some defining characteristics, some distinctions, some uniqueness that may be important in understanding the dream. Freely associate to such characters to discover their symbolic meaning.

Animals and Creatures

Our dreams are not always populated only by people. Other living things often play important roles. These living things may be recognizable domestic, farm, or wild animals, insects, and such. Or they may be creatures unknown or uncommon in the waking world. Whatever they are, consider them as metaphors. Especially interesting and meaningful is when such animals represent people we know. In this case, the dreamer's mind relates some of the animal's characteristics to the person. A dream of this type was related by Len.

> *I was in the dream together with my two younger brothers. We are on my dad's farm and have a white-horned bull to ship away. This must have been 5 to 8 years ago, because the red barn was torn down then. Anyway, my brothers are making mistakes and I yell at them telling them where to go. Finally, we get the bull into the barn when the older of my two brothers grabs it by the tail and is knocked out. I drag him away. My youngest brother then grabs the bull by the horns and is knocked silly and falls flat. I drag him away. Then the bull gets away and we start all over again.*

The weekend before, Len was told by his brothers that they wanted to take over control of the family farm. However, their father does not want to retire. Len, as the oldest brother feels like he is caught between the desires of his brothers and their stubborn father. By now, it was obvious to Len (and to us) that the bull symbolized his father and how he might react to his attempts by his sons to retire him.

Animals and creatures may also be symbolic of situations, principles, or institutions. The associations such animals or creatures produce may help bring out their meaning.

Houses

To me, some of the most fascinating metaphors found in dreams are those using houses and other buildings. In most cases, these buildings are symbolic of ourselves (or a person we know who is associated with the building in real life), our personality, our lifestyle, or our outlook. At other times, such buildings are symbolic of the dreamer's marriage or family relationships. Is the house large or small, simple or complex, dark or sunny, new or old, in good repair or not, and so on? The possibilities are numerous and provide a wealth of information. A common dream involves going back to one's childhood house, perhaps because a current life situation is a reminder of the childhood. Again, it is the associations that provide the meaning here.

There are two examples of house dreams - one was dreamed by Bonnie and the other one by Eveland.

> *I had a child with me, and we were walking around this old "haunted" house where I think "crazy" people lived. We had to find a bathroom for the child, and someone told us to go down these stairs where many rooms were located. As I looked into each room, I half expected to find something very frightening within. Yet, all I discovered were messy rooms with unmade beds. Then someone told me that there was only an outhouse, and I asked if they thought this would be safe to enter. By that, I think I was wondering if something evil would be in the outhouse.*

After spending some time struggling with the meaning of this dream with seemingly little success, Bonnie came to realize that the child was herself and the house was her current struggle to "find out who she was." As a child she was scared of big, dark houses because she was afraid that some creature would jump out of a room and scare her. This dream showed her that she was afraid of what might "jump out" at her as she began to explore unknown aspects of herself. What she discovered was not frightening but minor messes and things begun but not completely finished ("unmade beds"). The reference to "outhouse" she interpreted as needing to also get out side of herself in spite of her fears of the evil that might be out there.

> *My brother moved out of my parents house the other day, to a place he's sharing with two others. My dream deals with this event. I guess I was visiting my brother at his rented house and he was going to show me around. This house was some sort of*

Victorian mansion or something, and it was also located in Mason City for some unknown reason.

When I got to the house, I stopped on the sidewalk to look at it. It was on a knoll, some distance from the sidewalk. It was a dark, dreary day and I guess it was Fall because leaves were blowing all over the yard.

The house was white but looked gray because of chipping paint. It was a tall, long and narrow house, two stories high.

Once inside the house there are only a few things I remembered. The lighting was soft and glowing warmly. I was given a brief tour of the house. At the far end of the house were two huge rooms, one on first floor and one on second floor. He told me these were once used as classrooms for a school. I kind of got the impression that this was a school house and private home combined. Now the classrooms were shut off and that part of the house was without heat or any maintenance. The doors were usually locked, I guess. Next, I was taken up a narrow back staircase to the second floor living quarters.

There in the apartment the only room I was shown was the living room. It was now dark outside and everywhere else, except for a warm glowing light in the living room. I only remember looking at it from one direction, and that was "straight on." Ahead was sort of a low couch (grouping) into a square shape with all kinds of blankets, clothes, etc. thrown onto it in a heap (like you would do on moving day).

I remember telling my brother he should ask my friend in town if he wanted to live with them in the house, also. Then I reflected a minute and thought it wouldn't be such a good idea after all. But the next thing I remember is that my friend was in the house and I was going to show him around like my brother showed me around. At this time, I wasn't aware of anyone else's presence in the house until I asked someone to get something for me, I don't remember what. They had to dig through all the stuff on the couch to find it, but finally did come up with it, whatever it was.

As I was showing my friend around, I remember seeing a large wide staircase which led up to the living room. Apparently everything was taking place upstairs in the living room and the rest of the house was a black void. He wanted to go down the staircase but I told him "no", there is another stairway in the back of the house we will use instead. We went through a cold wooden door and into a cool grayish blue and also light red hallway. There was plaster on the floor and the walls were foggy like. I wanted to show my friend the two classrooms at that end of the house, but it seems like the door to the one on the second floor was locked. We went down the old narrow stairs to the lower floor and the door to this room was open, although it was dark everywhere else, so we didn't have to turn any lights on to see anything. The room was empty except for a few rows of desks, and I distinctly remember that the whole room was surrounded on three sides by windows, sort of like the drawing room in Loyalty Hall here on campus (in the art building). At this time I could also place myself outside the house looking up at the blackness inside those huge rows of windows.

This long dream had a lot of meaning for Eveland, but we won't go into all of it. Mainly, the dream represented her feelings about her brother's present lifestyle. First, the house was large but the living only centered in one area. Otherwise, it was dark and gloomy. The classroom part was especially empty and unheated. Eveland felt this made her realize that she did not totally approve of her brother getting a job and an apartment rather than going on to school. There was much potential in his life, but he was locking himself out from it.

Vehicles

Another fascinating source of information comes from vehicles in dreams. Vehicles may represent themselves, a lifestyle, or the direction of a relationship. They may also represent an institution or instruments of power and energy. It is important to note the type of vehicle, its speed, its direction, and whether the dreamer is the driver, passenger, owner, or whatever. For example, the way the driver controls their car may tell the dreamer how they see impulse control. Associating to these and similar aspects of vehicles in dreams often is very fruitful.

Tony's dream

I'm driving in the Indi. 500 Grand Prix. Someone is next to me. Maybe a coach or my girlfriend. We are on the highway going very fast; I can hardly see anything. We need to stop soon.

Next, we are inside a Casey's General Store for a pit stop. There are lots of people there - other drivers and coaches, etc. There is a lot of mixed talk. Free pop and other things are available. I am in forth place and I knew it. It was some kind of a race. It was crowded - I really did not want to be in there.

Now it is night. Rita (my girlfriend) and Karen (the best friend of one of Rita's girlfriends) are there. The dad of the best friend is on a motorcycle. Rita hops on it and they take off. I crowd into the driver's seat over Karen. It is her car, a Maserati or Ferrari - a slick car.

Tony, an all-american diver on the swim team, had this dream about the time things started getting serious with his girlfriend, Rita. (He wound up marrying her a few years later.) The dream reflects his ambivalence about what is happening to him. Although he is in the driver's seat, things are moving so fast that he cannot see clearly and he knows that he needs to stop soon for a rest. Yet it is exciting and it is a "slick" vehicle - although not his own. When they do stop to refuel (a pit stop), they are in the midst of other drivers (divers) and (swim team) coaches. He knows that he is not doing as well as he would like to (4th place) and feels uncomfortable and wants to leave. When they do, there is some confusion about who is traveling with whom as the dream ends.

Tim's recurrent dream.

It is the time of graduate school. I am riding in an elevator but unsure of which floor to get off on. I feel a lot of anxiety about what was there and the other people. In the most recent version of the dream, I went all the way to the top. It was painted ivory white and had a lot of windows looking out all ways.

This dream reflects Tim's ambiguity and anxiety about choices in life and what to do about them. In the end, he decides to go all the way to the top where he finds an ivory painted room ("Ivory Tower") that gives him a view of many things, and he is reasonably satisfied.

One common dream involves missing a vehicle, especially a bus, plane, or train. Most often this comes out of a fear that we may miss out on something in our present lives. It is not unusual to have such a dream before an important event or occasion.

Looking Inward (Personal Truth)

Parts of our personalities often come into conflict, or we may have aspects of our personalities that are weak and ineffectual, inappropriate, or even dysfunctional. Perhaps we are ignoring or neglecting parts of our personalities. We attempt to deal with aspects of our personalities in our dreams. How we feel about our private world is present in our dreams. Often these problems are a result of our past history that are causing us problems currently. The basic assumption at this level is that all dream images, in addition to whatever else they may be, are parts of ourselves - the parts that are threats to our conscious image of ourselves.

The method used here is Fritz Perls' Gestalt dialog (Perls, 1969). In a Gestalt dialog, the dreamer has various parts of the dream engage in a dialog. This is done by alternately sitting in two chairs that face one another. The dreamer sits on one of the chairs and assumes the role of any dream image. The dreamer begins to talk as if they were this image addressing another dream image. The dreamer then responds to what the first image said by changing seats and assuming the role of the other image. The dialog proceeds as the dreamer continues to alternate seats and talks as one, then the other image.

The aim of the Gestalt dialog is to bring out an existing conflict between two parts of the personality and then resolve it. In this way, the alienated parts of the personality come together to become a whole. It is sometimes awkward and uncomfortable to do a Gestalt dialog. It may even seem downright silly, but seems to work. Once a person gets into the flow of it, conflicts start emerging. Often it is not only what is said, but facial expressions and changes in body posture as one changes from chair to chair that convey a lot of meaning. Faraday believes the Gestalt method to be especially effective for recurrent dreams or the same character showing up in many dreams.

Where to start? The choice can be difficult, especially in a long and complex dream with many different images. Often it does not matter, though. A good idea is to start with the most obvious pair of images in the dream. If nothing seems to develop, switch to another pair of images. Keep doing this until a conflict develops, then stay with it until it is resolved. The dreamer, even if not a character in the dream, may be one of the dialog pairs. Inanimate objects of the dream can also participate and speak for themselves.

Often during this dialog, the "two clowns" emerge. The first clown is called **TOP DOG**. The top dog is righteous and authoritarian. It is a bully, making perfectionistic demands. You "ought" to do this. You "should" do that. "Never do" this. You "should not" have done that. It is usually assumed that top dog is right. Sometimes top dog is right, sometimes not, but it is always righteous. Top dog manipulates by using demands and threats of catastrophe. "If you don't do this, then..." People use top dog's perfectionism to browbeat themselves and berate others. Yet, top dog's demands are too ideal and can never be achieved.

The other clown, **UNDER DOG**, is very much different, but not much better in its own way. Under dog is defensive and apologetic, wheedling, and a cry-baby. "I didn't mean to." "It'll never happen again." "I couldn't help it." "I'll try to do better." Under dog does not come off as being powerful, but often tries to get the better of top dog in the long run. Under dog wants top dog's approval - sometimes almost desperately - but wants his own way, too. So, when under dog gives in it is still looking for a way out. Top dog's authoritarian attitude attempts to dominate but without total success. Under dog can never totally win approval, yet get its own way too. Something has to change.

Henry was a second semester freshman at the time of this dream. It was his first time away from his parents for any length of time, and he wasn't sure how it was going. He was enjoying the independence but was a little anxious and wondering if he was heading in the right direction for his life.

> *We were on a family skiing trip to Colorado on a warm, clear day. I took off without ski poles, sun-glasses, or sun-screen. My dad didn't get mad. But my mom showed raccoon eyes she was so angry. She gave me some broken sun glasses and sun screen. The broken glasses were his old ones and she threw them at me.*

The following Gestalt dialog between ski poles and Henry was productive. In this example, Henry becomes the under dog and the poles the top dog.

Henry: You could have told me I would need you. I never should have skied without you.

Poles: We could have told you, but we decided not to. You learn by making mistakes. You may fall down, but you can do it without us.

H: Ye,s but it's so hard and dangerous. I really need you.

P: (with an air of self righteousness) Well, now you know. If we had tried to tell you before, you would never have believed us. Now you know that you must never ski again without us. Promise?

H: Yes, you are right. I promise. *(Aside to other members of the group)* But it was kind of exciting...

Make under dog stand up to top dog. It should simply and openly state its needs. Top dog should try to accommodate those needs. The two should come to an agreement as equals. By doing this, the dreamer can understand the problem in their personality, usually something being avoided, and begin to correct it. Try to make oneself whole instead of divided and conflicting.

More recently, Faraday has described another, but more subtle, occurrence at this level - the secret saboteur. It never directly appears in the dream but is manipulating its content. It can be recognized as being at work when a goal or desire is repeatedly frustrated by the events of the dream. The very common missing the vehicle dream may be an example of the secret saboteur's work, especially if "everything seems to go wrong" when trying to catch a plane or bus. It's as if there is a conspiracy against you. That's because there is - the secret saboteur.

The secret saboteur may be either a top dog or an under dog. The only way to find out is for the dreamer to have a Gestalt dialog with the saboteur. Find out what he wants and why. Then relate this to your present life.

Other examples of the secret saboteur being at work can be suspected when in the dream you arrive late or are unprepared. Again, suspect the saboteur if a series of mishaps are the cause. But, first examine the dream at the first level (looking outward) to see if the dream is a warning dream. If it is not, then seek out the saboteur.

Sometimes people too easily misinterpret such dreams with the simple conclusion "you really didn't want to..." The secret saboteur - whether a top dog or a under dog - is more subtle than this. The underlying motivation is more complex. If the "you really didn't want to..." explanation does not set well with the dreamer, then suspect and look for a hidden saboteur.

Jill related this dream to us and then went on to discover the secret saboteur. She was a senior about to graduate and get married to her long-time boyfriend, Jim.

> *The dream begins with me going to class unprepared to give a dance demonstration. The class is held on the 2nd floor of Main in one of the classrooms. I didn't recognize the instructor, but the person was male, medium to heavy build, dark hair and probably in his late 40's or early 50's. A classmate was asking me about my presentation because she was supposed to be giving one too, and she wasn't ready either. I didn't recognize the girl, but I knew I knew her. I can't describe her, but she was around 20 years old.*
>
> *The instructor walks in and tells us he has so much to lecture on today that all he wants is a good write-up of the presentations that were supposed to be given. I didn't have mine written-up and I couldn't do it without my book, so I left the class and went to my room to get the book so I could write it up.*
>
> *When I got back to class, the instructor had started lecturing and I realized I didn't have my notebook so I could take notes, all I had was one piece of paper, so I told a fellow student that I was going back to my room again to get my notebook. On the way back from my room I stopped at the cafeteria, and there was a man there talking to these people on how to behaviorally control their bodies. The cafeteria was full of these people listening to this man. All the people had babies with them. I stood towards the back next to this lady and her baby. When the man gave instructions what to do with the babies, I followed these instructions using the lady's baby. The man was giving instructions on shaping behavior. I left the cafeteria and continued to Main.*
>
> *I went inside the doors, but the stairs were gone and there was a big net people were climbing up. I was required to climb the net to get to class. I made it to the top once and was pushed down, so I had to climb the net again. When I got to the top, my roommate from last semester was there, and told the instructor*

I shouldn't have to climb the net again. He didn't make me climb the net again.

Jill went through Faraday's first two stages without discovering anything major and she said that everything was fine with her dance class, so she next used the Gestalt dialog between herself and the secret saboteur.

Jill: Why did you make it so hard for me to participate in class in this dream?

Saboteur: Oh come on, you didn't really want to go to class. You didn't really want to go through with dancing in front of all those people and the strange instructor. I was just helping you get out of it and giving you a chance to review your decision. You know I'm right about this.

J: But I've been preparing for this class for a long time. People expect me to do it. I can't back out now.

S: Oh come on, who is in control of your life anyway?

J: I'm . . . I'm not really sure.

S: See. I told you that you did not really want to go through with this. You might stumble and give yourself away and ruin everything. All the practice in the world will not make it better. Why not just admit that you really don't want to go through with it?

J: But I have to! Everyone is expecting me to graduate. I don't know. (Long pause). Why did you delay me with the behavioral control of babies lecture?

S: That's obvious. You're about to get married and have kids. You need to know something about controlling kids. You are going to have lots of kids, you know.

J: Wait a minute, Jim, I don't . . . (Here the audience laughs and Jill smiles, then frowns. She then turns away from the chair, looks down at the floor, and continues). I don't know if I want to get married; I'm not sure I'm ready. I guess I have known this, but I have been trying to ignore the obvious.

And Finally

What do you do if you have diligently gone through all of the steps, yet the meaning of the dream continues to be elusive? Faraday

Summary of Faraday's method for Analyzing Dreams

I. *Objective Truth*

A. Source: Information about people or situations in the real world subconsciously perceived during the day

B. Method: A common sense look at the dream

C. Types
1. Reminder: specific events that have been forgotten
2. Warning: show what might happen if dreamer continues to ignore something
3. Revealing People: show the truth about a person that was not realized by the waking mind
4. "Clairvoyant": show present situations of which we were only subconsciously aware of
5. "Precognitive": "predict" the future through the mind's abilities of detection and prediction of logical outcomes

II. *Subjective Truth*

A. Source: the world as seen by the dreamer's personality

B. Method: look for obvious meanings and metaphors and/or associate to the details of the dream

C. People
1. Current intimates: usually represent the real person (Ask, "What does the dream tell me about my present feelings and thoughts about this person?")
2. Intimates from the past: may represent parts of ourselves that remind us of the person in the dream
3. Friends and Colleagues: either:
   a. our feelings about the actual person
   b. or our feelings about a "similar" person
   c. or represent a part of our personality

4. Public Figures, Historical Characters, and People from Fiction: either represent:
   a. someone else
   b. or a part of our personality. (Also ask: "Why this particular metaphor rather than another?")
5. Strangers: must be a metaphor

D. Animals and Creatures
1. usually metaphors
2. may represent a person with some of the characteristics of the animal or creature

E. Houses:
1. usually metaphors about ourselves
2. or our lifestyles
3. or our marriage
4. or our family relationships
5. or our personality

F. Vehicles:
1. usually metaphors about themselves
2. or dreamer's lifestyles
3. or direction of a relationship
4. or an institution
(5. the missing the vehicle dream: fear that we may miss out on something in our present lives. Note who is in control of the vehicle)

III. *Personal Truth*

A. Source: Conflicts between parts of our personality

B. Method: Gestalt Dialog

C. Find top dog v. under dog and have them resolve conflict

D. Especially effective for recurrent dreams or characters

commends continuing to look at it. Perhaps viewing it from a different angle or point of view will help. Talking about it with friends and listening to what they think of it may yield a clue or two. Allowing your mind to drift when thinking of the dream sometimes yields new associations. If all else fails, before falling asleep, ask your dreams for help in understanding a particular character or image or scene or even the entire dream.

Ullman's Method

Montague Ullman is a psychiatrist and psychoanalyst at the Albert Einstein College of Medicine in New York City who first became interested in dreams because of their possible clairvoyant content (see chapter 6). Subsequently, he began to work with dream interpretation, even to the extent of giving up other aspects of his practice. He describes his methods in a non-technical format with many examples in *Working with Dreams* (Ullman & Zimmerman, 1979).

He begins with the belief that dreams tell the truth about the dreamer - especially the state of relationships with others. Thus, it is important to realize that dreams come from our immediate life situations. But they do so as visual metaphors. Thus, in order to understand the meaning of a dream, the dreamer must interpret the meanings in the visual metaphors. Although reproductions of real events may occur in dreams, all aspects of the dream are symbolic and nothing is unimportant.

We should not expect to be totally successful in understanding all aspects of all of our dreams. Ullman makes the analogy of examining a fish out of the water. We cannot in this way totally understand its way of life in the water. So too with dreams. In our waking, rational state we have only what is remembered of the dream and can only work on it out of its natural sleeping environment.

Ullman's method requires a group of people in addition to the dreamer. The members of the group help give support to the dreamer during the process. Other people may be able to interpret the dreamer's metaphors better than the dreamer, because they are less affected by the consequences and do not have the same biases which often block interpretations. Yet, the dreamer, throughout the whole procedure, remains the ultimate authority over their dream.

Ullman`s procedure involves three stages. First, the dreamer tells the dream to the group, then the group suggests their interpretations, and finally the dreamer responds to these interpretations.

The method starts with the dreamer telling the dream as remembered, without interpretation. The dreamer may use any notes to help remember the dream and accurately relate it. Meanwhile, the rest of the group listens and takes notes. When the dreamer has finished, then the group can ask questions, but only to clarify not to interpret. For example, questions about the color of an object, the sequence of events, and who a character was are allowed, but not questions such as, "Who does that remind you of?"

Next, the dreamer remains quiet and takes notes as each member of the group treats the dream as if it were his or her own. That is, the comments are not directed to the dreamer using "your dream" but are directed to the group saying, "my dream." First, the overall feeling or mood of the dream is addressed. "I feel my dream is a very happy one." "This dream makes me feel sad in the beginning, then angry, but ends up very hopeful." Second, the members of the group tell what the images (as metaphors) mean to them. Anything goes. Group members may talk about any part of the dream, from the main characters or images all the way down to the minor details. This should continue until everyone has had a chance to say everything they want to. Someone in the group should be responsible, though, for seeing that no major character or image is left unattended and that the sequence of images is explored. (I do this by using a series of colored pens - one color for writing down the dream and another for writing the meanings suggested by the group written next to the appropriate place in the description. If I later see a place where there are no entries in the second color, I then give my associations for them or prompt the other group members to focus on them. I use a third color for recording what the dreamer says during the next stage.)

It is important for group members to treat the dream as if it were their own. Think of using phrases such as "my dream..." or "In this dream I..." Another thing to keep in mind is to avoid directing comments only to the dreamer; the whole group should be addressed.

Likewise, it is important for the dreamer to remain absolutely passive during this stage. The dreamer should try to avoid cueing the other members about their responses. Non-verbal cues are likely to occur here and are as important as verbal ones to keep under control.

At times, different members may have entirely opposite views of the dream's meanings. That's O.K. at this stage. Critical comments about the views of another must be avoided. Everyone must feel free to say whatever they think.

Now, it's the dreamers turn again. The dreamer now interprets the dream as they see it. The dreamer can (and usually does) respond to many of the suggestions made by the group members accepting those that feel right, rejecting those that do not, and ignoring any or all. It is important for the dreamer to recall events of a day or two that preceded the dream and to relate them to the dream as appropriate. The dreamer must have all the time they need without interruption.

When the dreamer is finished, a dialog may begin where the group members ask questions to help the dreamer explore the dream and its images more. The purpose here is to further help the dreamer explore the feelings and images and to direct attention to any aspects that may have been overlooked. The dreamer remains the authority, though. Group members must not try to convince the dreamer of the "rightness" of any interpretation. The final interpretation must feel right to the dreamer, and they must feel comfortable with it. No one should try to force any interpretation. At the end, someone should summarize the interpretation, often with "purposeful exaggeration."

The dreamer must always feel in control. The dreamer decides how much of theirself they wish to share. The dreamer may decide to stop at any point. No one should be forced to share a dream.

Sometimes returning to the dream again in a few days helps to bring new insights and to sort out the original ones. This is especially true for long, complex dreams or if the first analysis attempt was unsatisfactory.

It is also possible to use this method alone on one's own dreams. Treat the dream as if it were someone else's. Try to see it from a distance. Be as objective as possible. Next, try to see its feelings and metaphors as someone else's. Finally, look at the waking events that may have led to the dream. Overall, though, the method works best with a group.

The purpose of dreams is to heal us emotionally. The purpose of dreamwork should, likewise, be healing. Our dreams are honest. The goal of dreamwork is to discover and use this honesty. In the process, we can bring more personal resources into our daily lives. We may, for example, discover parts of ourselves of which we are not aware. Often, this stems from any unresolved problems remaining from childhood.

Summary of Ullman's Method of Dream Analysis

Stage 1.

a. DREAMER TELLS DREAM as if occurring right now They do not try to interpret it yet. Others only listen and take notes.

b. Next, GROUP MEMBERS may ASK QUESTIONS intended only to clarify details.

Stage 2.

Each GROUP MEMBER treats the dream as their own (while dreamer listens and takes notes). Use the first person ("I") when doing this.

a. Group members tell their FEELINGS from the dream.

b. Then the group members tell what they see as the meaning of IMAGES and METAPHORS in the dream.

Stage 3.

a. Now the DREAMER talks about the FEELINGS and METAPHORS of the dream in whatever way they desire, all the while attempting to relate it to recent events in their life. The dreamer may at this time accept, reject, or ignore any of the suggestions from other group members that were presented in stage 2.

b. Finally, GROUP MEMBERS may ASK QUESTIONS to help the dreamer explore the feelings and the images more.

REMEMBER: THE DREAMER ALWAYS REMAINS THE FINAL AUTHORITY OVER THE DREAM!

Through dream recall and subsequent dreamwork, we can recognize these subconscious parts and begin to integrate them more fully with the rest of ourselves in order to become more whole. Likewise, through dreamwork, we can see how dreams are relevant to recent problems and concerns in our lives and, at the same time, see how dreams relate these problems and concerns to our past. Dreamwork also shows how dreams reflect our relationships with others and how we represent problems and relationships to ourselves. In these ways we grow.

An Example of Ullman's Method

On the last day of a week long summer academic camp for high school students at Luther College, we studied dreams and did some analysis of group members' dreams. Lisa volunteered a dream that totally mystified her. She was unable to understand any of it. Lisa was heavy set and not very stylish. She had scabs and marks on her arms. During the week, she was always talking about how frightening our recreation activities were to her, although she participated in everything the group did. She was afraid of tipping in the canoe. She was afraid of heights when hiking in the hills, and so on. The rest of the group neither pandered to her neurotic fears nor ignored her. They all encouraged her to participate without belittling her and offered her a lot of support. Gradually, as the week progressed, her self-depreciation lessened and she began to interact with the others on a more open and adult level.

Stage 1a. Lisa tells her dream to the group:

> *I'm in a white room that is hopeless and sorta big. I don't know where it is - sort of a hospital or lab. Some people are there with gray or black hair. Their skin is kinda gray, too. I'm laying on a stretcher in a corner of the room. I'm all in white. Six or seven others are there too - one is my mom, but she is standing 10 feet away talking to a nurse. Mom walks up to me and starts to cry. "I'm really sorry this has to happen." I don't understand what she means.*
>
> *The nurse has a needle and says, "It's time for you to die." My mom is crying. I don't know what is going on, but I sort of know. She shoots the needle in. Then I am floating out of my*

body. I am about 10 feet up. Two people are there looking at me. I feel so light floating there. Then the dream ends.

Stage 1b. The groups ask clarifying questions:

Tim: Is your body floating?
Lisa: No. I can see my body below me still on the stretcher.
Paula: Can you describe the nurse?
L: She is 35 or 40. That's all I know.
Terri: What about the rest of the people?
L: Nobody distinct. Just some people.
Bill: What was the needle like? Can you tell us more about it?
L: It was just a big - extra big - injection needle loaded with some kind of fluid and ready to be injected.

Stage 2a. The group members treat the dream as if it is their own and talk about its feelings.

P: I'm uncertain, unclear, scary. Felt like indecision.
Joan: This is weird. Real scary and spooky.
Toby: Real nervous and shaky. Its scary.
Ron: I feel the spacelessness of the room. Kinda timeless too. I'm confused and uncertain. I can't seem to get my bearings.
B: The whole white tile thing is so cold and sterile. It's so white and sterile like an exaggerated attempt to be clean. Everything echoes. Even though there are other people there, I kinda feel like I'm in a tomb and almost dead.
J: Yeah. This is a real somber thing that is happening.
Terri: I'm not dead yet, but they are getting me ready for some kind of surgery - serious surgery and nobody is sure how it's going to come out.

Stage 2b. Again the group members treat the dream as if it is their own and now make associations to the images.

T: The nurse is cold, ominous, and featureless. It's like she is some force or something.

P: I'm laying on a stretcher; I'm not in control; I've lost control.

B: The needle is dominant, the only distinct thing in the dream other than my mother. It's the needle that has control - or rather the drug in it. After the injection, I change and float above it all.

Hillary: My mom's crying. She is helpless in this situation too. I need her and she wants to help, and yet she can't help me. It's like I'm in this all by myself.

Stage 3a. Now the dreamer analyzes the dream using her own interpretations of the feelings and images and adding background information.

B: Lisa, now its your turn.

L: This dream never made sense to me until now. I have been in drug treatment twice. My mom has had to commit me both times. This dream is about all of that. It's scary and hard to go through it. I felt so alone and rejected.

B: So just as in the dream, the drug has been a turning point in your life - both causing you to need treatment and then during treatment going without it was another turning point?

L: Yes. It changes things but only for a little while. I still don't know where I am going.

B: Do you feel kind of like you are floating above everything, looking down at yourself wondering which way to go? What's going to happen?

L: Yes, that makes a lot of sense. That's what it is about!

Definition Dream Analysis

Gayle Delaney is a Ph.D. psychologist in private practice in San Francisco. She specializes in dream analysis and has made numerous TV and radio appearances, as well as given lecture/demonstrations to live audiences around the country. She describes her technique, Dream Interviewing, in her books *Living Your Dreams, Revised Edition* (Delaney, 1988) and *Breakthrough Dreaming*(Delaney, 1991). Her method is the newest of the three techniques and perhaps the simplest.

It is based not so much on a theory as on an analogy plus a lot of experience.

The analogy is that of a motion picture. Each of us is the producer, writer, director, and star of our dreams. Our consciousness during sleep is more direct and immediate in its perceptions, with more wisdom and more access to information. Thus, our dreams are translations of our waking consciousness. Like a movie, the story, images, events, etc. are carefully picked to portray as well as possible the original theme, but yet not overdo it. Like movies, some dreams are better and more successful than others. The original theme may be something about your self (mind, body, or spirit), your relationships with others, or your unused potentials. Your dreams may also be trying out various possible future outcomes of potential actions.

Delaney's view of dreams and their interpretation is very positive. Our dreams are good for us and their interpretation can only help. Even frightening, embarrassing, or horrible dreams can be very good, and we should not avoid analyzing them. Such dreams force us to look at ourselves with the intent of helping. Even nightmares can bring pleasure in the same way that horror movies can. Most turn out to be interesting or even funny.

Our dreams come to enlighten us, but they do not relate to what we already know. They may be about things we fear knowing or do not fully appreciate. And although we create them, their meanings may not be immediately clear. Thus, the need for interpretation.

The method is called Dream Interviewing because the dream producer in you is interviewed. This can be done by yourself but is best done by a friend or a specialist in dream interpretation. The interviewer must have an attitude of acceptance and interest. Maintain a tone of light conversation, not heavy inquisition. Enjoy. Maintain eye contact. Give brief simple statements ("Oh my!" or "Uh huh.") during long responses by the dreamer to let them know you are paying attention. The dreamer should try to maintain an attitude of playfulness, exploration, and adventure, and avoid working too hard at it. The interviewer should try not to push interpretations because they may be wrong or be met with resistance on the part of the dreamer. The interviewer may *suggest* possibilities, however. The dreamer's interpretations are the ultimate authority, however. Both the interviewer and the dreamer must be aware of the metaphoric nature of dreams and the prevalence of puns.

There are several points Delaney wishes us to keep in mind:

- Things such as top dog, under dog, and secret saboteurs may be useful.
- Images that change probably represent past, present, or future changes in life, attitude, or feelings of the dreamer.
- The mood, feelings, and reflections of the dream - both during the dream and when interpreting it - are as important as anything.
- Even if there is an obvious, literal meaning in the dream, you should still look for a deeper, metaphoric meaning.
- "The dream itself says it best." Thus, any interpretation should always lead back to the dream.

The Interview Technique

The procedure starts with the dreamer telling the dream to the interviewer in first person, present tense. This encourages the dreamer to relive the dream again and to feel and express its emotions. Give the dreamer some kind of feedback and reward for telling the dream such as, "That was quite a dream!"

The dream interview technique is composed of four elements: Description, Recapitulation, Bridge, and Summary in addition to first retelling the dream.

DESCRIPTION: The heart of this technique is to ask the dreamer to **define** and **describe** elements of the dream. Usually, this will allow the dreamer to explore associations almost effortlessly and with less resistance than with other techniques. To elicit description, ask variations of, "What is _____ like?" Have the dreamer answer the questions as if they were talking to a person from another planet who understands nothing about planet Earth. Why? Often what we think is obvious to others is really our own perceptions, understanding, and feelings. Also, we may not be totally conscious of what these are until we have to explain them to someone else. Good descriptions always include feelings and value judgments. Remind the dreamer that these descriptions need not be fair or accurate.

Delaney's Dream Interview Technique

Retell
the dreamer retells the dream
in the present tense

Description
by dreamer
What are the ________ like?
SETTINGS
PEOPLE
OBJECTS
FEELINGS
ACTION

RECAPITULATION
by interviewer
using dreamer's own words

Bridge
by dreamer
to real life
UNPACK if necessary
(when dreamer says there is a
connection but does not say how)
ask, "How so?"

SUMMARY
by interviewer or dreamer
of dream and its bridges

After Delaney, G (1991). *Breakthrough Dreaming*. New York: Bantam Books.

Delaney suggests six basic kinds of things to ask questions about:

1. What are the major moods and feelings in the dream?
2. Describe the setting. How does it relate to your waking life?
3. Who is each dream person and what is he or she like? Also, the feelings about the person from the dream itself.
4. What is each dream object and what is it like?
5. How does each feeling, person, or object relate to your waking life?
6. Describe the dream events. What do they remind you of in your waking life?

The summary of the Definition Dream Analysis on the previous page provides a good set of initial specific questions. You don't have to use them all - or any of them for that matter - but they do give a start and may help focus the questioning.

Assume that the dreamer has associations just below the surface of consciousness and the right questions will bring them out. It is best to use the words and images of the dream when asking the questions.

RECAPITULATION: Now repeat the description back to the dreamer using the dreamer's own words as much as possible. Invite the dreamer to pick up, elaborate, and correct this recapitulation. Be careful not to lead the dreamer off course by trying to force an interpretation on them.

BRIDGE: Then ask the dreamer if it reminds them of anyone or anything in their waking life. If the dreamer says that aspects of the dream remind them of something in real life but does not spontaneously say how, ask, "How so?" Delaney calls this **UNPACKING,** as if unpacking a suitcase carried over the bridge. The aim is to help the dreamer understand her dream, not to convince her of any particular meaning the interviewer sees. However, the interviewer can make suggestions in the form of hypotheses to speed things up. Ask things like:

"Try this on for size."

"Does that fit?"

"What do you think about that?"

Summary of Delaney's Definition Dream Analysis

Both you and the dreamer should approach the dream and its analysis with an attitude of playful adventure. Allow the dreamer to discover the meanings in the dream.

I. Have the dreamer retell the dream as if describing what is happening right now using first person, present tense ("I am...").

II. Ask questions about the dream using, as much as possible, the dreamer's own words and phrases. Have the dreamer pretend that you come from another planet when giving you the answer to these questions.

Ask questions such as:

1. "What are the **FEELINGS** in the dream?" "How might they relate to your waking life?"
2. "What are the **SETTINGS** in the dream." "What is the mood or feeling of each setting?" "How do they relate to your waking life?"
3. "Tell me about the **PEOPLE** in the dream." "What is each one like?" "How do you feel about each one?" (If there are strangers in the dream, then ask what each ***seems*** to be like.) "Who or what do these people remind you of in your waking life?" "Do any of them remind you of yourself?"
4. "Tell me about the **THINGS** in the dream." "What are they doing in this dream?" "What do they remind your of in your waking life?" For animals in dreams, ask, "How would you describe the personality of this animal?"
5. "Tell me about the **EVENTS** in the dream." "Are they similar to any events in your waking life?"
6. (Finally), "What do you **UNDERSTAND** about the dream?" You may make suggestions here, but allow the dreamer to freely agree or disagree with your suggestions.

Aim to help the dreamer uncover the meaning of the dream, not to gather evidence to prove your hypothesis. At the same time, try not to deprive the dreamer of the joy and benefits of discovering the meanings for themselves.

Silent times during the interview may not be all bad. They may be times when things are falling into place or rising to the surface. Likewise, seemingly unrelated thoughts may be important. They should also be fully explored.

What Delaney calls the "aha" or esthetic experience shows that the dream has been successfully interpreted. The dreamer feels good about the results. Another indicator is when the dreamer has learned something they did not know before. Throughout the whole interview, the interviewer should encourage the dreamer's sense of play and exploration. Sometimes returning to the dream a few hours or days later helps things make more sense.

SUMMARY: Finish by having the dreamer put the pieces together by reviewing the dream and how its images bridge. Have the dreamer include background from their waking life. Then ask what is understood and what remains unexplained. Do the pieces fit together and are they appropriate? Do not lose sight of the larger picture by focusing too much on details. The flow of the plot can act like a directional compass.

Partial summaries may also be done periodically throughout the procedure. This may be especially useful if leading up to difficult or sensitive bridges. End by having the dreamer "relive the dream" to integrate the various things learned about the dream.

An Example of Definition Dream Analysis

Bill: Any volunteers today? (Ann raised her hand enthusiastically.) OK, Ann, first tell us the dream as if it is happening right here and right now.

Ann: I am back in my high school. The band is playing in the Gym with lots of people in the bleachers. We were told to be dressed up; we could wear anything as long as it was dressy. I am wearing a sun dress. It looks really nice on me. It has patterns and circles. There are lots of high school girls running around the floor. It's some kind of celebration. Some have instruments, others have a long cloth they're twirling around in a kinda' figure eight.

We're done playing and I am carrying my flute. I have to leave, because I have the feeling that I have to be somewhere else. I go through the door to the left and go left again toward the band room. The band room is carpeted in orange and yellow, which is pretty.

I am alone, but four guys are following me. I wonder why. I start to walk faster, then I get scared and drop my flute and run. I lose my shoes, too. I am running hard but I feel like I'm not going anywhere, even though these guys are running after me. I run right up the stairs, then I go left from the band room into Mr. Bergland's office. (He's the band director.) It takes me a long time to get there. Mr. Bergland's room is different than usual. This time it's in the storage room with lots of green shelves. But he's not there, so I turn around and these guys are right behind me. I recognize them as guys I know from school - as guys I like, but I would not want to get involved with. I get even more scared. Then I wake up.

B: That's quite an interesting dream. Now the essence of this procedure is that I'm going to interview you about your dream. You were the creator, you are the person who knows best why you created the dream this way, so I'm going to ask you questions about your creation, your dream. Pretend that I am an interviewer from Mars and I don't know anything about the Earth. Just think that you have to give answers to someone that doesn't know anything about what's going on here.

First of all, let me ask you if you have any ideas already about the meaning of this dream?

A: Not really.

B: Okay. What is a band?

A: A band is where a group of people are together and they play instruments that make sounds and they are all coordinated so that the sounds don't clash and it sounds pretty. They play for other people's entertainment.

B: What does a band remind you of? Did you like to play in the band?

A: Yah, I like to play in the band and I guess it doesn't remind me of much other than it's fun and it's a skill.

B: Why do you think in your dream that you start out in the band and then leave? You are with a lot of people and then you are alone.

A: I really don't know. It is like I have to go to work or something; like I am going to be late for work, because I am always leaving to go to work. But yet, this is in the evening and work ends at seven at night.

B: Okay. You're saying in real life that often you have to hurry from band practice to get to your job; from one situation to another.

A: Yah, or from job to band, like marching band at night.

B: What does that feel like?

A: Rushed and tense. I don't like it very much, but sometimes I've got to do it.

B: Okay. You described your sundress. What is a sundress?

A: It's a piece of cloth that you wear - that you can wear during the summer; it's thin and it keeps you cool during the hot weather of the summer; usually sleeveless.

B: And when you are describing it and talking about it, it sounds like you really like it, that you felt dressed up or something. Is that right?

A: Yah, it is a pretty dress on me.

B: So it makes you look pretty, prettier? Right?

A: Yah.

B: But it seems that you don't feel comfortable being dressed like this.

A: Yah.

B: Why is that?

A: Well, because when I dress up guys usually look at me, and I get afraid when they look at me.

B: Why is that?

A: I'm always afraid they are looking at me for a certain reason, for kind of sexual purposes, I guess.

B: Okay. Did you recognize any of the four guys that are following you?

A: Sort of. They aren't exactly the same faces as a few of the guys I like in high school, but they are like Mike Schwartz and Bob Bewder and Travis somebody-or-another but they are kind of real jerks too and I don't know why I like them, but I do anyway.

B: How about saying a little something about each one of them as they are in the dream, or as they are in the dream and in real life. What are they like?

A: In the dream, I don't really notice who they are until I am up in Mr. Bergland's office. And they all simply pile in the door and are kind of waiting there with intent it seems like. And there really is no characteristic about any of the three that I recognize. They just look like they want to say something or do something.

B: But in real life you say they are kind of jerks. What do you mean by that?

A: Well, I guess they drink and party and they have philosophies that they don't act on, and I guess I don't like that. And Travis like to play jokes and he throws things across the hall. And Bob, he's normally a jerk. I don't know how to describe it. It's like he talks to people but he doesn't mean anything by it. He just, you know, talks to them so that he has something to do. And Mike is nice except he goes out and drinks too and parties and stuff like that.

B: Okay. You said that the guys have philosophies that they really don't act upon. What do you mean by that?

A: Well, like they rag on other people for not being nice to somebody and then they're not nice to other people in the same situation. It is like they don't remember that.

B: So kind of two-faced?

A: Yah.

B: Okay. Do you think there is some part of you that is like those four guys or any one of them?

A: I don't know if there would be any part of me, but sometimes I have this desire to actually be mean to someone. You know, I don't know why, maybe to be like the rest of them 'cuz I am not really very different from everybody, but different enough that I don't fit in.

B: So, what I'm hearing you saying is that you feel different from them, those four guys, and the type of people they are. Is that what you're saying?

A: Well, they kind of... Everyone at school always thinks I am a Goody-Two-Shoes and that I don't do anything wrong.

B: You describe pretty well the band director's office modified into a storage room in the dream so I won't ask you to describe it again. But does that remind you of anything? Why do you use that set in your dream?

A: I suppose because it's like Mr. Bergland. His office is safety from everyone else, but having it in the storage room - having his office in the storage room would be like - I guess I think of storage rooms as places where anything can happen, where you can't really escape and you can't yell for help because there is no one around and I guess combining the two, going there for help, there is really nothing there. It's scary and I feel helpless.

B: I'm curious about something. When you describe everybody in the band who are down on the floor you said they are ladies, other high school students, other female high school students. Were there no guys in the band in the dream?

A: It isn't just band members. It's all women down there and there aren't any guys playing. It's just like we are just roaming around. It's Midsummer's Night Dream with all the fairies roaming around in the pasture.

B: Kind of idyllic and free and no problems and kind of paradise. And it's all female, so when you leave there and you are alone and there are four guys following you, do you see a connection there?

A: I don't know. It kind of seems like there is one, but I can't put my finger on it.

B: Flute. What is a flute?

A: It's a woodwind instrument and it has a hole on the top, or on the sides of the top and you hold it horizontally to your right and you blow through that hole. And there are a whole lot holes on the body of the instrument and you play it by moving certain fingers and opening up certain holes.

B: In real life you play the flute, not just in your dream life?

A: Yup.

B: When you think of a flute, what do you think of other than just describing it. What does a flute mean to you?

A: Beautiful, springtime and I guess that's about it.

B: And then when these guys are chasing you, you drop your flute. Why did you drop your flute?

A: Probably - I probably drop it so that I can run away faster. I suppose that could mean that I am giving up something in order to get free.

B: Do you think it means giving up something?

A: Yah.

B: Well, what would you be giving up?

A: Kind of my identify, I guess. Dropping part of my identity away in order to survive.

B: Survive.

A: Well....

B: What do you mean to survive?

A: To survive whatever those guys would do to me, I guess. To try to get away and if I didn't get away, I don't know.

B: Okay. Why are you afraid of guys?

A: Well, I guess I want... When I look nice I don't want them to look at the body, whereas sometimes they do. And I want to be seen as an intelligent person.

B: Okay. Let me try to exaggerate this dream a little bit and put some pieces together and see how they resonate with you, okay? This is a time in your life that you, like most teenagers, are experiencing a lot of changes. In the past, you were a little girl with little girl interests and enjoyed being with other girls and life with a lot of play and a lot of fun. You could play your flute and things were simple and happy. But now things are changing for you. You are noticing boys, boys are noticing you and your life is changing a lot. You have to leave behind a lot of the younger girl things, but you are a little bit afraid of boys and what they might do and things like that. As you run you drop your flute and your shoes. (Your Goody Two-Shoes maybe?) Even the place that you run to, that should be safe, is not. This dream kind of reflects the uneasiness of transition that you are feeling. How does that resonate with you?

A: Well, one thing, I have always been interested in guys since I was in grade school but I guess I am just uneasy around guys that show that.....that aren't my type, I guess, you know, drink and party and go for sexual relations and that stuff. And I guess I am beginning to be uneasy because they are noticing me whereas they never did before, but I have always been interested in guys.

I guess there is something. The day before the dream I talked to Scott Bjork in Dairy Queen. He seemed really interested in me and what I was doing and stuff. But since then, he hasn't talked to me anymore.

B: Let me change it just a little bit then. These guys are noticing you and maybe there is a part of you that is a little bit attracted, curious, wondering what you are missing, but yet repelled that those guys represent something scary to you.

A: Yah, that's it! I guess I am curious about what a boyfriend is like cuz I never really had one. And I guess that is kind of what that is all about. But I'm afraid of what having a boyfriend means; that I might be expected to do things. There might be expectations of things I really don't like or what people would think I am. I feel kinda' trapped. I'm afraid to be myself and dress up when I want to and things like that. And if I dress up, I'm afraid, that they will take notice. I'm afraid of being noticed - I'm afraid of what they think. Yet I want to be. I can see now that's what the dream is all about.

When to Analyze Dreams

Contrary to Faraday, Ullman, and Delaney, I do not believe that everybody should record and analyze dreams regularly. It takes a lot of time and effort to do even a single dream of average length and complexity. If you were to do this for several dreams each week, it would be very costly in time and effort. For most of us, that time and effort may probably be better used in other ways. And yet for some people, regular dream analysis may be useful; for others, occasional dream analysis may be a good idea.

I do, however, think that there are four situations in which the time and effort to do dream analysis is worth while:

1) For people who are undergoing psychological therapy or otherwise having psychological problems, regular dream interpretation may be advisable and very beneficial. The insights gained by both the dreamer and the therapist can be very good. Here the time and effort pay off well.

2) If you are having the same dream over and over again, dream interpretation is definitely called for. Recurrent dreams suggest that the emotional source of the dream is still present and unresolved and that there is a real need to do something about it.

Successful interpretation can break the cycle and help the dreamer deal with the underlying emotional source.

3) A third situation in which dream interpretation is worth the time and effort is for recreation and intellectual stimulation. Just as people enjoy mind games, such as Trivial Pursuit, for recreation, so too dream analysis can provide intellectual stimulation for fun. The general fascination that most people have with dreams can stimulate curiosity. As with other mental recreations, dream analysis for this purpose may also provide helpful, useful benefits.

4) A fourth situation is when a person is writing a book and needs examples for illustration. Serious scientific investigation of dreams and dreaming makes dream analysis worth the time and effort.

Conclusion

In my experience, most people who have seriously tried these methods of dream interpretation are impressed with how well they seem to work. Insights about themselves as well as people and events in their lives are commonly gained. Yet, the question remains if the interpretation uncovers the actual reason the dream was put together or if it is a projective, yet meaningful, response to the dream (Crick & Mitchison, 1983; Hunt, 1989).

Psychologists have long used projective techniques such as Rorschach Ink Blots and the Thematic Apperceptive Test (TAT) to gain insight into a person's personality. The comparison of the TAT to dream interpretation is particularly relevant. A person is shown an ambiguous picture and is asked to tell a story about it. People can easily do this. The stories vary considerably from one person to another because each individual "projects" their own personality into the story. That is, they tell the story in terms of things that they are familiar with and that are personally relevant to them. Perhaps we do the same thing when we interpret our dreams. The dream is a vague stimulus onto which we project our personalities and concerns when we do dream interpretation. The outcome may yield valuable insights but may have little to do with why we dreamed the dream in the first place.

I think both arguments may be partially correct. It does seem that our own dreams are related better to us than dreams from another person. There are people, things, and events from our waking lives that frequently are a part of our dreams. They are not totally random and abstract. The same seems to be true of the themes and story line. Yet, when we interpret our dreams we may read in more than was there originally. We embellish and expand. The end result may be very useful but not entirely faithful to the original intent of the dream.

Will we ever know if this compromise view is correct? Or if one of the other views is correct? Probably not because we have no way to know the original intended meaning (or, using Freud's term, latent content). There is no way to conclusively determine why our dreams are formulated the way they are and if interpretation accurately uncovers this formulative cause. The fact that dream interpretation "works" and we believe that it really leads to the actual source of dream content are inadequate for conclusive proof. So, we must make our decision based on intuition and incomplete facts, with a dose of skepticism thrown in. For me, the resultant choice is that the compromise is probably that true dream interpretation helps us discover the real meaning of the dream, but we also embellish and add meaning. The result can be very useful.

Sleep, Dreaming, & Sleep Disorders

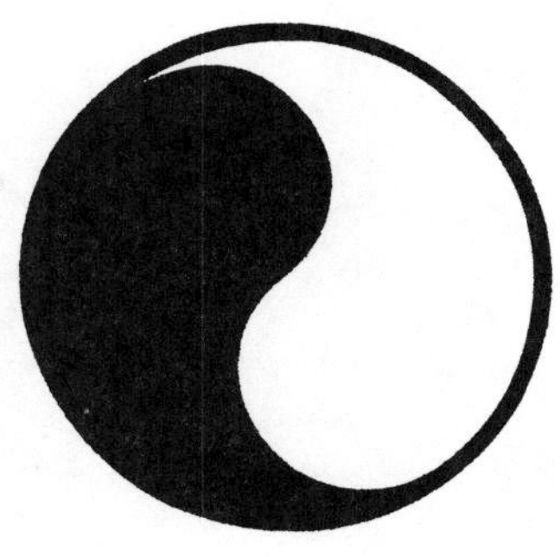

Section 3

Sleep Disorders

Chapter 9

Disorders of Sleep[1]

In the 1970s a new aspect of medicine evolved - sleep disorders. Previously, physicians, as well as lay people, knew that sleep could be problematic; however, knowledge of both the kinds of problems and the extent to which people suffered from them was limited, as was the knowledge of effective treatment for these problems. Insomnia, for example, has been well known for centuries, but knowledge of the number of different contributing factors to insomnia was minimal and treatment consisted primarily of prescribing sleeping potions and pills.

As researchers in sleep laboratories around the world began to learn more and more about normal sleep, interest in abnormal sleep grew. This knowledge of normal sleep provided necessary background for the study of the abnormal aspects of sleep. Thus during the decade of the 1970s sleep disorder centers were developed in many medical centers for the purposes of learning more about the disorders of sleep and to providing clinics for accurate diagnosis and effective treatment. The typical sleep disorders clinic in many ways resembles the sleep lab described in the prologue, since it contains the facilities to measure the nighttime (and daytime, if necessary) sleep of patients. In addition to the standard EEG, EOG, and EMG measurements used to assess the

---

1Thanks to Mark W. Mahowold, M.D., A.C.P., Director of the Minnesota Regional Sleep Disorders Center in Minneapolis for his very careful reading of an early draft of these chapters and many helpful suggestions.

states of sleep, other bodily functions during sleep are measured to aid in effective diagnosis.of sleep disorders. These additional measurements, and what they indicate, will be described as we progress through this chapter.

The typical sleep disorders clinic has technicians, just as the research lab does, and clinicians/researchers who are typically Ph.D.s and MDs. The Ph.D.s are most often psychologists or psychobiologists and the MDs are usually neurologists, psychiatrists, internists, and other related specialists. They meet regularly as a team to review and discuss patient histories and to confer on newly admitted patients about possible diagnosis and potential treatments. In addition, they usually meet once a week for about an hour with other interested professionals to discuss specific topics or patients in depth. These case studies, or "grand rounds" as they are sometimes called, provide a forum for sharing knowledge and ideas among the participants. In this chapter as several of the major sleep disorders will be presented as grand rounds case studies. Preceding this is an overview of the disorders of sleep.

Classification of Sleep Disorders

People show up at sleep disorders centers with one (or more) of three kinds of complaints: not being able to sleep, being sleepy during the day, or abnormal events that occur during their sleep. However, any one of these symptoms may have very different underlying causes. For these reasons, sleep disorders are usually classified and discussed by causes. There are three main categories of causes: dyssomnias, parasomnias, and sleep disorders associated with medical or psychiatric disorders. Unless otherwise noted, information for this chapter was obtained from the following sources: Anch et al, 1988; Association of Sleep Disorders Centers, 1979; Guilleminault, 1982; Guilleminault & Lugarsi, 1983; Hauri, 1982; Hauri & Linde, 1990, ICSD, 1990; Kryger, Roth, & Dement, 1989; Williams & Karacan, 1978.

Dyssomnias are problems with sleep that result in difficulties in initiating or maintaining sleep or result in being excessively sleepy. People with disorders of initiating or maintaining sleep are typically called insomniacs. However, that term is too vague. Some people have

The International Classification of Sleep Disorders

1. Dyssomnias
   A. Intrinsic Sleep Disorders
   B. Extrinsic Sleep Disorders
   C. Circadian Rhythm Sleep Disorders

2. Parasomnias
   A. Arousal Disorders
   B. Sleep-Wake Transition Disorders
   C. Parasomnias usually associated with REM Sleep
   D. Other Parasomnias

3. Medical/Psychiatric Sleep Disorders
   A. Associated with Mental Disorders
   B. Associated with Neurological Disorders
   C. Associated with Other Medical Disorders

From ICSD, 1990.

trouble getting to sleep, but once this is achieved, they sleep reasonably well. Others have no problem getting to sleep but have problems remaining asleep - either awakening many times during the night or awakening too early in the morning. Some people suffer from a combination of these problems. Those who suffer from being excessively sleepy do not complain of problems with sleeping at night, but rather of sleepiness or sleeping too much during the day. They spend much of their waking life fighting off sleep and suffer greatly in the process.

There are three subcategories of dyssomnias. *Intrinsic sleep disorders* have their primary source from within the body - either physiological or psychological. The *extrinsic sleep disorders* result primarily from causes outside the body. Removal of the cause usually resolves the sleep problem. *Circadian rhythm sleep disorders* are primarily related to a problem with the timing of sleep in the nychthemeron.

The parasomnias are problems resulting from things that occur during sleep that should not occur at this time and often cause distress when they do. Sleep walking, sleep talking, bed wetting, teeth grinding, and head banging are examples. Other parasomnias include problems like nightmares and night-terrors. Parasomnias have four subcategories. *Arousal disorders* are a result of partial (incomplete) arousal during sleep. It is as if parts of the brain mechanisms for sleep and wake are activated simultaneously or out of sequence. *Sleep-wake transition disorders* occur primarily during sleep stage transitions or transitions to wakefulness. *Disorders associated with REM* are parasomnias that occur in or start in REM. *Other parasomnias* are those that do not fit in the first three categories.

The sleep disorders associated with medical or psychiatric disorders occur in cases where sleep is a major component but is not the primary problem. Included in this category are people with major mental disorders (such as Schizophrenia, depression, anxiety, and alcoholism), neurological disorders (such as Parkinsonism, Alzheimer's, and Huntington's disease), or other medical problems (such as sleeping sickness, peptic ulcers, and emphysema).

A word of caution is in order here. As we examine these disorders and sample cases of them, you may recognize some of these problems as occurring in yourself or someone you know. Indeed, your observations may reflect a genuine sleep disorder that should be evaluated by professionals at a sleep disorder clinic. However, more often than not, you may be suffering from the medical student syndrome. Medical students sometimes begin to see, in themselves and others, many of the diseases and disorders they are studying, although in reality there is no problem. This happens because often there is no clear distinction between health and disease, but rather the difference is one of degree. So too with sleep disorders; everybody has had trouble sleeping sometime in their life or has had occasional sleepiness during the day without having a dyssomnia. Likewise, jet-lag is a frequent occurrence, but usually it is not severe enough to require a visit to a sleep disorder center. Only when the problems become excessive and debilitating do they become sleep disorders.

Dyssomnias: Intrinsic Sleep Disorders

Narcolepsy

It is 9 am Friday morning. About 15 people are seated around a conference table, most of them with lab coats on. In front of each place at the table are Xeroxed sheets of graphs and charts of data. At the end of the table, in front of one of the doctors, is a patient's record folder and a very large stack of polysomnograph paper containing the results of an all night recording of sleep. The doctor at the head of the table begins,

> *Today's case is a very interesting one regarding a woman who has had a considerably long struggle with narcolepsy.*
>
> *L.I.*[2] *is a 35 year old female who entered the clinic complaining of an increase in the severity of her narcolepsy symptoms. Recently, she reported becoming more and more sleepy with increased eye-lid drooping. Her symptoms first appeared as a teenager when she noticed a weakness in the knees when shooting free-throws during basketball games or on other occasions when she laughed at something funny. Eventually, she began to drop things she was holding, and her eyelids would often droop. Gradually, the symptoms became more frequent and more intense. When thinking back, she stated that she was always somewhat sleepy as a teenager but she began to feel sleepier during the daytime approximately the time she started college. Even after a long night of sleep she would fall asleep in class, at movies, after dinner, and at other quiet times. This began to affect her functioning, especially in social situations. The symptoms became worse if she became emotionally aroused, such as she would "pass out" while kissing.*

---

[2] All of the names used in this chapter are fictitious. The case histories are based on real patient histories with embellishments and additions for clarity and completeness. Many of the case histories presented were derived from the case histories of several patients.

Frequent visits to physicians provided no relief. She was diagnosed in the past as having a variety of physical problems, such as hypothyroidism and psychological problems. However, neither medication (she was at various times placed on thyroid hormone, tranquilizers, and other medications, etc.) nor psychotherapy provided any relief, and her symptoms gradually became worse.

At the age of 26, she was diagnosed as being narcoleptic. Subsequent to that diagnosis, she did find relief from various doses and kinds of amphetamines, but found that eventually the symptoms would return and that she would have trouble sleeping at night. About 7 months ago she had been put on a very high dose of Ritalin which helped at first, but prior to her admission to the sleep disorders clinic her symptoms were returning. She was obliged to take frequent naps, after which she felt refreshed. If she tried to "fight off" the need to nap, she would subsequently fall asleep in inappropriate places, such as at the dinner table. She has tried "sleeping-in" in the morning but is unable to do so.

About once a week, usually when going to sleep, but at other times when awakening, she reports hallucinations (called hypnogogic hallucinations) that are strong and frightening, such as someone in the room holding a knife about to stab her. Usually at these times she is unable to move for 1-2 minutes, even after awakening. If during this time someone touches her, her sleep paralysis quickly disappears.

In the past, she has experienced blackouts. She reports having periods of time for which she has no memory of what she was doing. For example, she noted several instances of driving home then suddenly becoming aware of having driven many miles past her home.

Both her father and grandfather were "nappers" and were very calm "unemotional" men.

In spite of her sleepiness, she succeeded in finishing nursing school even though she frequently fell asleep in class. However, overall the quality of her life has suffered. L.I. is an unemployed nurse, recently divorced with two pre-teenage children who live at home with her. She maintains that child support and alimony do not provide enough money and she needs to find a job, but her symptoms of narcolepsy have prevented her from finding and keeping one.

At times, although totally awake, she complains that she has experienced muscle weakness and even collapse, especially during times of emotional arousal such as dealing with her two pre-teenage children. This has forced her to avoid confrontations with them and try to "control" her emotions. As a result she is usually "emotionally flat." She appeared slightly depressed and desperate.

L.I.'s sleep was assessed in the lab for one night. Her sleepiness and characteristics of sleep during the subsequent day using the multiple sleep latency test (MSLT) were also assessed. The MSLT consists of 5 twenty minute sleep periods (naps). The first starts at 9 or 10 a.m. with the subsequent periods beginning every 2 hours. Both sleep latency and REM latency are measured for each nap.

Figure 9-1 shows the results of her night in the sleep lab. Comparison with the typical night of sleep of the young adult (Figure 1-3 and Table 1-2 in chapter 1) show several characteristic things. First, she experienced a hypnogogic hallucination with some sleep paralysis within the first few minutes after the lights were turned out and just when the polysomnograph showed she had fallen asleep. She reported a vague awareness of someone "lurking in the shadows" of the room and feeling very frightened but being unable to call out. Initially she began to move her eyes back and forth vigorously, then was able to move her eyebrows, next her nose and eventually her mouth. At this time she was able to call for help over the intercom. When the technician touched her arm she was able to move freely and describe the incident.

Second, she fell asleep quickly after the second time the lights were turned out and went into REM sleep almost immediately. This was followed by a relatively normal cycle of REM periods.

Third, her sleep was fragmented with more stage 1 and less stage 2 and SWS than is typical, as well as a high number of awakenings. All of this is reflected in a low sleep efficiency for her age.

The MSLT (Figure 9-2) likewise showed some unusual characteristics.During each nap period, she fell asleep very quickly

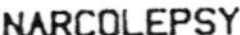

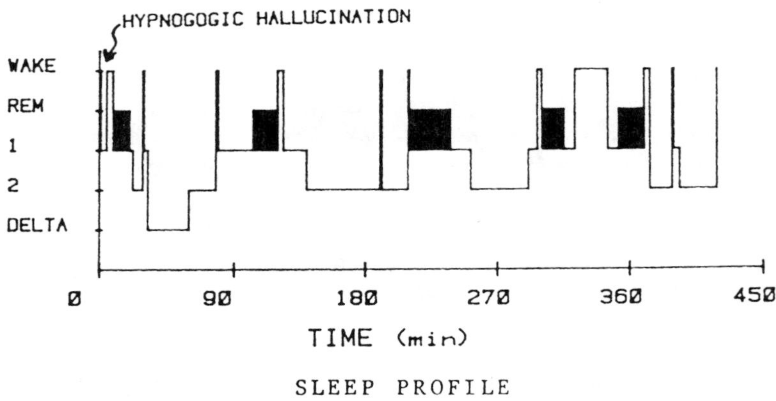

SLEEP PROFILE

Total Sleep Period(min)------------------- 351

Wake------	5%	Awakenings----------------	10
Stage 1---	20%	Sleep Latency(min)--------	2.5
Stage 2---	48%	Sleep Efficiency Index----	.81
Delta-----	8%	REM Latency(min)----------	18
REM-------	19%	REM Periods---------------	5

Stage Changes---------------62

Figure 9-1. The record of the sleep of L.I. - a person with narcolepsy.

quickly, in contrast to the normal pattern of taking over 15 minutes to initiate sleep. In addition, during three of her five naps she quickly went into REM. A normal young adult might, on a rare occasion, go into REM during one of the naps, especially an earlier one, but not during several of the naps.

These tests show that she is an excessively sleepy person who goes into REM prematurely, yet displays somewhat poor nocturnal sleep. These are all characteristics of narcolepsy.

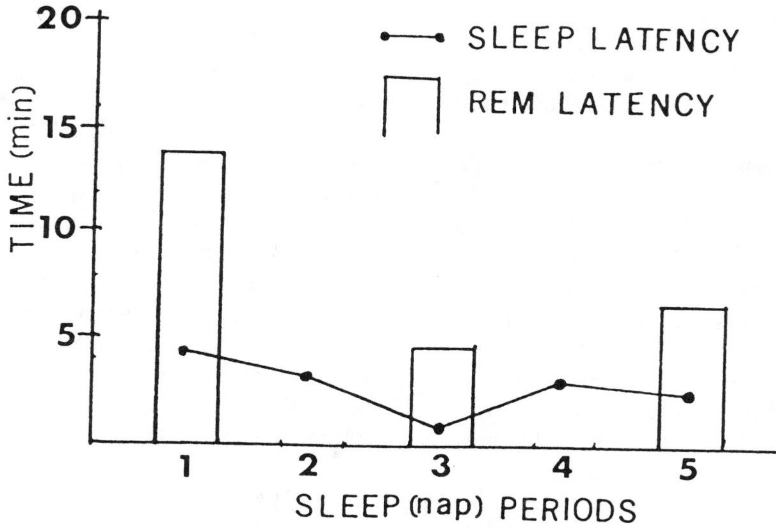

Figure 9-2. The results of L.I.'s Multiple Sleep Latency Test.

Treatment consisted of keeping her on amphetamines but more carefully following the changes in their effectiveness. In addition, instead of prescribing unusually high doses in order to continue to produce effects.. In addition, a second drug, imipramine, was prescribed to control her cateplexy (muscle weakness and collapse, and sleep paralysis).

Overall, this case is fairly typical of narcolepsy. The most common complaints are those of excessive sleepiness and sleep attacks that are irresistible even in arousing situations. The sleep may last up to an hour and be refreshing. People with narcolepsy report feeling perpetually drowsy. The next most common complaint is that of cateplexy, ranging anywhere from weakness in the limbs, face, or speech muscles to total collapse. Cateplexy is often triggered by emotions. During brief catepletic attacks a person is conscious, but longer attacks (over one minute) may quickly progress into sleep.

Hypnogogic hallucinations (or hypnagogic imagery) and sleep paralysis occur together or singly in almost one-half of people with narcolepsy. These hallucinations are vivid, brief, dream-like occurrences at entry to and from sleep that sometimes leave the person with a sense of fear or dread but may also be reenactments of a part of the past few hours. (Similar occurrences during emergence from sleep are called hypnapompic hallucinations.) Sleep paralysis is the inability to move that occurs on awakening or when attempting to fall asleep. Both of these types of hallucinations and paralysis these occur in normal individuals, especially children, but in much lower frequency than in people with narcolepsy. Other non-narcoleptic individuals may experience frequent occurrences of either hallucination or paralysis during sleep, although this is rare.

About one half of all people with narcolepsy report experiencing automatic behavior or black outs. During these episodes, a person may continue behavior associated with wakeful consciousness, but later have no memory of what they did. These episodes can last minutes or even hours. Naps, although inconvenient, are often refreshing to a people with narcolepsy.

Narcolepsy appears to be a problem of REM sleep. Cateplexy and sleep paralysis are the muscle paralysis of REM, while hypnogogic hallucinations are the dreams. REM occurring soon after sleep onset is not typical of normal adult sleep. The excessive sleepiness may result from overactive REM-on mechanisms in the brain or from the poor nocturnal sleep (frequent awakenings, less SWS, and fragmented REM) that has been shown to frequently (but not always) accompany narcolepsy. Blackouts are probably similar to sleepwalking.

Typically, narcolepsy begins to appear in the teens with sleep attacks as the first symptom, although onsets in younger and older people do occur. Over several years the sleep attacks worsen when cateplexy and other symptoms begin to appear and then become more frequent. Patients often report, however, that their problem has been unrecognized as narcolepsy for many years and that they were treated for many other problems or even called lazy.

Overall, narcolepsy impairs a person's life. Divorce is frequent, reflecting inter-personal complications caused by the symptoms. Likewise, the social life of people with narcolepsy is impaired, for they cannot go to movies, concerts, dinner parties, play cards, or participate in other "quiet" activities. The sleepiness of a person with narcolepsy even affects their participation in more active social events such as sports. Since catepletic attacks are likely to be triggered by strong emotions, people with narcolepsy tend to guard their emotions thus appearing dull and emotionally flat. Many have a history of being fired for falling asleep on the job, and people with narcolepsy frequently have had a number of accidents both while driving automobiles and on the job. They also complain of problems with their memories (which may really be a problem of paying attention). As a result of these problems they often are somewhat depressed, anxious, and frustrated. They are described by others as being unmotivated, withdrawn, and aggressive.

Many times people with narcolepsy, and people with other sleep disorders that render them sleepy during the day, are labeled lazy, bored, slothful, or depressed. They have difficulty getting sympathy and understanding from family, friends, teachers, and employers. Most of these people can relate stories of misdiagnosis and mistreatment by medical and psychological professionals that sometimes stretch out for years.

Narcolepsy occurs in over 5 out of every 10,000 persons. There are thought to be 250,000 people with narcolepsy in the U.S. today. There appears to be good evidence that it is at least partially inherited, but narcolepsy may also be caused by damage to the brain. At this time, control of symptoms with drugs - a stimulant for the sleepiness and other drugs for the cateplexy - is the only effective treatment. Monitoring of the person's drug levels by a physician is necessary. In some countries a drug called gammahydroxybutrate (GBH) is used to improve nighttime sleep, which lessens daytime symptoms. Several short naps (15-20 min.) also help reduce sleepiness. Psychological support and family therapy are also important.

Sleep Apnea

The subject of today's presentation is a 43 year old high school math teacher. R.P. came to the lab - or rather was pushed here by his wife (his third) - because of excessive snoring. During the interview he indicated that he has "always been a snorer." While in the service, his buddies kept threatening to throw him out of the barracks because of his snoring. His snoring got worse in his late 20's, coinciding with a 40 pound weight gain. He says that he is never aware of snoring because he is a very, very deep sleeper who awakens slowly and in a fog. The only time he doesn't sleep deeply is in a hot room. Even in a cool room, he will wake up with sweaty pajamas.

His wife reported that he sometimes snores so loudly that even when she goes to another part of the house in a desperate attempt to get her own sleep, she can still hear him "through closed doors and with a pillow over my head." She said his snoring has a gagging, choking quality separated by a minute or so of silence. She mentioned that he "flails around a bit" in his sleep sometimes hitting or kicking her. He blamed his snoring as part of the cause for his first two divorces and said he would like to get it under control before a third divorce happens.

When asked about his daytime alertness, he initially responded that he was about average. However, his responses to specific questions showed otherwise. During his teaching he found that he always had to be moving, such as standing at the blackboard. Even during tests he paced around. During teacher's meetings he often had to fight off the urge to sleep by sitting in uncomfortable positions. When grading papers he drank a lot of coffee, got up frequently, and sometimes splashed cold water on his face. Naps have never been refreshing for him.

He says that he doesn't attend movies, watch TV., or play cards, claiming to be bored by them. ("They must be boring because I always fall asleep!") He and his wife do bowl in a league once a week. He avoids long drives because of accidents he has had sleeping behind the wheel.

Interestingly, he later revealed that he used to coach basketball but had to give it up. "The practices were O.K. - I could keep moving around, but during the bus trips, in the locker room, and even during the games, I would drift off to sleep!"

R.P. is overweight by about 50 pounds. He appears to have no neck; rather his head continues straight down to his shoulders. He has a history of high blood pressure and heart problems (arrythemias). Otherwise, he appears to be in good health.

R.P. recalls that his father, who died of a heart attack at age 51, also snored heavily. In addition, his father appeared to be overweight and frequently napped.

R.P. reported trying several methods to stop snoring, including a special collar he purchased through the mail.

Nothing helped. He also related that he had tried hypnosis. When asked if that had helped he hesitated, showing a wry smile and replied, "Well, yes." When asked to elaborate, he continued, "The hypnotist gave me a post hypnotic suggestion - every time I would start snoring, I would turn over."

"And did it work?"

"Well, I spent the next three nights spinning!"

Subsequent to his first visit, we had his wife send a tape recording of his snoring. The tape revealed that he did indeed snore loudly, but that the snoring was intermittent, not continuous. Five or six snores were followed by a minute or so of silence. This continued over and over again with the first snore of each series having a gagging, gasping quality.

In the lab, R.P. was good-natured and even humorous. He fell asleep within 3 minutes of lights out (Figure 9-3) but awakened 62 seconds later with a gasping, snoring sound. This cycle continued throughout the rest of the night; as soon as he was in stage 1 or 2 sleep his breathing ceased then he would awaken a minute or so later gasping and snoring loudly. He woke 424 times in 433 minutes of the sleep period.

The profile of his sleep is very abnormal. In addition to the frequent arousals, he never reached SWS and had very little REM sleep. Most of his sleep was stage 1 with the rest stage 2. Time awake totaled about 1/5 of the sleep period. Sleep efficiency was low. Most of his arousals were accompanied by violent body movements.

Additional data on the breathing of this patient was gathered by electronically measuring the temperature of the air going into or out of his mouth. Exhaled air is much warmer than inhaled air. Further, breathing movements of the chest were assessed by measuring its expansions and contractions. The amount of oxygen in the blood was measured by a device called an ear oximeter that measures the color of the blood going through the ear lobe. Oxygen content can be determined in this way since oxygen makes blood more red. His sleep position was automatically recorded by placing a match-box size monitor on his chest.

These measurements confirmed that no air was entering or leaving his body between the bouts of snoring. This condition is called sleep apnea - the absence of breathing during sleep.

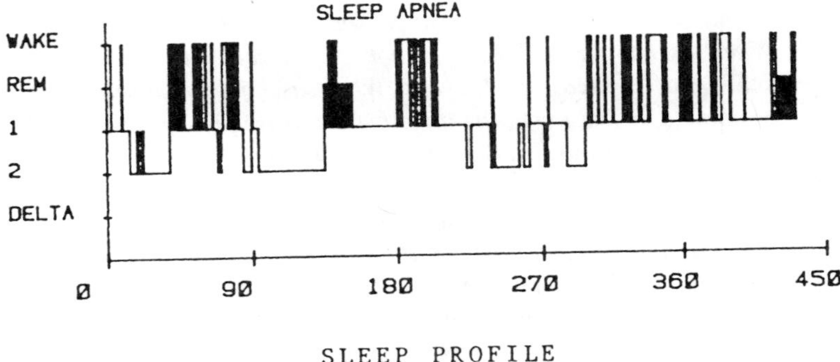

SLEEP PROFILE

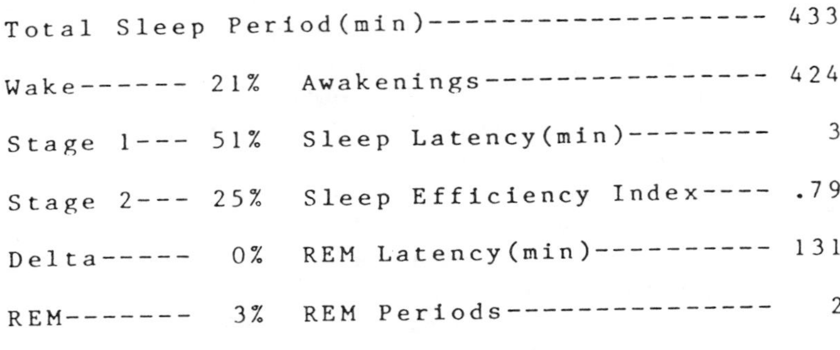

Total Sleep Period(min)------------------- 433

Wake------	21%	Awakenings----------------	424
Stage 1---	51%	Sleep Latency(min)--------	3
Stage 2---	25%	Sleep Efficiency Index----	.79
Delta-----	0%	REM Latency(min)----------	131
REM-------	3%	REM Periods---------------	2

Stage Changes---------------150

Figure 9-3. The record of the sleep of R.P. - a person with sleep apnea.

During most of these apnic episodes, his chest would be expanding and contracting - often more than when he was breathing successfully - but the air passages through the mouth and nose were blocked or obstructed. (At other times the air passages were only partially blocked, allowing some air to move in and out of his body but at well below normal levels. This condition is called sleep hypopnea - partial breathing during sleep.) The apnea plus hypopnea index (average number of apneas plus hypopneas per hour) was 57. The number of desaturations (when the level of blood oxygen fell 4% or more below what it was at the time of lights out) was 414 during the sleep period with a total duration of 108 of the 433 minutes of the sleep period. The average low value of oxygen saturation of the blood was 81% of its capacity with the lowest saturation reaching 58%. Normal percentages of saturation during sleep are in the high 90's and physiological consequences may occur at saturations of less than 88%.

R.P. stated the next morning that he had a typical night of sleep for him and thought he had awakened maybe 8 to 10 times. He did not feel refreshed and he had a headache. He asked if we could help him.

Treatment consisted of placing Mr. P. on CPAP (continuous positive air pressure). Each night he placed a small, soft plastic breathing mask over his nose. This mask was connected to a specially designed air pump placed close to the bed that was carefully adjusted so that air pressure would keep the throat open to allow normal breathing. A check with Mr. P. a few days later revealed a dramatic change. He said he felt alert and rested during the day. Although sleeping with the mask on was a bit uncomfortable, he loved it because of the rest he was now getting. And his wife said he was no longer keeping her awake with his snoring.

A few months later, R.P. spent another night in the sleep lab while using the CPAP machine. This time his sleep was essentially normal for his age. He showed few apneas and almost no oxygen desaturation. He stated his sleepiness during the day had almost disappeared. His blood pressure was also much improved.

R.P. displayed a severe case of obstructive sleep apnea. During sleep, the upper passages of the airways, typically the area around the base of the tongue, collapsed, thereby prohibiting the normal movement of air through them even though the chest was working hard. R.P.'s only recourse was to wake up regularly throughout the night in order to take several breaths accompanied by loud snoring as the air was forced through the narrow air passage, then return to sleep. Obviously, the result is very poor sleep. Little, if any, SWS occurs and REM is reduced, which thus results in excessive daytime sleepiness. Some people with sleep apnea complain of snoring, but only a few are aware of the frequent awakenings during the night. Those that do complain of the awakenings tell of the choking or suffocating sensations at such times which are accompanied by anxiety. Some patients show sleep apnea for only a part of the night or only in some sleep positions, such as on the back.

At least 1 of every 100 adults suffers from obstructive sleep apnea. Obstructive sleep apnea is at least 30 times more frequent in males than in premenopausal females and tends to run in families. Two thirds of sufferers are overweight and have thick necks. Sleep apnea is frequently accompanied in middle age patients by high blood pressure and various heart problems (arrhythmias). It gets progressively worse with time. The hypertension and heart problems may be caused, at least in part, by the fall in blood oxygen associated with the apnea, for the blood pressure increases dramatically during periods of apnea. Some people with long-term obstructive sleep apnea are in danger of dying in their sleep from heart failure during one of their apnic episodes. On the other hand, some people with obstructive sleep apnea, following successful treatment, show dramatic reductions of high blood pressure and heart problems.

People with sleep apnea may complain of other problems such as blackouts, automatic behaviors, night sweats, and morning headaches. They frequently maintain that they sleep deeply and are hard to arouse. They often awaken disoriented and "foggy headed". They may complain that they gag easily and that naps are not refreshing. Alcohol, antihistamines, tranquilizers, and sleeping pills make their symptoms worse. Some individuals may show symptoms only after having several alcoholic drinks prior to going to sleep.

Since sleep apnea has only been recognized since the mid 1970s, many people with apnea have a history of misdiagnosis and failed treatment attempts. Often they were simply called lazy or crazy. Because of the excessive sleepiness, they frequently have a history of divorce, multiple car accidents, and employment problems. It is not unusual for them to become depressed and irritable, because of the symptoms and also because of diminished sexual desires. Many also complain of concentration, judgment, and memory problems, as well as changes in personality marked by irritability and hostility.

CPAP has become the most commonly prescribed treatment of obstructive sleep apnea. In some cases other treatments are often tried first. Weight loss may be prescribed, especially in those patients who showed a dramatic gain in weight prior to the onset of the apnea. People who only have obstructive apnea when sleeping on their backs may be advised to try sewing a tennis ball into the upper back of their pajamas prevents them from sleeping in that position. Use of alcohol and other sleeping pills should be significantly reduced or eliminated.

Abnormalities of the upper airways, especially involving the throat, are sometimes found and surgically corrected in adults with obstructive sleep apnea. This type of surgical treatment is becoming more common for the treatment of obstructive apnea when other treatments fail, even if there is no outstanding abnormality. Abnormal constrictions of the respiratory passages are frequently found in children complaining of excessive daytime sleepiness. Surgery correcting the airway abnormality most often corrects the sleepiness at the same time.

Obstructive sleep apnea is not the only type of sleep apnea. Central sleep apnea likewise involves the cessation of respiratory air flow, but unlike the obstructive variety, the chest does not try to move air during the episode. In this type of apnea, the brain mechanisms controlling respiration seem to cease functioning until the person awakens briefly. Typically, people with central apnea do not snore excessively nor do they show the cardiac complications typical of obstructive apnea. Central apnea is much less frequent than obstructive apnea, but may be common in the elderly.

A third type of sleep apnea is called mixed. It is a combination of the central followed by the obstructive variety during each episode. It is treated as obstructive sleep apnea which, for some unknown reason, lessens the amount of both the obstructive and central components.

Sudden Infant Death Syndrome

A frequently asked question is, "What is the relationship between Sudden Infant Death Syndrome (SIDS) and sleep apnea?" That question cannot be completely answered at this time, but intensive research is ongoing to seek answers. What is known is that respiratory pauses and other irregular breathing patterns during sleep are typical of all infants. Some near-miss SIDS infants show more respiratory pauses and irregular breathing during sleep than is typical (Guilleminault, 1980). SIDS is viewed by some experts as a failure of the arousal mechanism to activate during sleep apnea. Further, some researchers have shown that adults with sleep apnea have a higher percentage of SIDS in their families. But SIDS may have many different causes, and sleep apnea may be but one factor. Near-miss SIDS and siblings of SIDS infants are sometimes evaluated in the sleep laboratory for sleep apnea. The risk of SIDS is highest after a few months of life and is virtually gone after the first year. Thus, the typical treatment for SIDS siblings and near-miss SIDS is to monitor the infant's breathing at home until 1 year of age with a device that sounds an alarm when an apnea occurs. The parents are prepared to deal with emergencies by training in infant CPR (cardio-pulmonary resuscitation).

Do near-miss SIDS and SIDS siblings tend to become adults with sleep apnea? Nobody knows, but long-term research on this significant question is in progress.

Idiopathic Hypersomnia

Some people are sleepier than others for no known reason. A few feel tired almost all of the time, and others sleep a great deal longer than the average. Some of these very sleepy people are classified as having Idiopathic (meaning not caused by something else) Hypersomnia. One such person is discussed in the following case study.

> *Today's subject, H.D., sought help at the Sleep Disorders Service because of excessive daytime sleepiness. She stated that she feels almost constantly sleepy, even though she averages about 8 hours of sound sleep per night plus a couple of short naps during the day. Life for her is a constant effort to stay awake. She always has to fight off sleep by keeping on the move and being active. As a single, self-employed beautician, she is able to both keep active and schedule a couple of naps per day for herself. She does little else other than work and sleep. Going to movies, playing cards, and watching TV. are impossible things. She first noticed the problem during her teens when she began to fall asleep in school and on quiet dates. Now 35, she has been maintaining her present schedule since her early 20's. She said her mother was sleepy a lot and napped frequently, too.*
>
> *She reports that she has had episodes of blackouts and automatic behavior. She states that she is a deep sleeper, seldom waking up during the night, and has even slept through a fire alarm, a breaking window in her bedroom, and a truck smashing into her apartment! When she does awaken in the morning, she does so spontaneously and with no problem. She*

suffers from occasional migraine headaches, but is otherwise healthy.

She kept a sleep diary for two weeks prior to sleeping in the lab. It showed a regular schedule of sleep of 8 hours per night plus frequent long naps. In the sleep lab she had about 8.2 hours of essentially normal patterned sleep. Latency to both sleep onset and REM were within normal limits. Her sleep efficiency was 0.91

During a Multiple Sleep Latency Test, she fell asleep during each of the 5 nap periods - very quickly on three of them - resulting in a mean MSLT score of 4.8. She showed no REM sleep during any of the naps. In short, she is a sleepy person during the day with normal sleep at night.

In the absence of any evidence of illicit drug use or known pathology, including narcolepsy or sleep apnea, not much could be done for her. Amphetamines and other stimulants were tried, but without success. In fact, some of these seemed to make associated symptoms, such as headaches and nausea, worse. Currently she is still taking naps and trying to fight off sleepiness by keeping active.

Idiopathic hypersomnia is not common, but it is striking when it occurs. It is not a result of insomnia, poor sleep, or other known sleep pathologies. It just happens. Most people with idiopathic hypersomnia resemble H.D.; beginning sometime between age 15 and 25, they feel almost constantly tired, but can resist naps. Short naps, when taken, are not refreshing, yet, without sufficient sleep, sufferers may begin to display automatic behavior, blackouts, and microsleeps. Most commonly, family members show a similar condition, although many report that they are unlike any relatives. They sleep deeply at night, but only slightly longer than average. They awaken easily and spontaneously in the morning.

Their sleep pattern is normal, but prolonged. However, they frequently are subject to fainting and migraine headaches. There is no known treatment.

Ideopathic hypersonmia needs to be distinguished from the long sleeper syndrome. Long sleepers may arrive at the sleep disorders clinic complaining about many of the same things as people with idiopathic hypersonmia, but careful history taking and polysomnographic testing reveal differences. Long sleepers need 10 or more hours of sleep per night. If they try to get along on less, they show the effects of continuous partial sleep deprivation (see Chapter 3), including excessive daytime sleepiness. This is shown both by their own subjective reports of a constant struggle to stay awake, multiple napping, blackouts and automatic behavior, and by a low average MSLT sleep latency. They usually report having difficulty arousing and often experience "sleep inertia" (foggy-headedness for a long time with confusions and commission of often impulsive and irrational, socially embarrassing or criminal acts; see chapter 10). They are hard to awaken and can be abusive and aggressive if awakened, even when they themselves have requested it. If they do get the 10 or more hours of sleep per night they require, the daytime sleepiness remits to normal levels. Prescribed treatment is usually simple - more sleep every night.

Periodic Limb Movement Disorder and Restless Legs

The next two cases present an interesting contrast. The problems that both patients complain about are caused by the same ailment, yet one complains of daytime sleepiness and the other of insomnia.

> *C.G. came to us complaining of lifelong sleepiness. He is a 54 year old insurance salesman who says he always remembers being sleepy - very sleepy. About 10 times per day the sleepiness becomes intense, with the most severe time around 1-2 in the afternoon. Naps, typically an hour in length, are not refreshing. When he awakens from either nocturnal sleep or a nap, his limbs feel heavy, as if he is still asleep. While some days are better than others, he never feels completely awake.*
>
> *As a self-employed insurance salesman, he is on the road a lot, but his sleepiness is beginning to cause him financial problems. While he has never been involved in a serious auto accident, he reports several near-misses caused by drowsiness. In order to stay awake, he almost constantly drinks coffee and colas. He reports that he is getting desperate and now must force himself just to do anything. His psychological tests support this. While not clinically depressed, he is very worried and anxious. When questioned about his night-time sleep, he did not report anything remarkable, saying only that he was a very sound sleeper.*

The second patient, E.C., is a 51 year old woman, who came to the clinic complaining of insomnia. She was without problems as a child but has had trouble sleeping as an adult, apparently getting worse in recent years. She has been a housewife much of her adult life, living with her husband and their youngest child, a 16 year old boy, and her 74 year old mother.

Her psychological tests show her to be depressed. She reports having to get up during the night to "stretch her legs" because of an uncomfortable feeling in them. When she does get to sleep, however, she says she sleeps very deeply, but awakens not feeling refreshed or rejuvenated. Her husband reports that she often shakes the bed during sleep and kicks off the bedcovers.

E.C. reports trying many things for her insomnia including many drugs, both prescribed and over-the-counter, but to no avail. Likewise, six weeks off caffeine was of no help. She exercises on an exercycle or plays tennis daily. She occasionally takes voluntary naps, which help. When trying to nap, she falls asleep quickly, but the creepy sensation in her legs awakens her every 10 minutes or so. Even when she is just sitting still, she feels the uncomfortableness inside of her calves and must get up every 15 minutes to walk it off. These sensations are getting worse as she gets older. They are also worse when she is tired.

She was not sure if her parents suffered from similar problems, but did remember that her father couldn't stand desk work and would rather have a job that kept him moving around.

The polysomnogram showed that Mrs. E.C. fell asleep quickly, but her sleep was punctuated with many, usually brief, awakenings. Most of these awakenings were caused by a series of leg jerks. These movements are very stereotyped (that is, identical to one another), abrupt contractions of certain lower leg muscles occurring about every half minute. The typical pattern was for early kicks in a series to disturb and lighten sleep, with only the later jerks causing actual awakening. Upon returning to sleep, the legs might be quiet for several minutes allowing sleep to proceed normally, but then the kicks would begin again, thus disturbing her sleep.

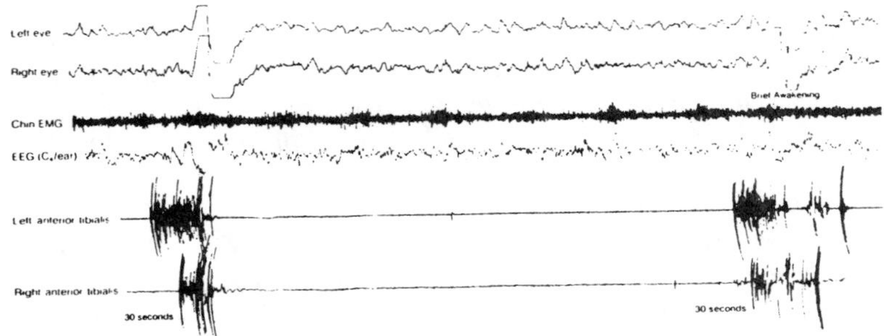

Figure 9-4. The polysomnographic record of an example of PLMD. (From Hauri, P., The Sleep Disorders, Kalamazoo, Michigan: The Upjohn Company, 1982. Used with permission.)

The pattern of kicks, measured by placing a pair of electrodes on the front of each leg half way between the knee and ankle, and the resulting sleep disruption, can be seen in Figure 9-4. The kick,s each lasting a few seconds, tend to come in bursts of 30 or more with 20 to 40 seconds between individual kicks. The quality and characteristics of the overall sleep pattern are not good, as can be seen in Figure 9-5. Note the high percentage of wake time and stage 1 accompanied by lowered amounts of stages 2 and delta. The number of awakenings is very hig,h as are the number of movements and stage shifts. Sleep efficiency was a very poor 0.70. During the 425 minutes of the sleep period, she had 353 kick,s with slightly more of them during REM. The next morning, she reported that her sleep was typical and that she felt tired and unrefreshed as usual.

Returning to the first patient, C.G., we see that his sleep showed a similar pattern (see Figure 9-6). Both the amount of time to get to sleep and the REM sleep latency were very long. This was caused by numerous awakenings and the poor quality of the sleep preceding REM (caused, in turn by many stereotyped leg and foot kicks). Thirty percent of his time in bed was spent awake and another 44% in stage 1 with only 10% in stage 2 and 8% in delta. Seventeen awakenings and 127 stage shifts punctuated his sleep, resulting in a sleep efficiency

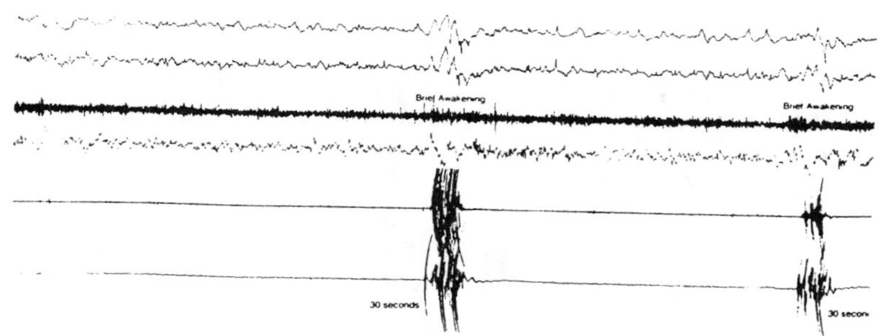

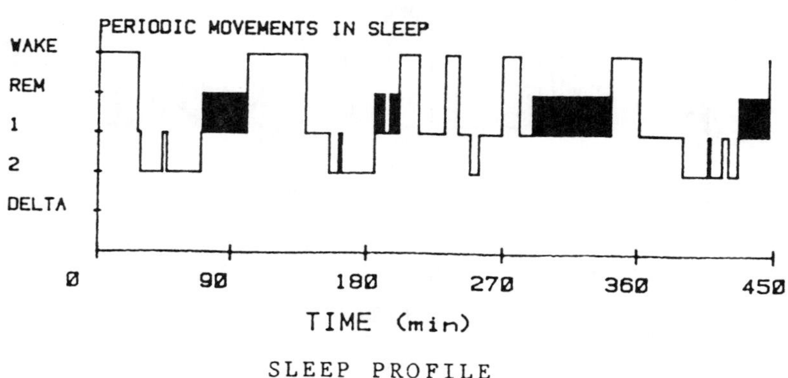

SLEEP PROFILE

Total Sleep Period(min)------------------ 425

Wake------	27%	Awakenings----------------	17
Stage 1---	24%	Sleep Latency(min)--------	26
Stage 2---	22%	Sleep Efficiency Index----	.70
Delta-----	0%	REM Latency(min)----------	46
REM-------	25%	REM Periods---------------	4

Stage Changes-------------- 82

Figure 9-5. The record of the sleep of E.C. - a case of PLMD.

of a very poor .52. He had a total of 228 leg jerks in his 439 minutes in bed.

When questioned the next morning, C.G. had no awareness of the many awakenings or leg kicks during the night and said that he felt about the same as on other mornings - needing to force himself out of bed.

Both of these patients suffer from periodic limb movement disorders (PLMD), formerly called periodic movements during sleep (PMS), or nocturnal myoclonus, but one of them complains of insomnia and the other of excessive daytime sleepiness. In addition,

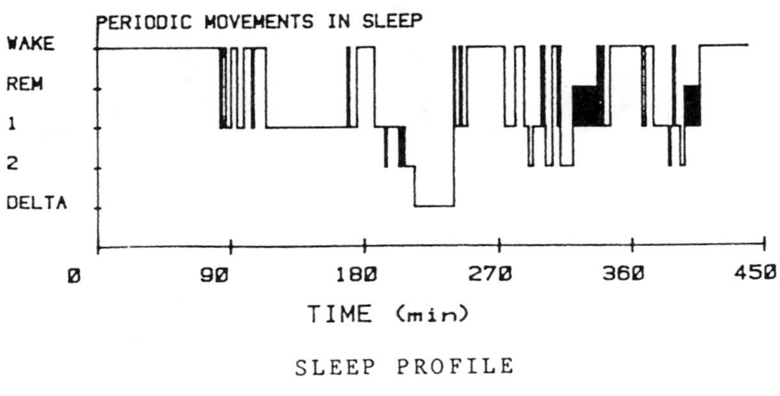

Total Sleep Period(min)------------------- 324

Wake------ 30% Awakenings---------------- 17

Stage 1--- 44% Sleep Latency(min)-------- 83

Stage 2--- 10% Sleep Efficiency Index---- .52

Delta----- 8% REM Latency(min)---------- 237

REM------- 8% REM Periods--------------- 2

Stage Changes--------------127

Figure 9-6. The sleep record of C.G. - another case of PLMD.

the second patient (E.C.) also had restless legs - the deep ache or "creeping" sensation in her calves. Restless legs often accompany PLMD. Neither patient was aware of the movements, and only the second was aware of the multiple awakenings caused by them. In both cases, however, sleep was seriously disrupted.

PLMD tends to run in families, where it is frequently associated with leg cramps. It is mainly seen in middle-aged and older persons, and tends to get worse with age, lack of sleep, stress or emotional upheaval. Over 40% of retirees have PLMD. A person may have PLMD every night or only occasionally. Although often occurring spontaneously, PLMD may be precipitated or caused by other medical conditions or drugs. Typically, both legs are involved, although it is not unusual for movement of other body parts to accompany the leg kicks. Kicks occur in clusters ranging from several minutes to hours, with individual movements of 1/2 to 5 seconds each occurring every 20 to 40 seconds. In some cases, only one leg kicks. Estimates have been made that PLMD accounts for up to 15% of insomnia and 7% of excessive sleepiness. PLMD tends to be more frequent early in the night, but it rarely occurs in REM. Yet,there are many people with PLMD that have no sleep problems.

People complaining of restless legs almost always also have PLMD (but many PLMD sufferers do not have restless legs). It is the creeping sensation inside the calves that occurs if the legs are stationary (sitting or lying) that necessitates the individual to keep moving and, thereby, may interfere with sleep onset. It is very disagreeable and relentless. The cause is unknown; no abnormality of the muscles, nerves, or blood has been observed in sufferers. Caffeine, warm rooms, exposure to cold, and pregnancy also intensify restless legs. Strangely, restless legs has been reported to disappear with fever.

The cause of both PLMD and restless legs is uncertain at this time. Exercise, stretching, and certain anti-convulsants have helped in some cases. More recently, drugs that deepen sleep, but have no effect on the kicks, have helped some sufferers obtain more satisfying sleep. Avoiding elements that intensify the conditions, such as stress or tiredness, is recommended.

Insomnia

Instead of a typical case conference, we will next attend a special symposium at the Association of Professional Sleep Societies (APSS) annual meeting, which has assembled a panel of experts on insomnia from 5 different sleep clinics (3 from the U.S., one from Vienna, and one from Denmark) to review and discuss insomnia. Rather than relating what each said verbatim, the following is a summary of the symposium. A moderator is asking the questions.

What is insomnia? Many have likened it to a fever. Just as a fever may be caused by many different things, insomnia is a symptom resulting from any of a number of causes. Just as a good physician would not treat a patient with a fever simply by prescribing aspirin, insomnia should not be simply treated with sleeping pills. Rather, it is important to discover, and then treat, the underlying cause or causes of the insomnia. Since insomnia may have various causes, it may be classified as a type of dyssomnia or as a type of sleep disorder associated with medical/psychiatric disorders.

How prevalent is insomnia? Surveys in the U.S. have shown that about 1/3 of all people report that they have some kind of trouble sleeping, with about 15% saying they have serious problems. Thus, about 35 million Americans label themselves as people with serious insomnia. But this varies with age and gender, with almost no complaints of insomnia in 8-10 year olds, but 90% in retirees and a greater prevalence in females than in males.

Is insomnia only having a problem falling asleep? No, insomnia may manifest itself in four different ways: difficulty falling asleep, difficulty staying asleep, awakening too early in the morning, and just generally poor sleep. Some people with insomnia may suffer from more than one of these four.

Figure 9-7a shows the sleep profile of an insomniac who has difficulty falling asleep. He or she lays in bed wanting to get to sleep, but remaining awake. Typically, we say that if a person takes longer than 30 minutes to fall asleep, **sleep onset** (long latency) **insomnia** has occurred. Less than 30 minutes is not considered insomnia.

Some people have no problem falling asleep, but are unable to maintain sleep throughout the night. Such a night of sleep is shown in Figure 9-7b, with several relatively long awakenings punctuating the sleep period. Specifically, we say a person has **sleep maintenance** (multiple arousal) **insomnia** if the person is awake for more than a total of 30 minutes during the sleep period and/or has five or more awakenings.

Others awaken earlier than desired from sleep, as shown in Figure 9-7c. In these people sleep onset is reasonably rapid and sleep continuity is good, but the length is inadequate. We say **early arousal insomnia** occurs when there is less than 6.5 hours of total sleep.

On occasion, a fourth type is seen. The problem here is not how much sleep is obtained, but how good it is. **Light sleep insomnia** is said to occur if the person has more than 12% of stage 1 sleep and less than 5% of SWS if 20 to 30 years of age, or less than 3% if 30 to 40 years old.

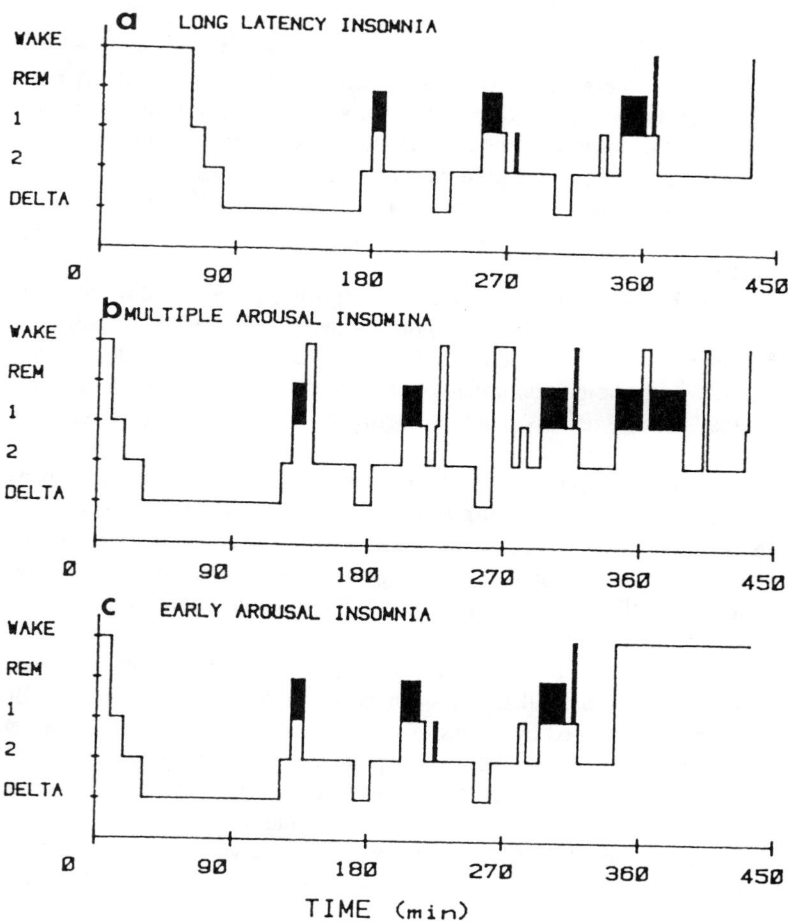

Figure 9-7. Sleep patterns of insomnia.

So, insomnia is a problem with sleeping? Yes, but it is also a 24 hour problem because, by definition, the person's waking life must also be affected by the troubled sleep. Usually this means complaints of depression, fatigue, or of being washed-out, as well as a lack of concentration and alertness. Some people think they are insomniac because they do not get the 8 hours of sleep per night that they have been told they need. However, rather than being insomniac these people are considered normal, naturally short, sleepers if they do not feel tired when awake.

Is anybody who meets these criteria is an insomniac? Yes, but duration of these problems also needs to be considered. Almost everybody has experienced a night or two of poor sleep, followed by a day or two of fatigue, some time in their lives. This may be caused by stress or excitement, hospitalization, sleeping in a different bed, or a host of other causes. This is called TRANSIENT INSOMNIA, because adequate sleep and alert days soon return. It is seldom a cause for treatment.

SHORT TERM INSOMNIA has a duration of several days to a few weeks. It often results from ongoing stress, such as school, work, or family problems, or a personal loss that takes some time to resolve. Usually once the person adjusts to the stress or the loss is adjusted to, normal sleep returns, but sometimes treatment intervention is beneficial.

When the symptoms of poor sleep with waking consequences persist for more than three weeks, it is labeled PERSISTENT INSOMNIA. In practice, many people with persistent insomnia have slept poorly and suffered the waking consequences for months or even years. It is these persistent people with insomnia that require, and benefit from, treatment.

Is persistent insomnia life threatening? Insomnia is not, by itself, dangerous. As compelling as sleep is for us, we are not seriously or irreparably damaged by a loss of it (see Chapter 2). It seldom causes physiological problems, yet it is frequently reported to be mentally and emotionally distressing, and can secondarily lead to grave consequences, such as automobile accidents and interpersonal problems in the family, on the job, and elsewhere. Usually, then, insomnia does not have as much of an effect on quantity of life as on quality of life.

Is there a simple treatment for insomnia? Insomnia is most often a symptom of some other problem. Thus, it should not automatically be treated as a disease, but rather used as an indicator that something else is probably causing the sleep disturbance, and the identity of that underlying problem should be sought and treated. On the other hand, in some cases, insomnia seems to be primary. But even in these situations, the treatment is similar to that used for secondary insomnia. Perhaps we should focus on the causes of primary insomnia and then on the treatments that can be applied.

What are the causes of primary insomnia? Typically, but certainly not always, the way insomnia manifests itself may give a clue to the cause. Sleep onset insomnia is associated with anxiety and/or over arousal of some kind. Depression, on the other hand, often results in early arousal insomnia, while maintenance insomnia is often linked with physical problems of some kind, such as sleep apnea or PLMD. The type of insomnia may thus give a clue to the most likely cause of the disturbance. However, insomnia can be caused by many other, more complicated, factors, which we will now explore. There are four major groupings of persistent insomnias - insomnia caused by medical problems, insomnia associated with psychological problems, insomnia associated with lifestyle, and primary insomnia.

Insomnia caused by medical problems. Some long term illnesses cause persistent insomnia because of pain and discomfort. But other relationships between illness and persistent insomnia are not so obvious. For example, sleep apnea and PLMD sometimes result in complaints of insomnia without any awareness on the part of the patient of their existence.

Psychological problems insomnia. One third to one half of people seeking medical help for persistent insomnia have a psychological problem as the primary cause. Both the more and the less severe psychological problems may affect sleep. Schizophrenics, for example, often complain of sleep onset problems and generally poor sleep. People with phobic disorders, anxiety problems, or those who are obsessive-compulsive, have sleep onset difficulties as well as some sleep maintenance problems. At the other end of the spectrum, continuing marital or job stress may also cause sleep difficulties. However, depression is the most common psychological problem causing persistent insomnia.

While about one out of five depressed people report hypersomnia, most of the rest complain of insomnia. Depressed individuals may have trouble falling asleep. However, they more commonly show sleep maintenance disturbances with multiple awakenings and early (premature) final awakenings. As a result, they feel achy and washed-out, although not really tired. Further, since REM predominates in the last half of the sleep period, depressed people are REM-deprived and show this by having much shorter REM latencies than normal. They also show reduced SWS, perhaps due to the REM pressure crowding out some SWS. The reduced REM latency is so dramatic in endogenously depressed individuals, that it is considered a biological indicator that a person is depressed, and may even be used as a very early sign of depression. Some of these disturbances of sleep tend to persist even when the behavioral indicators of depression are in remission.

Insomnia associated with lifestyle. For about one quarter of people with persistent insomnia, behaviors are the root cause. These are divided into two subgroups: persistent psychophysiological (about 15% of all people with insomnia), and insomnia as a result of substance consumption (about 12%).

Psychophysiological insomnia is often termed "learned" or "behavioral" insomnia because of the presence of maladaptive learning or behaviors incompatible with sleeping. There appears to be several subtypes.

Some people are chronically tense. When awake they tend to be restless, overactive, nervous, and apprehensive. It should not be surprising that such people also sleep poorly. Their general bodily tension carries over into sleep. In the laboratory, their sleep recordings may reveal higher than normal activity in the neck muscles, as well as other muscles, and their pulse rate tends to be high. They report and demonstrate numerous, sometimes prolonged, awakenings later in the night which are often associated with worried thoughts and anxious dreams. Often this results in reduced REM and SWS. Sometimes they also show sleep onset difficulties. They describe themselves as light sleepers.

These people are more fatigued than truly sleepy. They seldom nap, and when they do make attempts, they often fail to fall asleep. On the other hand, they tend to sleep better at the start of vacations. It is as if they feel they have permission to relax since they are on vacation.

Another subgroup of people with psychophysiological insomnia learn not to sleep! They have unconsciously learned to associate bedroom cues such as the bed, night clothes, etc., with not being able to sleep. Typically, these people will sleep better in a new and strange environment (such as a motel room), whereas most of us find we sleep a bit worse in a new situation. An extreme example of this was a student who, while mountain climbing, was forced to sleep on a narrow ledge tied to the rocks, yet had his best night of sleep in a year! This occurred because the sleeping situation was so different from his bedroom that he did not have enough learned associations to it to keep him awake. People with conditioned insomnia often report frequently falling asleep when not trying to, such as when reading, driving, or watching television.

How does learned insomnia come about? For most of us, the bedroom stimuli become cues to sleep. They are always present just before we successfully fall asleep, so we learn that when these cues are present, we will soon fall asleep. For the insomniac, however, something goes wrong. Perhaps, for a short period in their life something made sleep onset more difficult, such as excessive noise, poor weather, or emotional problems. For most people this is a temporary phenomenon and normal sleep quickly returns. But some individuals begin to unconsciously associate the bedroom cues with not sleeping. Even after the original cause is long gone, the learned insomnia remains because it is self-perpetuating. The bedroom cues lead to poor sleep onset and poor sleep onset occurs in the presence of these bedroom cues. So on and on it goes. Left untreated, learned insomnia seldom disappears on its own and usually gets worse.

In the third subgroup we find those people with insomnia who are their own worst enemies; they try too hard to fall asleep. When an individual consciously tries hard to do something, and works at it mentally, the brain is aroused. This arousal tends to oppose the brain mechanisms that bring on sleep. So, the person is trying to use the activated, wake brain to force the sleep control parts of the brain to induce sleep. Since the two oppose one another (see chapter 4), insomnia results. Frequent glances at the clock to see how long it is taking to fall asleep, calculations of how much sleep can be obtained before the alarm goes off, and concern about poor functioning the next waking day if "enough" sleep is not obtained, are often a part of this type of psychophysiological insomnia.

Substances and insomnia may be linked. Many psychotropic drugs (substances that affect behavior) also affect sleep. Almost without exception, the effect is to eventually reduce the amount, or disrupt the normal pattern, of sleep. Some substances may temporarily improve the amount of sleep (although they often alter the typical pattern of sleep at the same time), but their prolonged use has the reverse effect. It is like borrowing something now that has to be paid back later.

Sleeping pills are one type of substance that may cause insomnia. It seems a contradiction to state that substances advertised and taken to relieve insomnia actually are a major cause of it, but it is true. This is for two reasons.

First, by and large, sleeping pills work by reducing overall brain activity. In other words, they slow down the processes of almost all brain regions. But we know that sleep is not brain shut-down; rather it occurs when some areas of the brain become more active and dominant (see Chapter 2). At the same time these that substances are shutting down the wake areas of the brain, thus facilitating sleep, they are also diminishing the sleep control centers, thus *opposing* sleep, or at least normal sleep. The REM stage of sleep is usually the most severely affected.

Second, the brain, like the rest of the body, will attempt to compensate for the effects of some drugs that produce unnatural biological effects. Eventually (usually over a couple of weeks), a balance of effects - body compensation versus drug - will occur. This results in the drug losing its effectiveness. At this point, the person will typically do one of two things; either they will increase the dose, setting off a new effort by the body to compensate, or they will stop taking the now ineffective dose. If the person stops taking the sleeping pills, poor sleep usually results because the body's compensation mechanism is still ready to oppose the actions of the pill and reacts even though the pill is not there. Furthermore, whatever sleep is achieved becomes filled with vivid, intense dreams (REM nightmares, see Chapter 6), because the pill-suppressed REM is now rebounding. When the person is awake, restlessness and nervousness also occur. Often all of these effects are intolerable, and the person returns to the sleeping pill, if only to reduce the intensity of the withdrawal effects. (Perhaps you have noticed that this sounds much like narcotic addiction. You are right, because it is the same basic process!)

With continued, prolonged use, (say several months), the sleeping pill user has trouble with sleep maintenance and eventually even sleep onset difficulties. The maintenance problem occurs because the amount of drug in the blood is highest shortly after taking it, but this level gradually diminishes with time. Thus, toward the end of the night not enough is left to promote sleep, leaving the relatively stable level of the body's compensatory mechanisms to gain the upper hand.

The long-term user of sleeping pills may also experience many waking effects due to continued use of the drugs, such as poor memory, sluggishness, some loss of coordination, and speech slurring. These effects may take several days or weeks to disappear after the person is no longer taking the pills.

Finally, even when sleeping pills help a person to sleep better, the evidence that this sleep results in any benefits during the subsequent wake period is slight.

This is a very negative view of sleeping pills, as was intended, because these pills have been over-used and abused. However, prescription sleeping pills are safe and effective if properly used. First, they should be prescribed only for short periods of time or for only occasional use. They can be helpful for transient insomnia. At such times, use of prescription sleeping pills for a week or two is considered valid. Longer use should not be allowed, only for occasional use very special problems, such as persistent psychophysiological insomnia, PLMD, and insomnia from psychiatric disorders. They should never be used in patients with sleep apnea, in combination with excessive alcohol use, when pregnant, or by people who may have to be aroused and function during the night (such as firemen).

Second, preference should be given to a group of the newer prescription sleeping pills (the benzodiazpines) that seem to have less severe effects on the organization of sleep. These sleeping pills also have different lengths of time that they are effective, ranging from a few hours to a half a day or more, thus, the use of these pills can be more easily tailored to the needs of the individual.

Third, over-the-counter (non-prescription) sleeping pills are, at best, poor in producing sleep. In spite of the many different brand names and expensive advertising campaigns to convince us that each is unique and most effective, they are all very similar and relatively ineffective. A recent survey of drug store shelves shows that these sleeping pills all contain some kind of antihistamine, which is often also one of the main ingredients in cough medicines and decongestants. In some, the main ingredient is combined with other things such as aspirin. At best, they produce some drowsiness in some people, but at worst, they may easily produce troublesome side-effects. Side effects include constipation, a sense of weakness, and interactions with certain other drugs and alcohol. None are very powerful in producing sleep in any normal and consistent way. In carefully-worded advertising, the makers of these drugs do not promise that these drugs will make you sleep, but rather "induce drowsiness and assist in falling asleep" or that the use of them "relieves occasional sleeplessness." Most sleep professionals do not recommend them.

Finally, a word of caution: A person who is, and has been, habitually using sleeping pills, should seek medical advise and supervision before attempting to reduce or stop their use. As indicated above, the withdrawal effects can be severe and can cause real problems. Also, a physician may have some very good reason for wishing to keep a person on the medication. A person's personal physician is best able to determine this and to supervise withdrawal.

Alcohol is another substance that can produce insomnia. Alcohol severely disrupts the sleep of people who abuse it. Sleep will progressively disintegrate with continued, sustained alcohol use, resulting in a reduction of total sleep time, breaking up of REM periods, and less REM overall. Severe alcoholism can lead to a permanent, irreversible reduction of both REM and SWS. Sudden abstinence in alcoholics usually results in severe sleep onset problems, sharply reduced SWS, and a dramatic increase in REM. This withdrawal pattern typically lasts 10-14 days after the last bout of drinking. Even a single night of partying in anyone, alcoholic or not, that includes excessive use of alcohol, can disrupt sleep for several succeeding nights.

Even when not abused, alcohol can disturb sleep. For many people, a small amount of alcohol is taken either regularly or occasionally to hasten sleep onset, and it often works. However, the resulting sleep is altered, especially in the first half of the night. A person with alcohol in their blood will toss and turn more frequently during sleep. Additionally, alcohol reduces the amount of REM during sleep, with REM rebound following cessation of intake. Alcohol, however, does increase total sleep time.

People also use substances to keep themselves awake and alert - drugs such as amphetamines and substances such as coffee. Some weight reduction agents have the side effect, of increased arousal. Depending on the amount used, length of use, and individual susceptibility, the user may suffer various degrees of sleep disturbance. These include sleep onset delays, less total sleep time, reduced delta and REM, and, with continued use, sudden daytime sleepiness. Some coffee drinkers are so sensitive to caffeine, that even one cup in the morning may disturb the subsequent night of sleep.

Idiopathic insomnia. In about 5% of persistent insomnia cases, the cause is not easily attributed to medical or psychological problems, or to life style. In such cases, the insomnia is considered idiopathic. One example is childhood onset insomnia. The name is an adequate description: the person has had insomnia all of his or her life and for no apparent reason. However, it is presumed that there is a malfunction of the sleep/wake mechanisms of the brain. Sometimes hospital staff or parents note the remarkable lack of sleep in these people even as babies. Their memories of childhood are of long, lonely, sleepless nights followed by days of struggle, constantly fighting off fatigue. In many, neither sleeping pills nor stimulants are of much help. Extensive medical examination and testing during the person's life do not uncover any physical or psychological problems causing the sleeplessness. Often these people show both onset and maintenance sleep problems, and the sleep they do get is light (easily aroused, reduced delta, and reduced REM).

Sleep State Misperception. There is a final group (about 7.5%) of people that complain of persistent insomnia that need to be mentioned. While subjectively they think they have insomnia, they fail to meet criteria. Some are simply short sleepers who are worried because they have heard that healthy individuals need 7 to 8 hours of sleep per night, but they get much less. The key is that they do not suffer waketime sleepiness or fatigue. Their short sleep is adequate.

Others of this group have waketime complaints of tiredness and fatigue and all of the disruptions to life that result from insomnia. However, their sleep length and sleep profile are entirely within normal limits. Although it is typical for people with insomnia to underestimate their sleep time and sleep efficiency while overestimating their sleep latency, they, nevertheless, do not have normal sleep. With this group, however, there are no objective indications of poor sleep. In the past they have been labeled "pseudo insomniacs", but sleep state misperception is now the accepted label. Some sleep disorders experts have speculated that their insomnia is real ,but that we have not discovered what to look for or to measure in them. Another believes that, "they think all night long," and that such mental effort is fatiguing rather than restful. In any event, many of these patients report waketime benefit from the same treatments as other people with insomnia, even though such treatments make no change in their sleep as measured in the laboratory.

Just what are the treatments for insomnia? The treatment of insomnia depends on its cause. However, the cause of insomnia in any individual is usually some combination of factors rather than a single one. For this reason, the discussion of treatment for all causes of insomnia is combined. The final treatment package is put together by carefully selecting from among a number of possibilities and tailoring them to each individual.

First, any possible physical (medical) cause of the insomnia must be eliminated. We have not discussed the multitude of bodily ailments that can interfere with sleep, since that would carry us too far from our main purpose. However, the possibility of any of these being present must be eliminated when treating insomnia. This can be done by a routine physical exam, plus any special medical tests for suspected problems.

One or two nights of sleep should be measured in the sleep lab. This helps identify hidden problems, such as PLMD or sleep apnea. Further, the true (objective) nature of the person's sleep can be assessed and compared to the person's subjective analysis of his or her sleep. The pattern of the sleep problem can be objectively observed by experienced personnel. For instance, a rare, but important, insomnia occurs when the person awakens every time REM begins. This pattern can only be discerned in the laboratory. (Not all sleep disorders experts agree that polysomnography should routinely be done on people with insomnia. They believe that it is too expensive and often unnecessary, since the causes of the insomnia can be determined without it in many cases. Others counter that PLMD and apnea often cannot be discovered without overnight laboratory study and applying treatments appropriate for other causes of insomnia that provide little benefit for PLMD or sleep apnea is a waste of patient time and money, and only prolongs the misery until the real cause of the insomnia is discovered and treated.) A reasonable compromise is to do polysomnographys and MSLTs with patients that do not initial treatments for insomnia.

Second, the insomniac should be asked to tell what their sleep was like previously and to describe any differences between good and bad nights of sleep including differences in the wake period that proceeded such nights. Then they should wear an Actigraph (see Chapter 4) keep a sleep log or diary for a few weeks. An example of such a log is shown on the following pages. Most sleep logs include such things as time of going to bed, amount of time to get to sleep, number and duration of awakenings, quality of sleep, level of daytime wakefulness, naps, etc. There are two reasons for keeping the sleep log: it indicates to the sleep clinic personnel the sleep pattern, as well as the type and degree of insomnia from which the person is suffering. But more importantly, it also makes the sufferer more aware of their sleep patterns. Often people are not aware of how much they nap or of how irregular their bed times and wake-up times are. Sometimes this greater awareness is almost enough for the insomniac to realize what is necessary to sleep better at night.

Third, reduce personal problems. The major cause of insomnia is psychological. Direct treatment of psychological disorders or problems by a counselor, nurse, psychologist, psychiatrist, or other specialist is often the best way to improve the sleep of some people with persistent insomnia.

Fourth, educate the insomniac about sleep. Frequently, sufferers have poor knowledge about sleep. Some of the information in chapters 1 and 2 about sleep (especially its changes with normal aging and our propensity to sleep during certain parts of the nychthemeron) may be new to them. This information can lead to a change in attitude about sleep and then to a change in behavior.

Especially important is the knowledge that getting to sleep involves two brain circuits - one for arousal and one for sleep. Getting to sleep requires an increase of activity in the sleep circuit *and* a decrease of activity in the arousal circuit. However, the activity in the arousal circuit is easier to increase than that of the sleep circuit. It can quickly become active (by noises, thoughts, and so on), but only gradually quiets (taking several minutes). It is necessary to provide time and opportunity for the arousal circuit to become quiet. Many times people with insomnia need to focus their efforts here.

For some, a set of "sleep hygiene" rules to follow may be necessary and helpful. A typical set of hygiene rules can be found in the box on page 360.

Fifth, it may be necessary to change the insomniac's attitude about sleep. Some people have a "bad attitude" toward sleep:

"Everybody needs 8 hours of sleep per night."
"The best sleep occurs before midnight."
"I know I'll be a wreck the next day if I don't get enough sleep."

These are some of the misconceptions that people with insomnia often have. Changing these (and any others) will frequently ensure better sleep (by reducing the overall level of anxiety) and encourage a

SLEEP LOG

Day & Date	Bedtime Mood write a number from 1 to 10 where 10=very good & 1=very upset	Drugs Taken	Notes- important events of the day	Bedtime (the time you turned out the the lights

Name: ____________________

Estimate length of time to fall asleep	Number of awakenings during the night	Morning awakening time	Total sleep time	Wake-up mood, 1 to 10

Sleep Hygiene Rules

1) Provide for a safe, comfortable, and regular place to sleep that includes:
   a) a good mattress of ample size;
   b) measures to reduce noise and light. Loud noise or light may disrupt sleep even if you do not awaken;
   c) measures to provide appropriate temperature and humidity. A moderate - not excessively warm or cool or humid or dry - room allows the best sleep;
2) Use the bed only for sleep. (We will allow sex too, but in more severe cases one might have to move sex to a location other than that used for sleeping.)
3) Develop and use good presleep rituals such as reading, brushing teeth, putting on pajamas, and so on. They serve as a clear divider between waketime and sleeptime.
4) You might try eating a light snack before sleep. It may prevent hunger from disturbing sleep.
5) Lie down only when sleepy and desiring to sleep.
6) If sleep does not occur within a reasonable length of time, get out of bed and go to another room. Do something else, preferably something quiet like reading or watching TV, for a while. When sleepiness occurs, try the bed again. Repeat this as many times as necessary.
7) Get up at the same time each morning! This is both difficult and important. Difficult, because when one is finally asleep, one would like to get as much sleep as possible in order to not feel tired during the waking hours. But remember, the goal is a long-term one, to relieve the insomnia, not to get just a single night of good sleep. That is, the insomniac may have to live through some miserable nights and days now, in order to have better sleep in the future. Pay now, sleep later. Regimen is important, because a regular time of awakening is vital in helping the body acquire a good sleep/wake rhythm (see Chapter 4).
8. Sleep enough to feel refreshed but not more. Too much time in bed can cause problems with sleep quality and waking alertness.
9. Avoid "Sunday night insomnia/Monday morning blues" by not staying up late on weekends and then sleeping in.

positive outlook the next day, regardless of the length of the previous night of sleep. This may be accomplished by encouraging the person to talk to themselves about their own sleep. This is done by having the person record or write down their comments about sleep and then redefine the negative statements such as:

"I'll never sleep well."

"I cannot get to sleep the night before an important meeting."

"Sleep is a waste of time, but I cannot do without it."

to positive comments:

"Everybody, including me, can sleep well."

"Maybe it will take a little longer, but I can get to sleep and sleep well before an important meeting."

"Sleep takes time and is necessary, so I'll just enjoy it."

The person must practice these positive comments aloud several times during the day.

Sixth, make changes in daytime activities. For some people, what they do (or don't do) when awake has an effect on how they sleep. There are a number of things that may be hindering the sleep of individual people with insomnia - many of which may not effect the sleep of other people. They may exercise too vigorously prior to going to bed. Or they may not get enough aerobic exercise when awake. Perhaps they are too tense and on the go all day long to be able to relax enough when they desire to sleep. Maybe there is too much unmanaged stress in their lives. They may nap too much. Their eating or drinking habits may hinder sleep. Maybe they take in too much caffeine, alcohol, or nicotine. The goal is to discover, and then to alter, those things unique to the individual that may be contributing to the sleep problems.

Seventh, some people with persistent insomnia need to learn how to relax. In some cases this means to relax the body. In other cases, it means to relax the mind. Most people will find that they will need to learn both.

There are a number of relaxation methods: abdominal breathing, meditation, imaging, hypnosis, and so on. The following is a description of progressive relaxation that has been helpful for many. Essentially, you should find a quiet, comfortable spot where you can stay undisturbed for about 20-30 minutes. The exercise starts with controlled, rhythmic breathing. This helps relax your body and causes you to focus on relaxation instead of other concerns. Now do a series of tension-relaxation cycles in which a group of muscles (say, lower leg) are made as tense (contracted) as possible for several seconds, then are allowed to relax. For example, start at the head and work down to the toes, or vice versa. Concentrate on the muscle group, notice how it feels when contracted, then especially notice how it feels when subsequently relaxed. The purpose here is both to relax the muscle and to get you to feel what a relaxed muscle is like. Done correctly, you will not go back to the original relaxed state of the muscle, but beyond to an even more relaxed level. Repeat this with other muscle groups until the entire body is relaxed. After consistent practice with this technique, you should be able to automatically reproduce the relaxed state all over your body at any desired time without having to start with the tension. You will know what total relaxation feels like and be able to produce it. But this only occurs after several weeks of consistent practice. After learning this, you can produce relaxation whenever convenient, including when trying to get to sleep.

Once you have mastered body relaxation, you can begin mind relaxation techniques. Prepare ahead of time by picking two or three scenes that seem very relaxing to you. My favorite is lying on a seaside beach with a warm sun, a gentle breeze, and the sound of waves breaking on the sand. Go through one of these scenes in great detail, trying to notice all of its elements with all of your senses. When you have done this (it even helps to write them down) ,then you are ready for implementation.

Find a comfortable, quiet location. Totally relax your body and begin slow, rhythmic breathing while focusing on a single image. When you feel that your body is relaxed (don't hurry), then imagine one of your pleasant scenes in detail. Enjoy the relaxation that is occurring. When other thoughts intrude, don't worry about them. Let them drift away as you return to your scene. Likewise, go through your other scenes. After 20 to 30 minute slowly get up, stretch, and return to your day more relaxed and calm.

When you have mastered this during the day, you are ready to begin using it at night to help you fall asleep. As you imagine your scenes let them fade away as you drift off to sleep.

Another technique that may be helpful to some people is to schedule "worry time". For some people, problems and concerns seem to pop into their minds when they want to go to sleep. This keeps them awake. It is better to schedule a half hour or so in the evening (but not just before bedtime) to worry. During this time, first write each worry as it pops up onto a separate 3 x 5 card. This done, now make 3 to 6 categories of the worries by placing the cards in piles. Now, go through each group and write down a solution. If a solution is not possible, then write a comment such as, "I'll worry about this next week" or " I have no control over this" or "I can do something about this next month" or "This is now up to John" or "This is serious, so I'll seek help." Finally, put the cards away to look at in the morning.

If when attempting to go to sleep, a worry comes up, say, "I have worried about that. It's taken care of." or "I forgot to worry about this, but I can do it during my next worry time. Goodnight." The idea is to think of and deal with problems when the mind is fresh and can do something. This clears the deck for sleep.

Eighth, some individuals need extra help in order to learn how to control their bodies to enable them to sleep well. A special technique that helps them to do this is biofeedback.

Biofeedback requires two things in addition to yourself - first, special equipment. There are many things going on in our body of which we are not aware. Our blood pressure is a good example. We have no sensors in our body to tell our conscious brain what our blood pressure is. Without these sensors, our conscious brain has little ability to control blood pressure, since it receives no information (called feedback) telling it if it has been successful in its control. Blood pressure, however, can easily be measured by a machine, and the results of the measurement given to the brain via sight or hearing (such as a tone that gets higher in pitch as the blood pressure gets higher). Now the brain has information, or feedback, that it can use to change blood pressure. The whole procedure - a machine that measures changes in our body, providing this information to our brain in rapid succession, and allowing the brain to control what the machine is measuring - is called biofeedback.

The second thing necessary for biofeedback to be effective is a trained professional to operate the equipment. Careful placement of sensors on the body is required, as is attention to the setting and adjustment of the machine. The professional also helps the individual with the learning process - giving hints, assistance, and controlling the pace. Typically, it takes several sessions of one-half to one hour each to achieve mastery at a biofeedback task. Like many skill-learning tasks, we only need a lot of feedback information while learning, but eventually can perform the well-learned task with little feedback.

Biofeedback can help sleep directly. For example, certain brain waves (sensory-motor rhythm, or SMR, that come from the forebrain) are thought to be part of the process producing sleep, or at least are caused by the sleep-inducing process. Some people have learned to produce SMRs in a laboratory using biofeedback. Eventually, they could produce them even without getting feedback from the machine. These people then were able to transfer the use of this skill to the bed at night - again without being hooked up to the feedback machine - and found that they were able to get to sleep faster and better. However, SMR training is difficult to administer and tedious to learn.

Another example, that has a more indirect effect on sleep, is the use of muscle tension biofeedback. Some people need more than progressive relaxation techniques in order to learn how to relax their muscles. Muscle tension biofeedback can help them gain that ability, which they later can use when trying to fall asleep.

Ninth, an even more interventive therapy for persistent insomnia is called Sleep Restriction Therapy. The key is sleep efficiency. Insomnia means a lot of time in bed not sleeping, which results in lower than normal sleep efficiency (see Chapter 1). Sleep restriction therapy reduces time in bed to around five hours until a better sleep efficiency (.90 or greater) is captured. Then, while maintaining this good efficiency, time in bed is gradually increased in 15 minute increments until sufficient duration and quality of sleep is a regular occurrence. Sleep restriction therapy has proved to be very beneficial in the long run to those people with persistent insomnia who have stuck with it. They had to endure a few weeks of suffering from even less sleep than they had been getting.

Tenth, sleeping pills can play a helpful role in treating people with persistent insomnia, if used wisely. Having a few short-acting sleeping pills in the drawer for occasional (infrequent) "use after several miserable nights", can provide a great deal of psychological relief and support for the insomniac. And perhaps occasionally actual, beneficial sleep during difficult times. However, caution needs to be taken so that they are not used too frequently.

Finally, insomnia may be difficult to treat. The multitude of possible causes and interactions among the causes make it difficult to know which combination of treatments to apply and in what order. Further, it is often difficult for people with insomnia to completely follow through with the treatment because success normally takes several weeks, and the sleep problem may get worse for a while before improving. But successful treatment is possible and should, by all means, be attempted. A very helpful strategy is to enlist the aid of the patient in developing a treatment plan. Make them a partner (i.e. responsible) in, rather that a recipient of, the treatment.

Dyssomnias: Extrinsic Sleep Disorders

These disorders range from sleep problems resulting from poor sleep habits, sleep disturbing environments, and assent to high altitudes, to acute stress and food allergies.

Also, sleep disorders resulting from being dependent on alcohol, stimulants, or sleeping pills fall under this classification. They will not be discussed further here, because they are all fairly obvious and are similarly treated by removal of the extrinsic factor.

Dyssomnias: Circadian Rhythm Sleep Disorders

The following is a case of a man with a circadian rhythm sleep disorder.

W.N. is a 20 year old student living in the dorm at a nearby college. He was reasonably alert and energetic, yet looked tired. He was 20 minutes late for his 11 AM appointment.

He described his problem as insomnia. "I just can't get to sleep." The problem started this semester (he was midway through the first semester of his junior year) when he had to take a required course only offered at 8 AM. He said he was lucky when he started college to have no early-morning classes. He could "take advantage of college dorm life" at night without having to worry about getting up early. As a result, he typically went to sleep between 3 and 4 AM - later on weekends. After that, he carefully selected his courses in order to avoid those that met early in the morning - until this semester.

Because he could not get to sleep early enough at night, he had missed many of his 8 o'clock classes, since he "just could not wake up." He had repeatedly tried going to bed at midnight, but just laid awake for several hours. He had tried "everything", including: warm milk and graham crackers, sleeping pills, herbal teas, exhaustive exercise, alcohol, a dull textbook, and, on the advice of a friend, facing his bed due north to get the "proper magnetic pull" on his brain. Nothing worked. He was desperate because when he did get up after only a few hours of sleep, he was so "wiped out" that he got little out of the 8 o'clock lecture. He actually has fallen asleep in the class several times. He has missed so much that his professor is threatening to drop him from the course.

Upon questioning, he related how weekends and breaks were his salvation, because he slept in until mid-afternoon. When asked when he felt most alert, he immediately and emphatically stated "in the evening - once I make it past supper, I'm O.K." He scored 15 on the Smith, Reilly, and Midkiff (1989) questionnaire, which classifies him as a strong evening type. His psychological tests were within normal limits.

His polysomnogram showed a sleep latency of 233 minutes (lights out at 23:30 hours), but otherwise normal sleep for his age, other than a high normal amount of SWS, indicating a possible sleep deprivation. He awoke without much difficulty at 10:30 when called over the intercom by a polysomnographic technician who needed to analyze his sleep record before an 11:30 appointment. He said this was a typical night as of late.

It was apparent that W.N.'s problem was not insomnia, but phase delay disorder (see Figure 9-8). He could fall asleep only when his body was in it's circadian primary sleepiness zone (see chapter 4), which occurred after 3 AM. His body stubbornly refused to advance that zone when he went to bed earlier, thus he was unable to get to sleep. But he is not a sleep onset insomniac for two reasons. He falls asleep easily if he goes to bed around 3 AM, but he has much difficulty arising before 10 AM.

He was treated with chronotherapy. Chronotherapy consists of having the person go to bed 3 hours later each day or two, and getting out of bed after exactly 8 hours later, no matter what time of day or amount of sleep obtained. No napping is allowed until the next bedtime. This delay of sleep each "day" is greater than the person's typical phase delay, and thus, sleep onset is rapid and sleep is sound. This regimen seems to allow the person to recapture control of sleep onset an,d after about 8 days, the person is usually able to establish and maintain a normal, stable bedtime in the late evening and arise regularly mid-morning. The treatment was successful and he passed his course.

People with delayed sleep phase syndrome resemble people with insomnia in that they seem to have trouble getting to sleep. But unlike people with sleep onset insomnia, they fall asleep about the same time every night. Thus, if they go to bed at this time, they have no problem falling asleep, but if they go to bed earlier, their sleep onset problems occur. Furthermore, they tend to have problems awakening before a certain, relatively fixed clock time. Thus, they are on a stable 24 hour rhythm and their actual sleep times are at the same clock hours every day. It is just that these clock hours are delayed from those desired by the person or demanded by the person's environment.

These people can be considered extreme night owls. No amount of will power or sleeping pills are able to help. These people show peak alertness and efficiency only late in the day. The problem often starts in childhood perhaps with late-night study habits or illness. It does seem to run in families, suggesting that some people may be more prone to develop it. Chronotherapy is an effective treatment for these sufferers, as is the more recently developed light therapy.

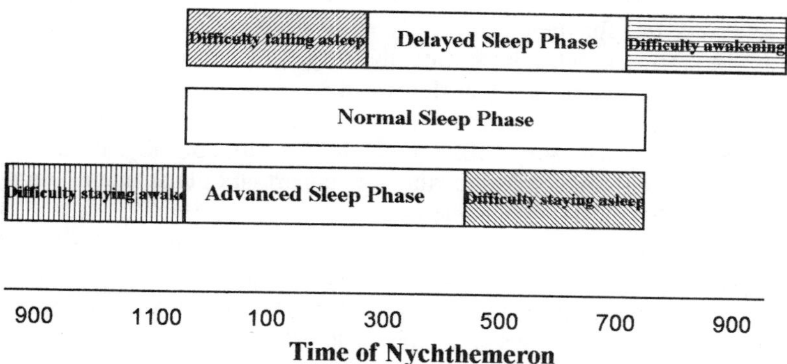

Figure 9-8. The differences between normal sleep, delayed sleep phase, and advanced aleep phase.

Light therapy takes advantage of the fact that bright light is a major zeitgeber for human circadian rhythms (see chapter 4). Light in the morning (before dawn) tends to phase advance circadian rhythms, while light in the evening (after dusk) tends to phase delay them. Thus, for phase delay syndrome, several days of 1 to 2 hours of bright (2500 or more lux) morning light is often sufficient to move the phase of the person's sleep cycle to the more desired and adaptive time.

Delayed sleep phase syndrome, such as in this case, is not the only kind of rhythm disruption that can occur. Others are the effects of shift work and jet lag (see chapter 4), and the more rare advanced sleep phase syndrome, non-24-hour sleep/wake rhythm, and irregular sleep/wake rhythm.

There are relatively few reports of people with advanced sleep phase syndrome. These are people with the inability to remain awake and alert in the evening and who typically go to sleep between 8 and 9 p.m. They then awaken at about 4 to 5 a.m. and are unable to return to sleep. Like phase delay persons, they are on a 24 hour schedule, but they are unable to modify the placement of their sleep period during the 24 hours. These people are true day larks. The reason so few cases of sleep advance syndrome have been reported is unclear. Perhaps it is not as troublesome to job and school schedules and no sleep loss occurs, so these people have no need to seek help for phase advance. Or perhaps the propensity for people is to phase delay (see chapter 4).

Non-24-hour sleep/wake rhythm is characterized by progressively later sleep onset and arousal times, that is, the person's body is on a 25 or 26 hour sleep/wake schedule. For part of each month, things are relatively fine for the person. They go to sleep and arise more or less as the world expects. But eventually, they drift out-of-phase with the world - desiring sleep when the world is awake and wake when the world is asleep. Chronotherapy or light therapy is used to treat these cases unless the person is blind. (One third of blind people have a non-24-hour sleep/wake cycle showing how important light is in entraining the circadian clock (see Chapter 4).

The final type of rhythm disruption is the lack of any well-defined rhythm at all. The person's nychthemeron consists of many daytime naps and shortened nocturnal sleep. Meal patterns also often become disrupted, and the person simply eats whenever they feel like it. Weakness, languor, and many bodily complaints typically also occur. These people usually complain of insomnia, not realizing that the inability to sleep well at night is caused by their disordered schedules.

Treatment is difficult for the absence of circadian sleep/wake schedule and may not necessarily be long-term. It consists of enforcing a more typical 24 hour cycle of rest/activity as well as regularizing other aspects of daily living, such as meals. Often, this requires someone living with the person to be responsible for establishing routines until the person becomes synchronized.

Parasomnias: Arousal Disorders

Generally speaking, parasomnias (Mahowald & Ettinger, 1990; Mahowald & Rosen, 1990) are occurrences during sleep that are undesirable. Either they do not normally occur during sleep (such as bedwetting) or sleep makes an existing problem worse (such as abnormal heart rhythms or arrhythmias). Hence, the term parasomnia is a kind of grab bag rather than a well-defined category. The key to understanding the parasomnias is to realize that sleep and wake are not always mutually exclusive states. Rather, they result from a recruitment of various components (see chapters 5 & 11).

Sleep Terror (Pavor Nocturnus, Incubus Attack)

Because of the large number of cases this week, the presentation of the next case is shortened to a summary. Parents of a ten year old child reported being suddenly awakened early in the night by their child's piercing scream. They rushed into their child's room and found her sitting up in bed in a state of near panic. Yet, in spite of the wide eyes, intense sweating, rapid breathing, and a look of fear on her face, the child did not quite, but rather had a glassy-eyed stare. For about 5 to 10 minutes the parents tried, but with little success, to console and comfort the child. After this time, the child might have described having sensed vague terror and an image of something frightening. Finally, the child returned to sleep and the parents, very much aroused by the event, attempted to do likewise. The next morning, the smiling, happy child had no memory at all of what happened the night before and could not understand what her parents were making the fuss about!

This is a typical sleep terror or pavor nocturnus. Such occurrences normally begin in children between the ages of 4 and 12, then usually gradually disappear by adolescence. The incidence of sleep terrors is about 1% to 4% in all children of this age group, it is more common in males, and it tends to run in families. Sleep terrors come out of deep SWS that quickly turns to wake-like alpha as breathing and heart rate double or quadruple. Thus it, is thought to be a rapid, but incomplete, awakening accompanied by body movements and other heightened basic body processes. It may be over quickly or last 20 minutes or more and progress to the child jumping out of bed and running, as if blindly fleeing some threat. Injury is possible at this time. Attempts at restraint may be met with increased efforts to escape, accompanied by violence.

The adult version of sleep terrors is preceded by impressions of dread, inability to move, feeling helpless, or even choking. It tends to emerge during the twenties or thirties, but seldom after age 40. In adults, it is usually chronic, but seldom progresses to other problems.

Daytime fatigue and stress tend to increase the likelihood of an attack the following night in susceptible people. In older children, disruptive family life may be implicated. Certain drugs taken at bedtime may also increase the chance of an attack. Attempts to awaken the child during the attack may only intensify and lengthen it.

Treatment depends on age. Since younger children usually outgrow the attacks and have no recall of them, usually nothing is done besides reassuring and educating the parents and family, since these witnesses are more affected than the sleeper! In older children and adults, some kind of psychotherapy is recommended only if obvious psychopathology is present. Hypnosis, and relaxation, and mental imagery have been shown to be beneficial. Drugs that reduce or lighten SWS may also be used. At all ages, steps should be taken to insure the safety of the sleeper, should the night terrors reoccur in the future.

Sleepwalking

The question was asked if, unlike sleep terrors, sleepwalking is more an acting out of a dream. One of the senior staff members replied that contrary to common sense, sleepwalkers are not acting out their dreams. It does not occur in REM, for the muscles necessary for walking are paralyzed in REM (see chapters 1 and 2). Sleepwalking usually begins when a person has been in high-amplitude SWS and unusual, but delta-like, brain waves continue during the episode. It is thought that sleepwalking is an incomplete or abnormal arousal from SWS - somewhat awake, but still somewhat asleep.

The behaviors that occur during sleepwalking usually take the form of persistent, continuing behaviors ranging from such things as simply standing up and returning to bed (most frequent), to going to the door, partially dressing, or going to sleep on the couch, to extreme actions, such as getting into a car or walking in the yard (least frequent). Sleepwalkers tend to be automatic or robot-like, with little real reaction to stimuli. Contrary to common belief, sleepwalking is not the acting out of a dream. Reports of any dreams at all from people awakened during sleepwalking are few, and even those reported are fragmentary and rarely contain no dream-typical plot.

Sleepwalking incidents may last from a few minutes to more than half an hour. Frequency may vary from once a life to every night, but tend to be more frequent if the person is fatigued, sleep deprived, taking sleeping pills, under stress, or (in some people) under emotional tension. Sometimes a sleepwalker may spontaneously awaken, but will feel disoriented. If no awakening occurs, the sleepwalker may return to bed or may lie down somewhere else. If not awakened, the person will probably have no recall of the event at all or only a vague awareness of it.

Until the 1960s, sleepwalking was felt to be pathological, indicating a serious, usually psychological, problem. It is now known that over half of sleepwalkers have no psychopathology. It is now looked upon as often benign, unless it occurs often, results in danger, or occurs in older children or adults.

It has been estimated that 10 to 20% of people have had at least one incident of sleepwalking which usually occurs during childhood, although sleepwalking is more common in adulthood than generally realized (2.5%). The incidence of repeat episodes is around 6%. Most sleepwalking in children develops before age 10, with peak incidences occurring in early adolescence (11-12 years of age), and almost always disappearing between 11-15. It may reoccur, or appear for the first time, during the 30's or 40's if the person has some kind of personality disturbance or psychopathology (Berlin & Qayyum, 1986) but may appear for no apparent reason. It may also be an early sign of temporal lobe epilepsy, as well as a medication side effect, if the first occurrence is in adults (Berlin & Qayyum, 1986). When sleepwalking occurs in adults, it tends to be more chronic. There appears to be a genetic base for the tendency to sleepwalk.

While sleepwalking, a person will have a dazed look on their face with their eyes open, yet they may be unable to avoid objects. Coordination is poor and the brain's rational decision-making capacity is deficient, thus injury and perilous situations are not uncommon. On the other hand, aggression and frenzy are rare. Sleeptalking may occur during sleepwalking.

The treatment strategy depends on the age of the sleepwalker and the past severity of the consequences of the sleepwalking. Little is done for children, the most common sleep walkers, who have no history of getting into danger while sleepwalking. The majority of children will out-grow sleepwalking, regardless of what is done.

If sleepwalking is very frequent, has resulted in dangerous circumstances, or occurs in adults, then more aggressive intervention is required (Berlin & Qayyum, 1986). This can range from steps to keep the person confined to a bedroom or other safe environment, to restraint of the sleeper, special alarms that go off when the sleepwalker jerks, and specially constructed bedrooms to minimize how far the sleepwalker can travel and the amount of harm they can cause. Hypnosis has proven to be effective as well as psychotherapy, when there are indications of psychopathology. Also, drugs may be used to try to reduce or lighten the stage of sleep from which sleepwalking emerges. In older children and adults, any underlying physical or psychological causes should be ruled out, or if found, treated.

What should you do when you encounter a sleepwalking person? First and foremost, try to ensure their safety. You may either gently guide the person back to bed or awaken them. Contrary to common wisdom, there is no danger in awakening a sleepwalking person. However, it may be difficult, and the person may be terribly confused or even hostile. (Imagine how you would feel if, while reading this book, you suddenly found somebody was shaking you in another room or even another building!) Thus, an awakened sleepwalker needs a lot of support and reassurance, but there is no reason not to awaken them.

Is sundown syndrome a form of sleepwalking? Sundown syndrome, or nocturnal wandering in the elderly, resembles sleepwalking but is different from it. Nocturnal wandering has its onset in the elderly and is most often associated with organic brain syndromes, such as Alzheimer's Disease (Berling & Qayyum, 1986). This is a nocturnal delirium in people who function reasonably well in the daytime but wander aimlessly while awake at night. It is classified as a sleep disorder associated with medical/psychiatric disorders. Treatment consists of low dosages of psychotropic drugs, institutionalization, and, if all else fails, physical restraint.

Parasomnias: Sleep-wake Transition Disorders

Sleeptalking

The topic of sleepwalking leads to discussion of sleeptalking (Arkin, 1981). Sleeptalking, like sleepwalking, is most common in children, but also occurs in adults. Unlike sleepwalking, it is classified as a sleep-wake transition disorder. It is estimated that 20 to nearly 100% of people have done it one time or another. It ranges from a few mumbles to a hundred or so intelligible words at a time. People may also sing, laugh, and so on. It usually only lasts for a few seconds. Although anecdotal accounts of two-way conversations with a sleeptalker abound, accomplishing this in the lab has only been partially successful. Secrets are seldom spoken, although occasionally used in literature such as Othello being convinced by Iogo's relaying the supposed sleeptalking of Cassio, nor has sleeptalking been successfully used to get a description of a dream as it is in progress. Many have tried, and failed, to use it as an avenue to the mind. The speech is usually too garbled or nonsensical to be of much use.

Sleeptalking can occur any time during sleep and out of any stage. Over half of it occurs out of stage 2 and only 10-20% out of REM. It may involve partial awakening. When sleeptalking does occur during REM, it tends to be more grammatically correct, more emotional, but without reference to the person's surroundings. In only a few cases has it been shown to be related to dream content.

Sleeptalking runs in families, is considered benign, and is not treated. I know of only one case in which sleeptalking may have had serious consequences - a sleeptalking fireman who was in danger of losing his job because he was keeping other firemen awake in the fire station dormitory!

Rhythmic Movement Disorder (Head Banging)

Another Sleep-wake Transition Disorder came up in the discussions. A rhythmic to and fro head rocking (or, less often, rocking of the entire body) just before or during sleep is called Rhythmic Movement Disorder. It occurs during early childhood (age of onset is usually during the first 9 months of life) and is outgrown usually by four years of age but may persist into adulthood. There do not appear to be any waking impairments that are associated with it, but it is more frequent in children of sub-normal IQ. and is related to the intensity of environmental stress.

Parasomnias usually associated with REM sleep

Nightmares

Since the earlier discussion of treatment of night terrors, one person has been waiting to ask if there was any treatment for nightmares (including REM Anxiety Nightmares, Stage 2 Nightmares, and Nightmares associated with Post-traumatic stress Disorder - see Chapter 6) beyond psychotherapy and drugs. Someone had just heard of a new treatment by Krakow and associates and relates it to us.

Barry Krakow and associates (Krakow & Neidhardt, 1992; Neidhardt, Krakow, Kellner, & Pathak, 1992) have developed a simple, but effective, way to treat almost all kinds of nightmares. It involves three steps: (1) learning imagery techniques, (2) recording the nightmares, and (3) changing the nightmares. In step one the person learns to imagine pleasant scenes. This is easily learned and improves with practice. Next, the person records each nightmares by writing it down as soon as possible after it occurs. This gives a clear picture of the nightmare for use in step three. Third, the person is to change the nightmare in any way they wish, then imagine the newly created dream. Repeat steps 2 and 3 after each new nightmare or, if awakened from sleep by a nightmare, imagine it with changes right then before returning to sleep.

REM Behavior Disorder

The following is a dramatic case presented at the start of one of the grand rounds sessions:

Mr. R.D. is a 73 year old male, retired librarian. He is a very pleasant, mild, and considerate person who came to us because of hitting, slapping, and even choking his wife "a couple of times a week" during his sleep. He has also bolted from the bed, breaking objects on dressers and damaging furniture. He has injured himself. These incidents are often accompanied by sleeptalking or more precisely, sleep yelling. The most recent event, which resulted in his hospitalization and referral to our sleep/wake disorders clinic, occurred when he dove from the bed into a dresser, breaking his nose. He said that he was diving out of the boat to escape ugly enemy thugs who were making threats and pursuing him.

When questioned, he said that some of his dreams have become very vivid and violent in the last decade or so. His wife of 47 years reported that he always jerked a lot during his sleep, but this kind of behavior only began around the time he was forced to retire due to age. She said she could awaken him during these incidents, but only after screaming his name many times for what seemed like several minutes. When awakened, he reported vividly dreaming of protecting himself and/or her from a variety of threatening criminals, terrorists, and monsters.

They both agreed that there were not marital problems or personality changes - only these sleep outbursts. His psychological tests showed no depression or pathology.

Mr. R.D. was only able to spend one night in the lab during which there was no incidents or vivid dream reports. His polysomnogram was normal except for (a) somewhat more SWS, (b) high REM density, (c) random, irregular limb movements and twitches in all sleep stages, and (d) brief loss of muscle paralysis during REM.

Mr. R.D. was diagnosed on the basis of these facts and findings as having REM Behavior Disorder (RBD) and was put on a daily dose of conazepam one month ago. Almost immediately he reported that the vivid, violent dreams had gone away, and there have been no incidents during his sleep.

RBD is a newly discovered parasomnia (Mahowald & Ettinger, 1990; Schenck, Bundlie, Patterson & Mahowald, 1987) characterized by unusual dreaming and nightmares whose content is vividly filled with a great deal of activity and violent confrontations. These are accompanied by actual complex, vigorous behavior including punching, kicking, grabbing, and leaping from bed, which are often accompanied by vocalizations. Usually the dreamer is experiencing fear, and the behaviors are defensive against what was subsequently reported to have been happening in the dream. Injury to the dreamer and sleeping partner is common.

Sleep laboratory studies confirm that these RBD events occur during REM. The typical rapid eye movements and characteristic EEG of REM are present and the events tend to occur in the latter half of the night. Muscle tone (as shown in the EMG) may be absent during non-eventful REM, but is sometimes present when these events occur. There is no arousal from sleep during the event.

Other changes in sleep have been noted in RBD sufferers. They have more SWS than typical and more rapid eye movements during REM. Limb movements in all stages of sleep are also common. Other aspects of sleep are within normal limits.

Most of the patients with RBD observed thus far are elderly, the average age of onset in the early 60's. However, it has been observed at other ages, including in children. Forty percent were found to have brain disease or damage of some kind, including Alzheimer's Disease. In other cases, no psychopathology is associated with RBD. In fact, most sufferers are very pleasant when awake and tend to be happily married. RBD sometimes runs in families.

The striking similarity in behavior between RBD and cats with damage to specific parts of the brainstem (see Chapter 2) has been noted. In these animals, just as in RBD humans, animated and violent behaviors occur during REM sleep. In RBD it appears as if something goes awry with the pontine REM-ON system (see chapter 2), such that the motor inhibition that is normally a part of REM, sometimes malfunctions. At the same time, cells that produce complex sequences of movement are activated, resulting in the behaviors. The cortex responds to these movements by synthesizing the dream content (see the Hobson-McCarley Activation Synthesis model of dreaming in chapter 6).

A temporary version of RBD may also occur in alcoholics going through delirium tremors ("DTs") and in other people following psychoactive drug withdrawal.

Effective treatment of both the vivid dreams and the behaviors has been achieved with low doses of clonazepam.

Sleep Paralysis

I've heard about something called sleep paralysis that seems to be the opposite of RBD. Does anyone know anything about it?

One of the psychiatric residents in attendance eagerly replied, "Around the turn of the century, people in England could order a coffin with a bell on top connected to a rope within. Should the coffin's occupant not really be dead, but just temporarily paralyzed, they could ring the bell (hopefully) before being buried alive. Perhaps reports of sleep paralysis contributed to the development of such a casket."

She continued to tell us that people with this inherited disorder feel paralyzed for several minutes, usually upon awakening, but sometimes at sleep onset as well. They are awake and fully conscious when it occurs. (Sometimes it is accompanied by hallucinations or dream-like thinking.) If touched by another, or if their name is called, the paralysis will immediately disappear. At other times, the person may find that they can still move their eyes and then, by making vigorous eye movements, can often control the muscles of the face, then work down through the rest of the body. Sleep paralysis may begin in childhood or adulthood and occurs mostly in females.

Impotence

Normal males have an erection of the penis during each REM period (see chapter 1). However, if something is physically wrong with the erection mechanism, then erections will be absent or quite diminished during REM sleep. If the impotence has a psychological base, then the erections will be obvious during REM sleep, even though lacking at times of sexual arousal. Since treatment of the impotence differs with the cause, biological vs. psychological, the evaluation of erections during REM sleep is important in determining the type of treatment to be applied.

Other Parasomnias

Sleep Enuresis (Bedwetting)

The discussion continued on to the category of Other Parasomnias.

Most children should be expected to have enough bladder control by age 3 not to wet their beds at night. Yet, 15% of female and 25% of male six year olds wet their beds frequently, with a spontaneous cure rate of about 15% per year. Most bedwetting occurs between ages 5 to 7, but is more common in adolescents than commonly thought (2% in 18 year olds).

Nocturnal bedwetting is a parasomnia that is more of an annoyance than a serious problem. It is no longer considered as pathological unless it re-emerges after several dry months. Although its frequency may increase in susceptible individuals when stress occurs in the prior waking period, it can also be increased by sudden changes in the sleep-wake schedule. Many causes for it have been found including genetic, delayed maturation, poor habit-training, and urological disorders.

It almost always occurs during the first half of the night in any stage of sleep. During bedwetting, the child may be very difficult to arouse and may be very confused and disoriented. Generally, bedwetters are very deep sleepers, and the bedwetting may occur during incomplete or partial arousal.

Treatment strategy depends on the cause. Any physical problem should be sought and treated if found. If that does not solve the problem, the parents should not overreact; usually the problem will simply be outgrown. Parents might try waking the child up to urinate after 1 or 2 hours of sleep. Instructing the child to take responsibility for his own wetting, by having him or her change the wet sheets and pajamas, helps in about 25% of the cases (Lamberg, 1985). Bladder stretching exercises, wetness alarms, and daytime rehearsal have also been beneficial, but results may take up to ten weeks (Lamberg, 1985). Relaxation mental imaging has also worked. Beyond these suggestions, help from a competent professional should be sought if bedwetting persists.

Sleep Bruxism (Teeth Grinding)

Ten to twenty percent of people (most prevalent in adolescents) may grind or click their teeth many times during sleep. For 9 out of 10 of these people bruxism is not serious, but for others it becomes problematic because it can cause damage to the teeth. It is not associated with any psychological problems, but may be more prevalent during times of stress.

It tends to occur in stage 2 sleep and REM but may also occur in other stages of sleep. It is usually accompanied by other body movements and an increased heart rate. Thus, it appears to occur during a partial arousal. The person has no awareness of it and seldom awakens. However, the sleeping partner or members of the family may be very aware of it because of the loud, unpleasant sound that is produced. In more severe cases, the person may awaken with an aching jaw in the morning and incur permanent damage to teeth and bone. A dentist is best consulted for treatment, which often involves sleeping with a guard over the teeth.

Medical/Psychiatric Sleep Disorders Disorders

Discussion of specifics of this category would take us too far afield, since the sleep problems in this category are not the primary problem. However, there is one example that is unique and worth discussion.

Alpha-Delta (Non-restorative) Sleep Fibrositis Syndrome

It is called alpha-delta sleep (from the patterns of EEG waves seen in this disorder) or non-restorative sleep (from the effect) or fibrositis syndrome (from associated complaints of stiffness and achy muscles). Whether these are different manifestations of one disorder or three different phenomena is unclear at this time. Persons with the complete manifestation of this disorder look tired with large bags under their eyes. They complain of light, restless sleep that is unrefreshing. They feel tired and washed out during the day and complain of stiff, aching muscles, but are not extremely sleepy. Their laboratory sleep is unique. The NREM sleep contains varying amounts of alpha-like waves superimposed upon NREM slow waves (such as delta). Also, numerous short arousals (alpha bursts plus EMG enlargement) occur. REM sleep, however, appears to be normal.

However, other patients may have only some of these symptoms. Some with the fibrositis component do not have alpha-delta waves when they sleep. Others with alpha-delta sleep waves do not complain of any of the other symptoms. Still other patients who complain of non-restorative sleep do not have alpha-delta sleep nor symptoms of fibrositis.

One interpretation of this disorder is that the brain's sleep-controlling mechanisms are malfunctioning, resulting in the simultaneous activation of slow waves (sleep) with alpha waves (wake), and thus the sleep is not restful, which causes or at least contributes to the other symptoms. However, there is some doubt that the alpha waves are true alpha (Weber, Bergan, Golden, Moorcroft, & Hansen, 1983). Alpha waves are 8-12 Hz in frequency and originate (are strongest) from the back of the brain. The alpha waves of alpha-delta sleep, however, are slightly faster and originate more toward the front of the brain. These faster, more anterior waves are characteristic of sleep spindles. If this is correct, then the problem is not one of a mix of sleep-wake but an unusual mixing of the stages or characteristics of sleep.

Alpha-delta (non-restorative sleep) fibrositis syndrome is sometimes successfully treated with low doses of anti-depressants, low impact aerobic exercise, and counseling (for the stress that accompanies this disorder).

Conclusion

Sleep/wake disorders medicine has a relatively brief history. However, since the first sleep/wake disorders center opened in the early 1970's many people have been assessed and treated. Many of these people were found to have serious sleep/awake disorders that were not even known to exist prior to research conducted at sleep/wake centers. Today, the majority of people with any kind of sleep complaint have a condition which is diagnosable and, more importantly, treatable. Many people now live better quality lives, as a result. The likelihood is for even more improvement of life for countless numbers of people, as they too are diagnosed and treated and as research finds out more about these disorders, how they affect our lives, and how they can be treated. Any support you can give to these efforts will help bring adequate treatment to many people and probably to someone you know and love. Perhaps you may want to enter the expanding field of Sleep Disorders Medicine yourself as a Polysomnographic Technician or, following earning a Ph.D. or MD., as an Accredited Clinical Polysomnographer. For more information on either of these careers contact, the Association of Professional Sleep

Societies (507/287-6006) 1610 14th Street Northwest, Suite 300, Rochester, MN 55901-2200. There is also a National Multi-Site Training Program for Basic Sleep Research involving six universities in the United States (UCLA, University of Chicago, Harvard, University of Pennsylvania, Stanford, the University of Texas) that provides interdisciplinary training for predoctoral and postdoctoral students with full tuition and financial aid. Contact the Sleep Research Training Program, Brain Research Institute, University of California, Los Angeles, California 90024-1746. Finally, The National Sleep Foundation, (310/288-0466) 122 South Robertson Blvd., Suite 201, Los Angeles, California 90048, is an excellent resource for anyone, professional and non-professional alike, who would like to obtain more information about sleep disorders.

Sleep, Dreaming, & Sleep Disorders

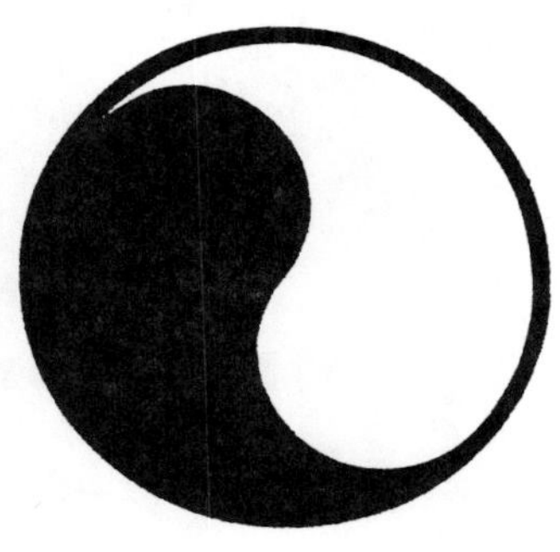

Section 4

Questions & Functions

Chapter 10

Questions and Answers

Can Sleeping too Much or Too Little Affect One's Life Expectancy?

A survey of more than a million adults over the age of thirty has led to the discovery of a relationship between length of sleep and mortality (Borbély, 1986). (The mortality rate equals the ratio of the actual number of deaths to the statistically expected number of deaths). The results are summarized in Figure 10.1.

This graph shows that for extremely short sleepers (those sleeping less than four hours) the rate of mortality was nearly two and a half times greater than for those who slept an average of seven to eight hours per night. Those who slept more than ten hours, the extremely long sleepers, did not fare much better. The mortality rate for these people was almost two times higher than for normal length sleepers. What were the causes of death in the two groups whose mortality rates were high? It was found that both extremely long and extremely short sleepers died more often of cancer, suicide, and heart disease. In fact, nearly all of the causes of death were more prevalent in these two extreme groups than in normal length sleepers.

Subsequently, several other studies have replicated these findings (Carskadon, 1993). These studies showed that factors such as diet, sex, exercise, age, use of sleeping pills, and smoking are not contributing causes to the differences in mortality between either long and short sleepers and average length sleepers.

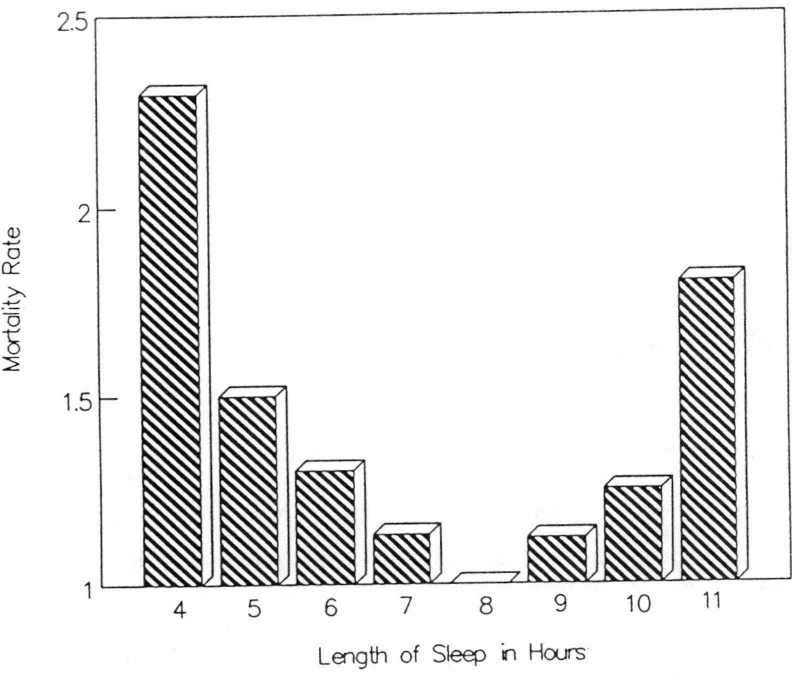

Figure 10-1. Mortality rates and the length of sleep in over one million adults. (After Kripke, Simons, Garfinkel, & Hammond, 1979. Short and long sleep and sleeping pills: Is increased mortality associated? *Archives of General Psychiatry, 36*, 103-116.)

One possible explanation for these data is that sleep length directly affects mortality rate. Other explanations are, however, equally plausible since these data are correlational, making it impossible to determine causation. Extremely short or extremely long sleepers may have a destructive lifestyle compared to that of normal length sleepers. There is also the possibility that internal factors, such as early stages of disease, as well as external elements, for example stress or night shift work, have a direct influence on both sleep and mortality rate. At the moment, the possibility that too much or too little sleep may be harmful cannot be discounted.

What is Sleep Inertia (Sleep Drunkenness)?

Sleep inertia, also called sleep drunkenness, has been defined as a condition of abnormally excessive confusion occurring during the transition from sleep to wakefulness (Carskadon, 1993; Dinges, Orne, & Orne, 1985) that lasts from a few minutes up to half an hour (Anch et al, 1988; Dinges, 1989). This period of confusion, which a person may or may not be aware of, is marked by a decrement in performance, the severity and duration of which seems to depend a great deal upon several factors prior to awakening.

There is a relationship between sleep stage immediately prior to awakening and the severity of confusion upon awakening, as measured by the levels of performance at various tasks. Awakening from REM sleep produces the least severe performance impairment. In addition, arousal from delta sleep during the first one-third of the night results in the greatest performance decrements. But other factors are also important such as depth of sleep, length of sleep, and phase of the circadian cycle. For example, there is a mid-afternoon peak in sleep inertia. Also, sleep inertia following naps is more severe the longer the nap. Sleep inertia is especially severe when awakened from a brief sleep (such as a couple of hours) following 24 or more hours of sleep deprivation. Surprisingly, sleep inertia is less common in the elderly. An explanation for this finding could be the decreased amount of Stage 4 sleep in the aged (see Chapter 1). Researchers have also verified a relationship between threshold of arousal and sleep drunkenness. The more intense the stimulus necessary to cause arousal, the more severe the decrement of performance upon awakening. Also, the more abrupt the awakening, the greater the sleep inertia.

Sleep inertia produces grogginess, confusion, and decrements in cognitive performance. Alertness is low and it is easy to return to sleep. Performance on mental tasks (e.g. mental arithmetic) is most severely compromised, while perception and movement performance is less severely affected. Memory is also severely compromised during sleep inertia; a person may not remember the contents of a phone call or even talking on the phone at all. Or a person might repeat without remembering, almost automatically, a simple behavior such as turning off an alarm clock.

Sleep inertia, and the decrement of performance associated with sleep inertia, has been the cause of concern in the military. The sleep schedules of such personnel, as well as fire and other emergency personnel, have been questioned. They must be alert and ready for quick action at any time of the day. Because the evidence has indicated that performance is not good following arousal from deep sleep, it can safely be assumed that soldiers and others, who are awakened during the night from sound sleep, are not able to perform to their fullest potentials, due to possible sleep inertia. Although some research has been done on the sleep schedules of these personnel, nothing conclusive has been discovered for prevention of sleep inertia.

How many kinds of tiredness are there?

One thing that becomes clear from the study of sleep deprivation, shift work, and other sleep disruptions (see Chapter 3 and 4) is that there are different kinds of tiredness (Anch et al, 1988; Dement, 1979; Dinges, 1989; Horne, 1988). Tiredness is reflected in subjective feelings, objective measures such as sleep latencies, and in decrements in performance. Surprisingly, these are not always related to one another. For example, Horne (1988) has shown that people exercising after sleep deprivation feel that they are not doing as well and are fatiguing faster, while objective measures show no difference from exercise following a normal night of sleep.

When a person says they are tired, they can mean one or a combination of several things. Lack of adequate amount or quality of sleep can lead to feelings of SLEEPINESS. Sleepiness can also be a result of a sleep disorder (see Chapter 9). MUSCLE FATIGUE may result from physical work or exercise. Prolonged concentration or other mental effort may cause MENTAL FATIGUE. PSYCHOLOGICAL FATIGUE has been reported to result from lethargy, boredom, and disinterest. It can also be a result of depression. ILLNESSES are frequently accompanied by feelings of fatigue (see Chapter 2), and certain drugs can induce fatigue.

Let us focus our attention on sleepiness (Carskadon, 1993). Sleepiness may creep up on you gradually but can grow to become very powerful in several hours. Interest in current endeavors is challenged by growing sleepiness. Stretching, deep breaths, rubbing the eyes, and so on, may bring temporary relief. Eventually, there is a growing conviction that you must close your eyes, lie down, and allow sleep to occur. Sleepiness may be pleasant if you are willing and able to sleep, but can be unpleasant if you need or desire to stay awake. Sleepiness is a function of the influence of several factors, which can be divided into two types - things that produce PHYSIOLOGICAL SLEEP

TENDENCY (the need of the body for sleep) and things that interact with physiological sleep tendency to produce MANIFEST SLEEP TENDENCY (how sleepy a person feels or how difficult it is to stay awake).

The major determinant of physiological sleep tendency is the amount and quality of prior sleep and the amount of wakefulness. The greater the deviation of obtained sleep from sleep need, the greater the sleepiness (see chapter 3). This includes too much sleep as well too little sleep. Also, sleep loss can accumulate over several nychthemerons of sub-optimal sleep. Time asleep is not a sufficient measure; the quality of the sleep is important also (see Chapter 3 and 9).

Circadian rhythms also have a major influence on physiological sleepiness. As detailed in Chapter 4, most people have two periods of peak sleepiness and two periods of peak alertness every nychthemeron. The circadian influence on tiredness interacts with other factors. An example of this interaction was shown in Borbély's model (see Chapter 4).

Age also seems to play a role in physiological sleepiness. Elderly persons, on the average, do not sleep as well as young adults and, as a result, may feel sleepier in general. Infants and children need more sleep and, thus, are more easily sleep deprived.

The conditions of the body also influence physiological sleepiness. Illness frequently results in sleepiness. Some drugs, especially those that depress brain functions, also can cause sleepiness.

Manifest sleepiness does not automatically parallel physiological sleepiness, because the amount of stimulation being experienced from the environment is also important. Enjoyable social stimulation may invigorate a sleep deprived person. On the other hand, a hot environment, boredom, uninteresting repetitious tasks, and a large meal all are reputed to make the effects of lack of sleep worse. (The effects of a large meal on sleepiness are commonly experienced, although little research appears to have been done on this effect.) As the physiological sleepiness increases, manifest sleepiness (both subjective feelings and objective performance measures) depends more and more on the environmental context, and the environment becomes more important in the success or failure of attempts to remain awake. A very sleepy person would easily remain awake at an exciting basketball gave and a non-sleep deprived person would remain awake at the most boring long movie. Furthermore, motivation and incentives can contribute to or "override" environmental effects when physiological sleepiness is high, but only temporarily.

The level of physiological sleepiness is measured with the MSLT (see Chapter 3). Manifest sleepiness can be assessed in a variety of ways, such as, the Maintenance of Wakefulness Test, Stanford Sleepiness Scale, and various performance tests (see Chapter 3).

Why Do We Yawn?

Yawning occurs in all humans at all ages and is easily recognized (Provine in Carskadon, 1993). It seems like we yawn when we are tired or bored. It also seems like yawns are contagious - when one person yawns, others also yawn. There has been some scientific research done on yawning, yet conclusions drawn from this research about the purpose and mechanism of yawns are still somewhat speculative. What is known has been summarized by Carskadon, (1993); Kleitman (1972); Lehmann, 1979; Provine (1985), and Provine & Hamernik, (1986).

Yawning occurs in both humans and animals, although comparative analyses are difficult, because yawning in animals may resemble the human yawn only because the movements of animal jaws may have less flexibility. Also, the situations that bring about yawning may be very different in different animals.

A yawn appears to be an "all-or-none" action. That is, once you begin a yawn, it is very difficult to stifle it, equally difficult as it is to stop a sneeze. However, the duration and frequency of yawns may vary; yawns are shorter and less frequent when experiencing interesting stimuli and shorter in females than in males.

It appears that yawning has both physiological and, especially in humans, psychological causes. It is a common impression that yawning occurs to increase the amount of oxygen in the blood, but recent research rejects this. High levels of blood oxygen do not reduce yawning. Nor does an increase of simple breathing through the nose stifle yawning. Rather, yawning seems to occur when there is a reduction in brain metabolism. Stretching of the neck and nearby muscles that occurs during yawning stimulates local blood flow to the entire head region, including the brain, which in turn promotes greater metabolism in the brain.

There are other bodily changes that occur during a yawn. For example, a temporary increase in heart rate is associated with the process of yawning. Additionally, less blood flows to the arms and legs during a yawn because the blood vessels there constrict. These findings may be due to indirect adjustments that help increase circulation in the lungs and brain. There is also evidence that yawning, like stretching, restores tone of the muscles involved. All of these blood flow changes may, in the end, serve to stimulate alertness. Yawning may also enhance alertness by reflexively causing stimulation of the arousal centers in the brainstem reticular formation (see Chapter 2) via stretch receptors in the jaw muscles (Garma & Aubin, 1989). It has been suggested that the completeness of a night of sleep is indicated by the stretching and yawning that occur on the following morning.

In animals, stimulation of a few specific brain regions induced yawning, whereas stimulation of areas in the rest of the brain had no effect on yawning. Other observations have shown that pathological yawning was the result of damage in parts of the central nervous system in humans. Such findings suggest that yawning must be important, since it is found in so many different animals and since there are definite brain mechanisms for its control.

One reason for studying yawning is its clinical aspect: yawning may be a symptom of any one of a number of problems, such as brain lesions and tumors, motion sickness, chorea, and encephalitis. On the other hand, yawning may signal the return of health following an acute physical illness, since yawning may not be evident when the condition is serious.

Yawning also occurs for psychological reasons that may be equal to, or even greater than, physiological causes. If you were to see someone yawning in a social situation, what would be your response? Most likely you would consider that person to be rude, because yawning is typically seen as an indicator of boredom. Indeed, in humans yawning tends to occur in situations of reduced stimulation, such as long waits or monotonous jobs. Some researchers have speculated that yawning has the psychological role of filling a void when we are tired or bored. Students in a calculus class yawned the most. Subway riders in near-empty cars yawned more than riders in packed rush-hour cars. Studies have shown that yawning increases before bedtime and upon awakening, indicating the relationship of yawning with drowsiness. Yawning has also been considered an expression of affect.

It is because of these social signals that many people try to block the gaping component of yawning by yawning with clenched teeth.

However, research found that clenching teeth did not block yawns or influence their frequency, although it may have slightly shortened their duration. But, the subjects indicated that they felt as if they had "got stuck in mid-yawn." This lack of satisfaction and unpleasant sensation when yawning through clenched teeth may indicate that some function of yawning has gone unfulfilled.

It is also obvious that yawns can be very infectious. People may yawn by simply noticing someone else yawning or by thinking about yawning. As a matter of fact, you the reader may have yawned already in response to reading this section (Carskadon, 1991). Fifty five percent of the subjects who were shown a series of videotaped yawns, yawned themselves within 5 minutes of seeing the first yawn. Reading about yawning produced actual yawns in over 1/4 of subjects and about 3/4 of the subjects either yawned or thought about yawning within 5 minutes of reading a passage about yawning. Even auditory recordings of yawns have been shown to stimulate yawning in blind subjects.

Because there are so many causes of yawning, both physiological and psychological, we cannot simply attribute someone's yawn to boredom or rudeness.

What is the significance of K-complexes and sleep spindles?

It appears that K-complexes and spindles are changes in the EEG in response to sensory stimuli (Horne, 1988; Anch et al, 1988). The stimuli may be external, such as noises, or internal, such as bladder contractions. K-complexes and spindles may represent the activity of the brain when processing these stimuli in such a way as to prevent awakening to them. That is, they reflect a process that helps preserve sleep.

Several facts lead to this hypothesis. First, K-complexes are easily induced in a sleeper during stage 2 by a discrete sound (such as dropping a pen on a desk near the sleeper); the louder the sound, the larger the K-complexes. Second, they increase in frequency as the night of sleep progresses, when the need for sleep is decreasing and arousal is easier. The absence of such an increase in K-complexes and spindles in the elderly as the night progresses corresponds to the fragmentation of sleep in this group. Third, K-complexes and spindles are accompanied by brief changes in vegetative functions (increases in pulse, respiration, blood vessel constriction, and galvanic skin responses) (see Chapter 2) that accompany changes in arousal to stimuli during wakefulness.

Can We Learn While We Sleep?

The idea of sleep learning has been a topic of science-fiction novels, as well as of laboratory investigation. Numerous investigations have been done to determine whether or not we can learn while we are asleep (Badia, 1990; Eich, 1990; Kleitman, 1972). In one experiment, sleeping subjects were presented ten Chinese words and their English equivalents. Later, when awake, they were tested for their memory of these word equivalents. The data showed that learning had not occurred. In another study, twenty-one subjects were presented with ninety-six sets of questions and answers at five-minute intervals throughout the night of sleep. The EEG's of all the patients were monitored and it was discovered that the percentage of items recalled during wakefulness decreased as alpha wave frequency (a sign of wakefulness - see Chapter 1) decreased. It was concluded that sleep learning is a very weak phenomenon at best and, therefore, an impractical way to acquire any new learning.

Sleep learning may possibly be state dependent learning. That is, what is learned when the brain is in one state of organization may be capable of being recalled only when the brain is again in that state. Thus, you would have to be tested during sleep to demonstrate what you have learned during previous sleep. For example, sleeping subjects were instructed to make a specific response (such as, "your nose will itch and you will scratch it") to a word (such as ITCH). Later, these words (mixed in with other new words) were spoken to the still sleeping subjects. Sometimes the suggested response occurred, but only if the suggestion was given during REM and only if the cue word was spoken during REM. Appropriate responses to the cue words were still seen five months later in some of the subjects. None of the subjects were able to recall any of the words or the suggested responses when awake.

There has also been some evidence that more elementary kinds of learning, such as classical (Pavlovian) conditioning and habituation involving things like heart rate and eye blinks, may occur during sleep (Carskadon, 1993).

The data from studies on sleep learning have been disappointing to those that expected useful, easy, and efficient learning during sleep. Most authorities in the Western world do not believe learning of any significance occurs while sleeping that transfers to the waking state. Neither explicit nor implicit (that is, without awareness) learning have been shown to occur during sleep and be manifested during wakefulness when adequate measures have been taken to not present the to-be-learned material when alpha waves are present. Russian researchers conclude that sleep learning is a hardy, viable, and useful phenomenon. However, their conclusions are based on highly trained subjects and no direct measurement of sleep. In fact, the information-to-be-learned was presented early and late in the sleep period when a lot of wake was likely to be occurring

(An implicit assumption of sleep learning is that nothing of value or use occurs during sleep, thus the unoccupied brain is available for learning. This assumption is unfounded - see Chapter 11.)

If I Wake Up in the Middle of a Dream, Will I Be Able to Get Back Into That Dream?

Probably all of us have been awakened in the middle of a dream. If the dream was a bad one, we were thankful to escape it. But if the dream was good, we may have closed our eyes in an attempt to get back into that dream to see how it would end.

Dement (1978) investigated the possibility of returning to a dream once one has been awakened. He discovered that in about 95-98 percent of all instances, once REM has been interrupted for a period of five minutes or longer, the next REM period will not occur for at least thirty minutes. If this is indeed the case, getting back into a dream after awakening would be nearly impossible if the awakening exceeds several minutes.

Nevertheless, some people report that they can, in fact, re-enter a dream after waking up. To date, there has been no documentation to support their testimonies.

Do Animals Dream?

It is difficult to discover the answer to this question, since dreaming is a subjective experience (see Chapter 11). We are unable to ask animals about their dreams and receive a direct answer, as we can with humans. Yet, many people have observed a pet making movements and sounds while asleep and have assumed that it was dreaming.

Allison and Van Twyver (1970) have articulated the arguments in favor of the idea that animals do dream. First, they say that active sleep (the animal equivalent of REM - see chapter 5) is the same in all animals, including humans. Since humans relate that they dream in this state, it is reasonable that animals do also. Second, they assert that animals have mental processes that are similar to those of humans. They cite Darwin's statement that all animal forms show emotional expressions which reflect their "states of mind." Subjective states such as "pain, hunger, and fear" are attributed to animals, even though they do not show these like humans. They also state that "it is reasonable to suppose that visual, auditory, and tactile imagery occur in animals" (pg. 64). Third, they cite the studies in cats with damage in the brain (near the locus coeruleus - see chapter 2). These animals, although in REM sleep, move as though reacting and interacting with something. That is, they appear to be acting out dreams. Fourth, the most direct evidence they cite (and the evidence most frequently cited by others as most convincing) is observations made by Vaughan (1963-unpublished dissertation). Vaughan was doing a study on the visual perception of monkeys. The monkeys were confined to a chair with a projection screen directly in front of their head. They had successfully learned to press a button at their fingertips when they saw patterned stimuli on the screen. Vaughan observed that when the monkeys were asleep in the chair they would sometimes press the response button, but only when the sleep was accompanied by rapid eye movements. The obvious explanation was that they were responding to the visual stimuli of their dreams.

More recent evidence comes from the observations of a gorilla who had been taught to communicate with sign language. The gorilla combined, on its own without coaching, the signs for "sleep" and "pictures" (Anch et al, 1988).

Foulkes (1983) has articulated arguments against the idea that animals dream. First, he maintains, on philosophical grounds, that only humans are capable of symbolic mentation and that symbolic mentation is necessary for dreaming. Second, he points out that the experiments involving damage to the locus coeruleus not only results in the "release" or movements during REM but also "release" waking locomotor activity. But, more generally, he questions the logical leap that behavior during sleep reflects underlying symbolic processes. Evidence show that sleepwalkers are not acting out dreams since they are in NREM sleep and have no dream recall. In short, REM behavior does not equal dream behavior. (Subsequent to this article, REM behavior disorder - see Chapter 9 - was discovered during which people do act out their dreams.) Third, the experiment by Vaughan contains many problems. No polysomnographic measurements were done to see if the monkeys were actually asleep. The signaling periods bore no relationship to normal REM cycles and length of REM periods (many hours apart and sometimes very long such as over five hours). There were no control subjects. It was during this visual deprivation that the button responses in question were made. This procedure was very stressful for the monkeys , Foulkes maintains, and this stress may have triggered the responses. Also the monkeys made many errors when awake - button presses that did not follow patterned stimuli. Foulkes concludes, "Vaughan's results themselves clearly are far too equivocal to be viewed as offering any consequential evidence of subhuman dreaming."

What Kind of Music is Best to Sleep To?

Researchers from Northwestern University in Evanston, Illinois have reported that static "white noise" is more conducive to good sleep than is rock music (Sanchez & Bootzin, 1985).

Ramiro Sanchez, then an undergraduate at Northwestern University, tested forty-eight students during a two-hour evening nap. The students were told they could listen either to nothing, white noise, classical music, soft rock, or hard rock. The results of the experiment revealed what many would have suspected. Those who slept with white noise had a sleep latency of 15 minutes and had the greatest total sleep time - 103 minutes. Classical music produced the next highest total sleep time - 66 to 73 minutes. Soft rock listeners were next, with a total sleep time of 38 minutes. And, not surprisingly, individuals who chose hard rock got the least amount of sleep - 5.4 minutes. Data for those choosing to listen to nothing was not given.

Sanchez and Bootzin offered an explanation for these results. They believe that the key factor in the disruption of sleep is the unpredictability of the sound, and suggest that heavy metal lovers who choose to fall asleep to screaming guitars and drum solos are cheating themselves out of a good night of sleep.

What Have Sleep Arrangements Been Like in Other Times and Places?

The contemporary Western cultural norm of a home with a traditional master bedroom and separate children's rooms has not always been the customary household sleeping arrangement (Borbély,

1986). In fact, it was not until after the 19th Century that private bedrooms for the sole purpose of sleeping were commonplace.

During the late Middle Ages in Europe, the conventional bedroom was a large room shared by several people. This room was not only a bedroom, but was used for other purposes as well. And it was not uncommon for servants to sleep near their masters, readily available to perform tasks at all hours.

One of the first to have his own separate bedroom was Louis XIV, Sun King of France. This room was anything but private, however. Located in the center of the palace, it was the site of a ceremony which the king held every morning while still in bed. In fact, this ceremony was said to be the most important event of the day.

Many German spas of the 17th Century had a quite unique arrangement for sleeping. Because there was an insufficient number of beds, half of the guests slept until midnight, at which time the other half was allowed to sleep in the beds. Another group with an interesting sleeping arrangement was the farm community of Breton in the 19th Century. Family members and their servants slept together in one bed. Hospitality offered to travelers was in the form of a place in the same, shared bed.

With the increased social segregation of men and women came an increasing desire for a bedroom with privacy. Wealthy families built houses with separate bedrooms for the master and mistress and sons and daughters were given their own private rooms. Today, this custom is practiced in middle and even lower class households.

Ideas have also changed about the appropriate time of day for sleeping. During the Middle Ages, it was not uncommon to catch people sleeping during the day next to houses or in fields. This practice of sleeping outdoors in the daytime is still commonplace in countries such as India. However, in the contemporary Western World we equate sleeping during the day with laziness, and we tend to frown on this practice. We prefer that sleeping occur at night in the privacy of our own bedrooms.

Should babies and infants sleep with their parents?

James J McKenna, an Anthropologist from Pomona College, has researched the topic of babies and infants sleeping with their parents (Carskadon, 1993).

In our Western industrialized culture infants and babies have their own sleeping area separate from that of their parents. This may be a crib or (later) a bed that is often in a separate room. This is considered natural and normal. However, from the perspective of total human existence (and in the majority of the world's cultures today, including modern industrial countries such as Japan), such solitary sleep in infants is an aberration and is perhaps unnatural (Carskadon, 1993). For 99% of human existence, hunting and gathering has been the norm. The industrial emphasis prevalent in the developed world today is a relatively new phenomenon of only the last 200 years. Hunters and gatherers not only sleep with their babies and infants (up to around four years of age) but also carry them (often in "back packs") when awake. Thus, there is a very large amount of physical contact between the infant and parent for the first several years of life.

Affluence, attitude, and fear have combined to make solitary sleeping the norm in the Western industrialized world. Separate beds in separate rooms became affordable to the majority of people. More importantly, the importance of individualism in the Western world led to the belief that the infant quietly sleeping alone was good and desirable. In many other parts of the world, interdependence is more the ideal of human existence and, thus, infants sleeping with parents is viewed as good and desirable. Finally, there is a fear in the Western world that the infant sleeping with its parents may be the victim of suffocation if it rolls under a sleeping adult.

From an evolutionary standpoint, sleep and its physiological regulators evolved in an environment of co-sleeping during the early life of the individual, and this might be the environment that is best for early brain and psychological development. Humans are born with very immature brains that slowly mature during the first several years following birth. Normal development of the brain requires that it be stimulated and activated by light, sounds, smells, and so forth (Kalat, 1992). Perhaps the stimulation (touch, temperature, and arousal) that an infant receives as a result of co-sleeping is helpful for brain maturation. For example, co-sleeping results in more arousals in the infant as the parent moves. This may give the developing nervous system practice to arouse the immature organism. It is also possible that there are important psychological factors involved with co-sleeping also. There is ample evidence that near total absence of human contact has devastating psychological effects.

At this point, these arguments are highly speculative. Research is going on to assess the effects and possible benefits of co-sleeping.

What is the Sleep of Astronauts Like?

All human beings are under the influence of the biological clock ticking inside us (see Chapter 4). But astronauts, it seems, feel the control of this internal timing device even more strongly than do those of us on earth. Early astronauts complained of sleep loss and of poor sleep while in space. They encounter new environmental stimuli, weightlessness, long hours of work, interruptions from continuous radio transmissions, and a complete absence of environmental time cues. All of these may disrupt the biological clock (Carskadon, 1993; Coleman, 1986).

Interestingly, studies measuring the brain waves of sky lab crew members have revealed that although these space travelers claimed they slept less while in space, in actuality the majority of them slept essentially the same and for the same amount of time as they did on earth (Anch et al, 1988; Coleman, 1986). In fact, data has suggested that it is possible for the astronauts to maintain a 24 hour nychthemeron by following a regular 24-hour work-rest schedule. However, if this schedule is not maintained, the space traveler will invariably experience some internal imbalance. Therefore, it is now considered crucial that the astronauts be entrained on a 24-hour schedule and that they be synchronized with each other to insure maximum performance from each crew member.

What is Sleeping Sickness?

There are two distinct types of sleeping sicknesses. The first is encephalitis lethargica. This disease involves inflammation of brain tissue. Von Economo (1916, cited in Ward, 1986) was the first to describe the disease as a relatively rapid lapse into extended sleep, or a state that was clinically indistinguishable from sleep. The symptoms also include incomplete paralysis of the eyes. As yet, there has been no conclusive evidence about the cause of encephalitis lethargica, and so far an effective treatment has evaded researchers (Ward, 1986).

The other form of sleeping sickness is African trypanosomiasis. Patrick Manson (1898) was one of the first to describe this disease. He defined three stages of the disease, the first of which included puffiness of the face, listlessness, and occasional attacks of vertigo, and heat flashes. The second stage, for which this disease was probably termed "sleeping sickness," found the patient suffering from extreme drowsiness. It was also during this stage that victims were likely to fall asleep at inappropriate times. It is now apparent that this sleep does not correspond to normal sleep (Carskadon, 1993). Finally, during the third stage of the disease, patients were comatose, and usually remained so until death.

Is it true that some animals sleep standing up? (with Amy [Barribeau] Lang)

The positions assumed by animals for sleep vary tremendously (Carskadon, 1993). Cats and dogs generally curl up, but often assume other lying positions for their sleep. Hooved animals are capable of sleeping standing up, but lie down occasionally. For example, deer sleep standing or lying. Wild herd animals (e.g., zebra and buffalo) sleep lying down, but the whole herd never sleeps at the same time. Cows always lie down on their stomach or side to sleep, although they are usually not asleep when lying (see Chapters 5 and 11). Horses have been observed sleeping in four different positions: 1) standing with head hanging, 2) standing with neck resting on stall partition, top of fence, or gate, 3) lying on stomach, and 4) lying on their side. There is some suggestion that the sleep while standing is "lighter".

Animals can, and do, change their sleeping positions as circumstances require. For example, laboratory rats normally sleep lying down, but have been observed sleeping while hanging by their upper teeth from the wire ceiling of the cage when the cage is so crowded that there is no room on the floor. Another example is the canary, that normally sleeps with one foot on a perch and the other tucked into its feathers, but will assume the roosting position of a chicken on the floor of its cage, or even sleep on its side, when there is no perch.

Why Don't Birds Fall Out of Trees When They Sleep?

The sight of a bird asleep while perched on the limb of a tree has been a subject of awe to many a bird watcher. The question, "Why doesn't the bird fall off the limb the instant it falls asleep?" has been posed on many occasion and without a satisfactory answer. Hediger (1983) offers an explanation. Birds, he claims, have quite unique legs. Their design enables the birds to remain perched on a limb without muscular effort. A ratchet-like mechanism, which causes the toes of birds to curve and clutch the limb, is activated as the birds squat down to sleep.

Is Hibernation sleep?

Hibernation (Carskadon, 1993; Heller, 1979; Horne, 1988; Krilewiez, 1991) is characterized by periodic immobility accompanied by regulated, yet greatly lowered, level of both metabolic rate and body temperature. Hibernation occurs in six of the thirty-four families of mammals and in one bird, the poorwill- each of which may have evolved its hibernation independently. In some animals, hibernation is seasonal; for example, hibernation every winter regardless of the weather (squirrels, marmots). Other animals hibernate in response to environmental cues such as cold, lack of food, or less daylight (hamsters). During hibernation, animals drop their body temperatures from over 25° C to between 10° C & 2° C. Their EEG is flat, indicating an absence of activity in the cortex. There is still activity in the brain stem, but it is different than when the animal is not hibernating.

Hibernation is not a continuous, uninterrupted state. Rather, there are repeated bouts of waking during the period of hibernation, lasting several hours to several weeks each. Even within the periods of hibernation, there may be brief periodic arousals at about twice per hour, with increases in muscle tension and brain stem cell activity. The animal may take several breaths during this arousal. Hibernation may be terminated by either warm or extremely cold weather.

Table 10-1

Relationship of Hibernation to other States

(after Walker & Berger, 1980)

Wake with Inactivity	← →	Sleep	← →	Torpor	← →	Hibernation
no change in body temperature		slight temperature drop (2°C)		moderate temperature drop (10°C)		great temperature drop (25°C)
immediate arousal		rapid arousal		slow arousal		very slow arousal

A related process in mammals and birds is called torpor. Torpor is a process of reduction of body heat and metabolic rate for part of a day. In some animals, torpor occurs only during certain times of the year. The drop in body temperature and metabolism is not as great as that during hibernation.

Although some consider hibernation a unique and separate state from sleep (Kalat, 1992), the widely held notion is that sleep, torpor, and hibernation are all points on a continuum (see Table 10-1). Shallow torpor consists mostly of QS (NREM-SWS) but with a lowered amplitude of EEG. Brain waves cannot be recorded and scored during hibernation using traditional methods and criteria, but hibernation is usually entered through slow-wave sleep and then torpor. Some animals may go directly into hibernation from sleep without going through shallow torpor.

Although hibernation may be related to sleep, it is not the same as sleep. When animals arouse from hibernation, they sleep for a long time. The longer the hibernation, the longer they sleep and the greater the power of delta waves during this sleep. These are the same characteristics of recovery sleep following sleep deprivation, suggesting that hibernators are deprived of sleep as well as being deprived of wake.

What is the "First Night Effect?"

Often times, sleep on the first night in the sleep lab differs in research subjects from sleep on subsequent nights and also from age-related norms (Browman & Cartwright, 1980b). There is more stage 1, but less REM and SWS. Also, the latency to REM is longer, there are more stage shifts, more wakefulness after sleep onset, and less sleep efficiency. Sleep researchers have termed this the first night effect. Data acquired on the initial night in the sleep laboratory are usually discarded in research studies to control for this effect. In contrast, this control is usually not necessary when doing sleep disorder assessments with patients because their disordered sleep overwhelms the first night effect.

The first night effect is really a special case of a more general response to a novel environment (Browman & Cartwright, 1980b). Whether it is a general curiosity, fear of the unfamiliar, or some other process, a persons mental state is, to some degree, affected by novelty. Sleep disruption is but a part of this more general process. There may also be some performance anxiety about sleeping knowing that sleep is being assessed.

The first night effect can be ameliorated by making the sleeping rooms of the lab more familiar and less lab-like. It is, of course, not possible to duplicate each subject's home bedroom. But making the lab sleep rooms resemble a typical American motel room has been very successful in reducing the first night effect to insignificant levels (Browman & Cartwright, 1980b). However, even in these motel-like rooms, the first night in the lab still influences dream content. This is evidenced by the large number of incorporations of the laboratory into the content of the dreams. More recent technology has allowed sleep to be recorded in a person's own home, which has been reported to eliminate the first night effect (e.g. Dunhan, Broughton, & Hoffmann, 1991).

My own sleep laboratory bedroom looks very much like a motel room. Yet, the first night effect frequently occurs when a student volunteer sleeps for the first time with 10 to 40 members of my sleep and dreams class staying up all night "watching." (Actually, they are in a separate room watching the polysomnogram via closed circuit TV.) The next morning, the subjects talk about being aware that their sleep was being observed for class and wanting very much to sleep well. In this case, the first night effect results from the subjects trying too hard to sleep. This seems to occur only on the first night, since those who volunteer for subsequent nights show typical-for-age sleep.

Is Hypnosis Sleep?

During the process of hypnotizing a person, the hypnotist often refers to sleep or sleep phenomena. "Your eyelids are getting heavy. You can't keep them open." "Deeper and deeper asleep." And so on. And in some ways, the person appears to be asleep (Fromm & Shor, 1979). For example, the hypnotized person is usually unresponsive, unmoving, and relaxed. Later, the person may describe the whole experience as being sleep-like and vivid dreams may even be reported. Sometimes people go into a deep sleep after hypnosis.

Yet, there are far too many differences between sleep and hypnosis to say that hypnosis is sleep (Atkinson, Atkinson, Smith, & Hilgard, 1987; Oswald, 1974). Most importantly, there is no physiological way to determine if a person is hypnotized. No changes in brain waves or other bodily physiology have been observed in a hypnotized person. In contrast, a vast number of physiological changes are readily observable in sleeping people (see Chapter 2). Even the contents of the dreams of hypnotized people differ from those of sleepers (Fromm & Shor, 1979). Sleep is necessary; hypnosis is not. Nor is hypnosis a replacement for sleep.

What is snoring?

Snoring (Carskadon, 1993; Coleman, 1986) is a result of the narrowing of the air passage during sleep, allowing the soft palate to vibrate. If the passage is considerably narrowed, then the snoring is loud and continuous and respiration is insufficient. This, in turn, results in low oxygen levels in the blood and high blood pressure during sleep. Snoring is usually made worse by obesity, smoking, alcohol, high altitude, sleep deprivation, and colds or sinus infections. Although people with sleep apnea snore (see Chapter 9), not all people who snore have sleep apnea. Nevertheless, even non-apneic snoring may contribute to heart disease and stroke.

About 25% of all men are regular snorers. After 40 years of age, 30% of males and 20% of females snore. The percentage rises to 50% of males and 40% of females after 60 years of age. One third of overweight people snore (because of fat deposits in the throat) compared to 10% of normal weight people.

There are many alleged treatments for snoring. Hundreds of patents have been issued for devices to stop snoring. One is the Thomas collar; a padded collar that stretches the neck and therefore keeps the mouth closed. Weight loss is often effective, as is reduction in the use of alcohol. Surgery on the air passageway has also been successful.

What is known about depression and sleep?

Several changes in the sleep of depressed people have been universally observed (Buysse, Reynolds, & Kupfer in Carskadon, 1993):

a) too little sleep - with frequent awakenings and early morning awakening well before the desired time predominating. (About 15% of depressives sleep excessively, however);

b) fragmented and shallow sleep;

c) a decrease in the amount of SWS sleep;

d) a short latency to the first REM period (more evident in primary depression - depression without obvious cause - but may also be present in secondary depression - depression as a reaction to something that emotionally affected the person).

e) much longer first REM period with more frequent rapid eye movements;

f) increased dream activity, often with themes involving physical harm, abandonment, or pursuit.

Sleep deprivation (or REM deprivation) has been used with some success to temporarily relieve depression. One night of total sleep deprivation, or even just half a night, has been shown to be effective 60% of the time. The effect is quickly, although not entirely, reversed with subsequent sleep (often only a nap). REM sleep deprivation (see Chapter 3) produces similar effects that last a bit longer.

During either REM deprivation or total sleep deprivation treatment, the patients are reported to be more active and animated. They take part in more activities and appear more cheerful and outgoing. They are energized. Sleep deprivations (total, partial, or REM) do not have parallel consequences on mood in non-depressed individuals (see Chapter 3).

Chapter 11

The Functions of Sleep and Dreams

"If sleep does not serve an absolutely vital function, then it is the biggest mistake the evolutionary process ever made" (Rechtschaffen, 1971, p 88). Surely something as unique and universal as sleep must have physiological and/or psychological importance. Yet there is no complete understanding of, much less complete agreement about, the functions of sleep. While there are some points of general agreement, there are also many ideas that have been offered that seem to stand alone without many supporters or detractors. There are also some outright controversies and fundamental disagreements. It seems as if we are on the threshold of understanding what sleep is for. It is like being in a room with several doors that are just a bit open allowing us a peak of what is inside. With a bit of effort, we can open those doors wider and get a clearer view. In this chapter we will review many of the theories of sleep, especially those that remain active and viable or that are new and exciting.

First, let us be clear on what is meant by function (Webb in Carskadon, 1993). Function means purpose. Function means the effect or effects accomplished. But there are different levels of effects and purposes, ranging from essential to trivial to detrimental. Consider your nose. It is a vital component of the respiratory system, a convenient place upon which to rest glasses, an enhancer or detractor of facial beauty, and a most annoying place of irritation when you have a cold. A purpose may be but a component of a larger system or sequence. Again, your nose is a part of the respiratory system and a component of your face. Its function is in relation to the greater whole. Some functions of things are absolutely necessary; the system would fail without them. Other functions may not be necessary, but the system works better or faster with them. Still other functions may be convenient but could be easily replaced or done without. Finally, other functions may be superfluous or even detrimental.

Often the search for the functions of sleep has concentrated on the first type - that which is essential. The organism has no other way to accomplish these functions and would suffer from their loss. Yet the next two levels of functions are also important and are worthy of search and research efforts and should not be "belittled". We may find that the functions of sleep are of these types more than of the first type. We also must realize that it is more difficult to seek and find a non-essential function. Simply by its very nature, it can be done without. Yet it is possible to determine such functions by careful research and reasoning.

Often the question is put too simply: "What is the function of sleep?" Turn the question around and ask, "What is the function of wakefulness?" There is no one, simple answer to either question. Thus we must ask, "What are the functions of sleep?", and seek answers on many levels, from molecular to behavioral (Hauri, 1979). Furthermore, we need to remember that "sleep and wake are mutually interacting and cyclic phenomena" (Hauri, 1979, p. 252), and thus a theory of sleep necessarily involves wakefulness, too.

Before we present the theories, we need to review the kind of things for which a complete and adequate theory of sleep must account.

- sleep is unlearned, inherited, or innate (Webb, 1979);
- sleep has systematic developmental patterns (Webb, 1979);
- sleep is species-specific, yet there can be a wide range of individual differences in it (Webb, 1979);
- sleep is more than just rest, since being awake in bed throughout the night leaves you sleepy and fatigued the next day (Coleman, 1986);
- sleep is adaptive, yet has limits; it is flexible, but only up to a point (Webb, 1979);

- sleep is universal, at least among higher animals (Horne, 1988), and includes:
- a reduced activity level, and;
- a lowered responsiveness to the environment (even when this might be dangerous for the animal);
- even insects and mollusks show rest/activity cycles from which sleep seems to have evolved (Borbély, 1986);
- sleep has component parts such as REM and NREM, PGO spikes, spindles, dreams, etc.;
- sleep is predictable;
- sleep is rhythmic;
- sleep is regulated, since there is rebound if it is missed;
- abnormal sleep produces negative consequences;
- sleep is physiological;
- sleep is psychological;
- sleep interacts with the wake that both precedes it and follows it.

Finally, a theory or explanation of the functions of sleep must be consistent with the other myriads of details that are known about it - many of which have been presented in the other chapters of this book.

There are several possible ways to organize the search for the functions of sleep. One is to separate its functions that are internal to the organism, such as bodily restoration, from those that are external, such as safety from predation (Borbély, 1986). In this chapter, we will divide the functions of sleep into 3 types: **restorative, behavioral**, and **mental** (McGaugh, Jensen, & Martinez, 1979; Meddis, 1983). Like most efforts to categorize phenomena, the boundaries between these three areas are not always clear.

When we say that sleep is **restorative**, we imply that sleep does something the opposite of wakefulness which results in an improvement of condition or a return to a more normal or ideal state (Webb, 1983). Most people probably have a vague notion of this as the primary purpose of sleep. Indeed, restorative theories have a long history and many variants (from Webb, 1983). For example, Aristotle stated that:

- if awake too long, one's sense perceptions weaken;
- sleep is a necessity for conservation of the body;
- nutrition and growth are best when asleep.

Around the turn of this century, various "humoral" theories abounded describing the accumulation of toxic substances in the fluids of the body which disrupt the nervous system; sleep was said to rid the body of them (see Chapter 2). Also at that time, theories of "inhibition" were proposed stating that sleep was needed to revive the parts of the nervous system that stopped functioning normally as a result of wakefulness. Throughout this century, variations and new versions of these theories continued to be proposed, seemingly incorporating each new neurological or biochemical discovery.

Sleep has also been viewed as a type of **behavioral** adaptation to the environment (Webb, 1983). Sleep is a state of decreased responsivity to the surroundings. But the daily amount, length, periodicity, and timing of sleep are specific to individual animal species. This occurs because sleep may increase the chances of survival for the animal relative to its niche and, thus, in evolutionary terms, the survival of the species. Theories about the behavioral functions for sleep are more recent, less specific, and more speculative than restoration theories. Supporting data comes more from the study of animal rather than human sleep. Some of the important data include (see Chapter 5 for details):

- most animals go to a specific site and/or assume a specific posture for energy conservation and safety;
- an internal clock promotes sleep during the part or parts of the 24-hour day in which it will be most beneficial for the animal;
- unconsciousness tends to keep the animal quietly in place until it is appropriate to go forth again.

It has also been proposed that sleep benefits internal **mental** functions. Included here are theories that view sleep as beneficial for emotional well being. Also included are ideas that sleep enhances information processing such as aiding in retention of the experiences of the day or in other ways promoting learning and memory. The functions of dreams are especially prevalent in this category.

For a long time, the theories in one category were usually presented in isolation and frequently even in opposition to those of another category. More recently, as we shall see, some theories have attempted to encompass more than one category or combine theories from more than one category to show how they are compatible. Also, the degree of importance of each category may vary in different species (Meddis, 1983).

We will begin our review by examining the overall functions of sleep, then look at the functions of its major stages, and conclude with the functions of dreaming.

You may ask, "Why is it important to seek out and understand the functions of sleep and dreaming?" We can never really know what sleep is until we understand its functions. This in turn influences our (Meddis, 1979):

- attitudes toward our own sleep;
- research endeavors (a good example of this is the dramatic change in sleep research that occurred when it was realized that sleep is active and not passive);
- treatments for sleep/wake disorders;
- and contributes to our basic understanding of human beings and the world in which we live.

The Functions of Sleep

Restorative and Conservative Theories

Restoration. An old and obvious notion about the function of sleep involves tissue growth and repair. According to this idea, sleep is a time of quiescence during which the body can, seemingly, more easily grow new tissue and/or repair the damage done to it when awake. For a while such notions were out of favor with scientists, but have shown a resurgence this decade. Kristine Adam and Ian Oswald of Scotland have been notable spokespersons for just such a theory (Adam, 1980;

Adam & Oswald, 1983; Oswald, 1980). The following is based on their writings.

Body tissues are in need of continuous repair. They are like a brick wall whose bricks are always falling out and need to be put back or be replaced with new ones (Horne, 1988). Animal studies show that mitosis of epithelial cells of many body tissues occurs preferentially during sleep. Also, there is an increase of protein synthesis at this time. Other data show protein synthesis to be enhanced in the brain of rats and cats during sleep and, Adam and Oswald speculate, probably also in recently exercised muscles. If an animal is deprived of its normal sleep, both mitosis and protein synthesis are reduced. When sleep is shifted to an unusual time the peak of mitosis and protein synthesis follow it to the new time. Other studies have shown that the healing of wounds is faster during sleep, as is bone growth. Additional supporting evidence includes a reinterpretation of Zepelin & Rechtschaffen's (1974) correlation of metabolic rate and the duration of sleep of animals (see Chapter 5). Rather than being caused by a greater need to conserve energy during sleep in the higher metabolically active animals (as Zepelin and Rechtschaffen proposed), Adam and Oswald see this correlation as a greater need for tissue repair in animals with higher metabolic rates. They also point out that growing animals sleep the most. Further, children with emotional problems which stunted their growth showed poor sleep during those times when their growth was only one third of normal.

Hormone cycles (see Chapter 2) compliment these events. Growth hormone is released in its highest levels in young, growing humans during sleep and only during the first SWS period of the night in adults. The level of other anabolic hormones (prolactin, leutenizing hormone, testosterone) are also highest during sleep. In contrast, catabolic hormones such as the corticosteroids are low during normally phased sleep periods (see Chapter 2).

A more detailed and specific aspect of Adam and Oswald's theory involves the general level of energy stored in the cells of the body. During wakefulness, the relative level of cellular stored energy falls because of a general higher level of "cellular work." The reduction of stored energy in cells results in an increase in cellular degradation as well as an inhibition of protein synthesis and cell division. During sleep, overall cellular work diminishes, allowing cellular energy stores to increase. This in turn stimulates protein synthesis and mitosis. (It is important to note here that protein synthesis itself does not really utilize much energy). Adam and Oswald cite laboratory evidence that shows the level of stored cellular energy does increase during sleep.

Adam and Oswald have presented additional support for their theory. The correlation between higher metabolic rate of wakefulness and the greater subsequent length of sleep indicates a greater need for restoration. In humans, the greater the metabolic demand because of the events of wakefulness, the longer the subsequent total sleep time with more SWS and more growth hormone released. (Meddis, 1975, cites data which seem to support these ideas. Sleep in mammals increases prior to hibernation, during infancy, during brooding, in very cold or very hot weather, after injury, following feeding, and after copulation.)

Rest alone is not sufficient to bring about the repletion of stores of cellular energy. While it is true that rest is a time of less depletion of cellular energy, only sleep has been shown to be a time of its repletion. Yet, Adam and Oswald realize that sleep may be a *convenient* rather than a *necessary* state for tissue restoration and repletion of cellular energy stores. That is, these events might be able to occur in some abnormal circumstances outside of the state of sleep. But under normal, and even most other circumstances, they occur best together during sleep. Thus, the function of sleep may not be to produce these results but to provide circumstances when they can best occur. It's somewhat like fertilizing human eggs - it can be done outside of the human body ("test tube" fertilization) but it is much simpler, more convenient, and usually more assured inside of the human body.

Horne (1983a; 1988;1989) has taken exception to the restoration hypothesis of Adam and Oswald. He carefully and methodically goes through the data used to support their theory and points out the limitations and weaknesses of them. In the end, he feels the theory does not apply to the body as a whole - only the brain - and not to all of sleep - mainly SWS. One of his counter points is that tissue restoration requires an abundant supply of amino acids. Sleep in humans is a time of fasting, during which the availability of amino acids to the body is low (but not to the brain, because it is uniquely provided with nutrients at all times). Adam and Oswald counter that many animals sleep after eating and, thus, are digesting a fresh supply of nutrients. Horne agrees that this is true for many animals such as rodents but not for humans. Adam and Oswald also cite evidence that suggests that protein synthesis is not locked to feeding.

Horne also presented several other criticisms. First, in spite of its name, growth hormone facilitates protein synthesis and mitosis only if amino acids are available but does other things in their absence. Furthermore, the release of growth hormone only during sleep is rare in other mammals.

Second, the data on cellular energy stores cited by Adam and Oswald are from studies of brain tissue and probably do not apply to the rest of the body. Furthermore, there are questions of a very technical nature with these data that call them into question.

Finally, the peak of cell mitosis during sleep is really secondary to the low levels of cortisol during sleep. Cortisol levels and cell mitosis tend to have their own circadian rhythm that does not easily follow sleep when it is delayed to previously awake times (see Chapter 2). Organ malfunction or damage is not readily observable during sleep deprivation nor are any indirect signs of bodily breakdown observable, such as changes in level of cortisol. The reason is that in humans (and other higher mammals), relaxed wakefulness, Horne maintains, is sufficient for such restoration, and higher mammals spend a lot of time in relaxed wakefulness. (This is not true of many small animals that are active when awake, since activity contributes to tissue destruction and they need sleep to enforce inactivity during which they can repair and restore. It is important to note in this context that Adam and Oswald's conclusion of increased tissue restoration during sleep is based on rodent research. Their conclusions may be correct for rodents but is not generalized to humans.)

In contrast, Horne contends that human sleep is for the good of the brain, rather than the whole body. Most of the conclusions based on sleep deprivation studies are limited to effects on the brain and to psychological effects. Whenever a person is awake, the brain is at maximal activity levels or very near to it. Even during quiet restfulness when alpha waves are dominating the EEG, the brain cells are still considerably active. This is rather like a computer whenever it is turned on - it consumes about the same amount of power whether it is running a program or waiting for instructions. In order for maintenance to be done, brain activity needs to be reduced. Only during SWS is this condition met. (This applies to the cerebrum but not to the brainstem. The functions of the brainstem are rigidly determined, with little possibility for adaptability or change. In contrast, the cerebrum is very plastic, allowing greater flexibility in behavior and learning. Such a system requires more upkeep and maintenance.) Thus, to Horne, at best the theory of Adam and Oswald applies only to the brain and, since the length of wake is related only to the length and intensity of subsequent SWS, it is limited only to this stage of sleep.

Hobson (1988) has some notions compatible with the conclusions of Horne. He speculates that small, neurons that use norepinephrine as their neurotransmitter and have large fields of influence on other neurons may deplete their levels of norepinephrine during wakefulness, but regenerate during REM sleep when they are relatively inactive. At the same time, other neurons that are not susceptible to fatigue are being stimulated during sleep in a stereotyped, redundant, and highly organized manner, thus insuring daily activation. They might otherwise deteriorate from disuse given the vicissitudes of external, waking stimulation. Thus, REM may function as a reliable, patterned circuit check that, additionally, may change and improve the functioning of the nervous system rather than just maintain it. During growth in the young organism, this same mechanism helps insure proper construction of the brain.

Both Horne and Hobson may be correct. REM and NREM may both be important for brain maintenance, but each for different aspects of that organ. REM may be beneficial for small, but widely influenced cells using noradrenalin (mainly in the brainstem) and NREM for the cerebrum. Additionally, REM and NREM may alternate for a good reason (McGrath & Cohen, 1978). REM may provide a regularized system check that can, in part, help determine the adequacy of repair done in NREM and locate where more maintenance is needed during the subsequent NREM episode. Early in the night, the need is for macro restoration and adjustment that requires only brief testing, thus NREM is long and REM is short. Later, however, the restoration and adjustment becomes more and more refined and delicate (micro restoration) which requires longer and more detailed evaluation possible only in REM, thus NREM is short and REM is long. REM may also be testing the rest of the nervous system beyond the brain also, hence the bodily events of REM such as irregular activation of the respiratory system, cardiovascular system, and others functions controlled by the automatic nervous system. (However, for safety's sake, it is necessary to prevent the muscles of movement from being activated while their nervous system controlling units are being tested.) Or perhaps REM is a way of warning the brain by activating it after the cooling quiescence of NREM. Allowing the brain to cool too much might not be a good thing. Or the brain might need periodic reactivation by REM following deactivation during NREM (Siegel in Carskadon, 1993). Or maybe you can come up with other hypotheses.

Feinberg and Floyd (1982) also have described a restorative theory. It is one version of what have been called bottle theories. When awake, the body is like a bottle that gradually fills up with a poison-like substance that lessens the ability of the cells of the body to function efficiently. Sleep rids the bottle (body) of this poison. According to Feinberg and Floyd, sleep, especially SWS, reverses the level of a "substrate" that is built-up during waking. They speculate that this substrate consists of "metabolic or macromolecular changes in neurons involved in the most plastic (or modifiable) perceptual-cognitive functions" (p. 186). The origin of their speculations comes from the decline in SWS with advanced age in humans (see Chapter 1) that parallels a decline in perceptual-cognitive functions. They do cite evidence that is consistent with their theory but also admit how speculative much of it is.

Other restorative functions for sleep have been postulated. One is the enhancement of the immune system during sleep (see Chapter 2).

Conservation. If sleep does not restore, perhaps it conserves. A prominent theory that advocates sleep as a time to conserve its resources is called the "Bioenergetic Theory." According to this theory, sleep occurs in order to conserve energy when little is to be gained from being awake and active (see below) (Obál, 1984; Webb, 1979). Evidence comes from the correlation of total sleep time and metabolic rate in warm-blooded animals (see Chapter 5). But the conservation of energy that occurs during sleep comes from more than a lack of activity, since a period of simple rest wold accomplish that. Rather, it is the decrease of body temperature during sleep that conserves considerable energy. The cost of maintaining temperature in warm-blooded animals is high, and a reduction of only a few degrees is cost-effective. Yet, the animal must maintain a high enough temperature to be able to quickly arouse. Sleep provides just such a circumstance (Walker & Berger, 1980). In addition, such a period of cooler body temperature may provide a cooling period for the brain; continuous periods of high temperature may be deleterious (McGinty & Szymusiak, 1987). Knowledge of the evolution of sleep in warm-blooded animals is consistent with this theory that sleep has a temperature regulating function (McGinty in Carskadon, 1993) (see also Chapter 5). Sleep, with its inactivity and reduced body temperature, may also simply reduce the physiological stress that would occur if the animal remained awake (Meddis, 1983).

Al Rechtschaffen and associates at the University of Chicago have been conducting a series of experiments (see Landis, Bergmann, Ismail & Rechtschaffen, 1992) on the effects of long term (up to 3 weeks) sleep deprivation on rats. The sleep deprivation was either total and continuous or selective for either AS or QS.

In these experiments, pairs of rats were placed in special cages. The floor of these cages was a plastic disk suspended over 3 cm of water. The disk was divided in half by a wall with one rat on either side. When the sleep deprived rat fell asleep (as determined by a computer monitoring the polysomnograph connected by fine cable to the rat) the disk rotated. This rotation forced the newly sleeping rat to awaken in order to move to avoid being shoved into the water. This successfully prevented the experimental rat from obtaining substantial amounts of the "forbidden" sleep. The control rat also had to be awake when the disk moved, but it could sleep freely as long as the experimental rat was awake. (Bonnet, [1990 personal communication] maintains that this is really sleep fragmentation in the experimental animal, not sleep deprivation, since it gets brief snatches of sleep before being quickly awakened.) The presence of the "yoked" control is important since the control rat is undergoing the same stress of moving to avoid the water, so any effects seen in the experimental subjects is most likely due to the loss of sleep itself and not the stress of the procedure used to produce the loss of sleep.

Total or REM sleep deprivation eventually was lethal to the experimental rats. The exact cause of death was difficult to determine, since most physiological systems in these animals were near normal except for:

1) skin lesions on hairless regions;
2) changes in the brain (inferred from changes in behavior);
3) a great increase in eating;
4) some decrease in body weight;
5) a large apparent increase in body heat production;
6) accompanied by a large increase in body heat loss (attributable to the loss of REM sleep);

7) and an increase in body temperature preferred by the rat (during total sleep deprivation but not REM sleep deprivation, thus attributable to SWS loss);

8) also, just prior to death, body temperature fell precipitously as theremoregulation deteriorated.

Subsequent studies have shown that the main effect of long term sleep deprivation in these rats is a breakdown of the ability of the body to prevent excessive heat loss. This causes an increase in energy expenditure to maintain body temperature in the face of this excessive heat loss. The body debilitation is secondary to the rise in energy expenditure and/or heat loss. When the body is no longer able to compensate, body temperature decreases rapidly and death ensues.

Recovery from near terminal sleep deprivation (12 to 20 days or more of continuous sleep deprivation) was also studied (Everson et al, 1987). With the return of uninterrupted sleep, recovery is swift. Energy expenditure and plasma levels of epinephrine ad norepinephrine all return to baseline levels within only 1 to 3 days. Although its course is more erratic, body temperature also quickly returns to baseline. Appearance and skin condition are near normal within two weeks.

A surprising finding involved the characteristics of the recovery sleep. Typically, with shorter periods of sleep deprivation (up to a few days) both QS and AS rebound (see Chapter 3), but in these long term deprived subjects only AS during recovery sleep shows high and immediate rebounds.

Related theories. McGinty (1985) has hypothesized that the amount of sleep at any time is the result of many physiological influences in addition to temperature including breathing, feeding, blood pressure, movement, and hormone levels. All of these have been shown to effect sleep and each is, in turn, affected by sleep. In addition, each is controlled by brain areas that are implicated with sleep. Thus, sleep may be a part of a homeostatic feedback control system that is both affected by and affects several physiological systems of the body. Perhaps this is like a large steel ring with several chains leading from it in various directions. Moving the ring affects the chains, but pulling on a chain moves the ring.

Another function might involve the synchronizing of the various circadian rhythms of the body. Some human beings who have irregular sleep/wake habits lose the synchronization of various rhythms, much to their detriment (see Chapter 9). Although this may not be a major, important function of sleep, it nevertheless may be a legitimate one.

But Meddis (1979) raises a valid logical point. Without sleep we become tired and our performance efficiency (at least for some tasks - see Chapter 3) drops. Sleep typically reverses this and, thus, we say our sleep was refreshing and recuperative. But it is just as possible that the need to sleep produces the tired feelings and inefficient performance rather than the other way around. That is, we need to sleep whether we are tired and inefficient or not. Feeling tired and inefficient are the means by which we are compelled to get the sleep necessary for other reasons.

Behavioral Theories

One of the behavioral theories of sleep can be summed up by the phrase, "It's safer to be asleep." There are times in the twenty-four hour day when an animal may be less safe. The danger might be from other animals attacking it when it is more vulnerable. Another threat might be from an accident when it is less able to perceive danger in its environment. For many animals, including human beings, nighttime is more dangerous. Our main sensory receptor - our eyes - are built to respond best during daylight. We can see at night, but not well. This makes us, and other animals like us, more susceptible to surprise attack or stumbling over a cliff, or other natural dangers. For other animals, daytime is the dangerous time. During such dangerous times, it is safer to be asleep (Meddis, 1983).

Another way of looking at this is sleep is "adaptive non-responding" during such times of danger (Webb, 1983). Sleep forces an animal to be inactive and unconscious. When awake, all animals are responding to their environment, and many tend to be moving much more than when asleep. Adaptive non-responding is under circadian control and resembles an evolutionarily developed instinct. It may be more important in more advanced animals (Horne, 1983c).

Paralleling the safety function of sleep may be a function related to food availability (see Chapter 5). It is not effective for an animal to be active during those parts of the day when its food is not as available (maybe because the food in the form of other animals is sleeping!). From a cost/benefit basis, it is better to be asleep if it takes too much energy and poses too great a risk to be awake and active with little likelihood of securing much food (Meddis, 1975).

Theories Involving Mental Functioning

Two types of mental functions for sleep have also been proposed. The first involves memory (McGaugh, Jensen, & Martinez, 1979). Short sleep prior to learning may result in poor retention, suggesting that brain processes early in sleep are not favorable for new information storage. In contrast, if sleep follows new learning, the memory of it is better than if sleep did not follow. Something occurs in the brain to convert the new learning into a stronger, more permanent form or at least make it easier to use later. (The effects of sleep on memory are explored more below in the section on the functions of REM.)

A second mental function proposed for sleep involves mood. Sleep may be, at least in part, for recreation (Horn, 1983c). The descriptions shared by many humans seem to reinforce this notion. Sleep has been described as a distraction and a pleasant one at that. It may function to restore a certain peace of mind.

But, sleep may even have a more specific mood related function. It may be an important mood regulator (Kramer, 1993). There are changes in mood from pre-sleep night to post-sleep morning. Some of these mood changes (dizzy [anxious], clear-thinking, and sleepiness) are due to the physiology of sleeping (especially total amount of sleep, stage 2, and SWS, as well as sleep onset latency, but not REM). Other mood changes (unhappy, aggressive, and friendly) are related to dreaming (see below).

Stages of Sleep

As we have seen, sleep is not a unitary state. There are clear differences between REM (AS) and NREM (QS). NREM is produced in response to prior wakefulness (Chapter 3), while REM is manifested on a circadian schedule (Chapter 4). Both have distinct evolutionary histories (although the exact nature of those histories is not generally agreed upon [Chapter 5]). Each is controlled by different brain structures utilizing different neurotransmitters (Chapter 2). Sleep deprivation causes "pressure" and subsequent rebound in both, but with important differences. NREM rebound usually takes precedence and is as much accomplished by increased intensity as increased length. REM rebound occurs primarily through increased length (Chapter 3). REM and NREM show different developmental sequences (Chapter 1). Cognitive processes occurring during REM and NREM differ (Chapter 6). Different sleep disorders are associated with each of these stages of sleep (Chapter 9). In light of such consistent and important differences, these two divisions of sleep must have different, but nevertheless necessary, functions.

A prevalent notion is that NREM is for the body and REM is for the mind. Hartmann (1973) clearly articulated such a position. REM is important for our psychological well-being by endeavoring to restore our intellectual and emotional functions following concerns arising during our waking lives. It does so by (a) consolidating (a psychological term for organizing and strengthening) memories and (b) elevating mood. Hartmann postulated that this was accomplished by providing for recuperation of specific neurochemical systems of the brain.

NREM, Hartmann continues, is important for the physiological restoration of our bodies, primarily by protein synthesis. Waking activities take a physical toll on our bodies which require periods of NREM to repair. He also specified that the protein synthesis of NREM prepares the brain for REM, because REM uses protein.

Support for theories such as this one comes from the comparison REM and NREM. In many ways, they are almost exact opposites of one another with regard to what is happening in the brain and the rest of the body. REM is a time of great activity in the brain and associated nervous system; NREM is not. NREM is a time of great steady relaxation of most body organs and systems; REM, apart from the paralysis of the muscles of movement, is a time of greatly irregular activation of most body organs. Restoration of the body would seem to require a relaxed, low level of functioning, but restoration of mental functions would seem to require an active, but off line, brain.

More recent theories have viewed the functions of NREM quite differently from Hartmann did have supported and extended his view of the function of REM. Horne (1988), in particular,thinks that the notion that REM is for the brain and NREM is for the body is too simple. While this notion may be true for some (especially smaller) animals, he states the functions of sleep have changed with evolution of larger, more complex mammals.

NREM

In April of 1990, an International Symposium was held in Santa Monica, California that brought together experts who had done extensive research and writing about SWS. The conclusion from this Symposium (Chase & Roth, 1990) was that the functions of SWS (and often the rest of NREM) have not been determined as of yet with certainty and precision, but speculations seem to fall into three main groups (see also McGinty & Szymusiak, 1990b);

1) to restore or recover some aspects of body functions worn down during wakefulness
2) to conserve energy by reducing body temperature, metabolic rate, and energy expenditure
3) to enforce safe inactivity while remaining easily arousable.

Let's take a closer look at each of these.

la) *NREM functions to restore or recover some aspects of bodily functions worn down during wakefulness.* This is a homeostatic notion that is old and very prevalent (see above). Many lines of evidence are marshaled in its support but not always without qualifiers or alternate explanations.

- The longer you are awake, the longer your subsequent SWS. Conversely, SWS intensity decreases proportionally to the length of sleep (Chapter 3). An explanation of these facts is that he longer you are awake the greater the wearing down of the body and/or using up of vital resources which can only be built back up during SWS. However this explanation is weak, because the relationship between length of wake and subsequent SWS (QS) is not found in all animals.
- During NREM there is a decrease of catabolic hormones and an increase of anabolic hormones in the body (Chapter 2). The catabolic hormones tend to wear the body out, while the anabolic hormones tend to build up and restore the body.
- Growth hormone is present only during the first SWS period of the night in adult humans. It is even more prevalent during SWS in children. However, it has been pointed out that

growth hormone may not always do what its name implies (Horne, 1988), and the relationship between SWS and growth hormone has not been found in most other mammals.

- Sleep deprivation (or deprivation of SWS, specifically) results in a rebound during subsequent undisturbed sleep (Chapter 3). The body has a need for SWS and will make an effort to obtain it even if the opportunity is delayed. This implies SWS has an homeostatic function.
- If deprived of SWS early in the night, there will be more of it later in the night than is normal.
- There is a high amount of SWS in children, with slow declines during adulthood and much less or none in retirees (Chapter 1). This decline parallels that of metabolic rate in humans. In other species with no decline in SWS with advancing age, there is no decline in metabolic rate either.
- However, the increase of SWS following exercise sometimes observed in the past is no longer viewed as supportive evidence, because these effects are mediated by the resulting increase in body temperature (Horne in Carskadon, 1993).
- There are increases in the capability of the immune system that occur during NREM (Chapter 2). Further, many illnesses cause enhanced sleepiness, and the resulting extra sleep has been shown to be beneficial to the recovery from illness (Chapter 2).

1b) More recently, it has been proposed that *SWS provides necessary benefits only for the brain* (see above). The body gets all of the restorative rest it needs during relaxed wakefulness (except in smaller animals such as rats that do not engage in relaxed wakefulness). The brain, however, needs "off line" maintenance that can only occur during SWS.

- The effects of sleep deprivation on mood and performance are reversed with subsequent undisturbed recovery sleep (Chapter 3). These disfunctions have been shown to be due to more than simply "lapses" caused by "microsleeps"; rather, they are also the results of cognitive deficits. It is the brain, not the body, that dysfunctions without SWS. However, such dysfunctions may be due to the disruption of the circadian rhythms that accompany sleep deprivation.

- SWS increases more following wakefulness filled with mental activity than it does following less stimulating periods of wakefulness (Chapter 3).
- Cerebral metabolic rate is high during infancy and childhood when SWS is also high (Horne, 1988; Wauguier, Dugovic, & Radulovacki, 1989) when there is more brain organization and information processing occurring.
- Horne (1992) seems to argue that SWS in humans is most important for the functioning of the prefrontal part of the cortex, dince sleep deprivation results in reversible deficits in functions typically associated with this area of the brain. Also, people with psychological disorders known to involve the frontal cortex have less SWS.

2a) *NREM functions to conserve energy by reducing metabolic rate, energy expenditure, and temperature.* Most of the focus has been on temperature reduction but, metabolic rate and energy expenditure are interrelated with temperature reduction.

- NREM is a time of regulated, controlled, active cooling of the body (Chapter 2) by a decrease in heat production coupled by changes in heat conservation mechanisms that allow increased loss of body heat. This is in contrast to REM, which is a time of uncontrolled body temperature regulation (see Chapter 4).
- Several studies in humans and other mammals show a high correlation between metabolic rate and amount of NREM sleep. However,critics say that these data are confounded by equally high correlations of these factors with body size and feeding habits
- One theory sees the development of NREM sleep occurring during evolution about the time that warm blooded animals evolved (see Chapter 5). This is not viewed as a coincidence, but rather a necessity to prevent negative effects of being too warm for too long.

- It has been argued that SWS is the first stage on a continuum toward hibernation (Chapter 10). While hibernation conserves maximal amounts of energy by minimal metabolic levels, SWS does so too, only to a lesser extent.
- Some animals increase SWS during times of fasting necessitated by a reduced availability of food.
- In altricial species (i.e., those born relatively immature), the development of metabolic rate and SWS parallel each other.
- The recent work of Rechtschaffen and colleagues at the University of Chicago show the major effects of prolonged sleep deprivation in rats (see above), which is eventually lethal, to be a disruption of energy metabolism and temperature regulation. (However, these conclusions are for all of sleep and not just for NREM.)
- Heating the body just a degree or two increases the amount of subsequent SWS (Chapter 2). It is as if the body is using the cooling that accompanies SWS to balance off the increased heating of the body earlier, in an effort to maintain a constant daily average body temperature.
- Heating the Basal Forebrain (including portions of the nearly anterior hypothalamus) increases SWS. This may be the mechanism by which average daily body temperature (just mentioned above) is regulated.
- Sleep is longest in free-running conditions (see Chapter 4) when it occurs during the peak of the circadian body temperature rhythm.
- Extended sleep (12 hours or more) often includes the return of some SWS. This occurs when circadian body temperature is again on the rise.
- To be sure, some of the decrease in body temperature during NREM is due to its typical co-occurrence with the low of the circadian body temperature rhythm and to the typical recumbent, reduced activity position typically assumed during sleep. However, a significant part of the decrease is due to NREM sleep itself and occurs whenever NREM sleep happens.

2b) It has been suggested that it is not the entire body that requires and benefits from this reduction of temperature that accompanies NREM, but this *reduction in temperature benefits just the brain.*

- Observations of the negative mental effects and consequences of brain temperatures just slightly above normal indicate that normal brain temperatures are very close to dangerous levels. Yet, other observations of sub-maximal performance that occurs when brains are cooler than normal indicate that such higher brain temperatures are necessary for optimal brain functioning. It follows then that the brain may not be able to sustain uninterrupted periods of normally high temperature without beginning to sustain dysfunction and even damage. NREM sleep provides the needed, regular slight cooling of the brain.
- Brain temperature drops on the sleeping half of the dolphin brain (Chapter 5).

3) *NREM functions to enforce inactivity during certain times of the nychthemeron.* There are times during each nycthemeron that an animal may be more vulnerable. If it has a relatively safe place to sleep and can get ample food while awake, it is safer for it to be asleep with its forced inactivity than to be awake and moving about. (See Chapter 5 for more elaboration and evidence.)

There is nothing to indicate that these functions may not all be occurring simultaneously during NREM sleep. It may also be true that some are more important in some species than others. Finally, nobody is willing to say that this list of functions as presented here is the last word. Further research and thinking may suggest modifying or eliminating some of them or adding more functions to the list. Indeed, Feinberg's "sleep cognition" hypothesis (Feinberg, 1976; Feinberg, Koresko, & Heller, 1967) described in the first edition of this book has fallen by the way-side due to a preponderance of negative evidence and criticism (Spiegel, Koberle, & Allen, 1986; Zepelin, 1983). Time will tell about further changes.

Little attention has been paid specifically to stage 2 sleep ("light quiet sleep" in cats and primates (see Chapter 5)), probably because it is harder to manipulate (see Chapter 3). However, Meddis (1975) has speculated (more than concluded from data) about the functions of this stage of sleep.

Slow waves, he says, indicate that the brain is not processing informational input that is complex. It is most difficult to awaken humans or animals from SWS and elicit behavioral responses. SWS is also a time of enforced behavioral inactivity.

Light quiet sleep (stage 2) is seen only in cats and primates, thus it is most likely of more recent evolutionary development. It is similar to SWS except for less amplitude of the slow waves (in cats). In primates, K-complexes are a kind of isolated slow wave with a characteristic shape. This accounts for the lower behavioral thresholds of light quiet sleep. Spindles and K-complexes have been observed to occur in response to stimuli and might serve to jam out stimuli not important enough to need or to cause arousal (see Chapter 10).

If these things are true, then it follows that light quiet sleep is a more advanced way of maintaining the behavioral quiescence of SWS while simultaneously sustaining a high level of selective vigilance than is present in SWS. Indeed, those primates who are more vulnerable while asleep have more light quiet sleep, which would keep them more vigilant.

REM

There has been more research and speculative focus on REM sleep than on other sleep states, probably because of its paradoxical nature (see Chapter 1). Unlike NREM, which is proportional to prior wakefulness, REM seems related to the circadian temperature rhythm, since the propensity for REM increases when body temperature is at its trough but shows the least likelihood when body temperature is at its peak and for a few hours thereafter (Borbély, 1986). Yet, this cannot be the entire explanation for REM. Rebound of this stage occurs following deprivation, suggesting that it is too important to be missed. Something is both necessary and uniquely, or at least most easily, obtained by this stage of sleep, yet there is no severe psychological deterioration if it is missed.

Cohen (1980) has emphasized that some of the functions of REM seem to be preparatory while others are adaptive. That is, some anticipate future needs and insure that the organism is ready, while others respond to what the organism has experienced and attempt to better or more efficiently utilize that experience. The preparatory functions he includes are the stimulation of the brain for proper growth, the repair and maintenance of the brain, and the exercising of genetically-based behaviors. These help insure that the brain is ready to respond appropriately in the future when called upon. The adaptive functions include memory work on new learning, modulation of emotions, and the psychological benefits of dreams.

Several theorists recognize that REM may serve a number of functions simultaneously (see for example Hobson, 1989, and Horne, 1989) although they may not agree on which of the above components to include and which to exclude from their lists.

REM As Preparatory

Growth and restoration. The most popular theory of REM function is that it is important for normal growth of the brain in the developing animal and for restoration of the brain in the adult (Roffwarg, Muzio, & Dement, 1966). These are related processes. Something as complicated as the brain with billions of active cells making trillions of interconnections (Kalat, 1992) needs to be carefully constructed and maintained. REM is proposed to do both of these by providing adequate, relatively controlled, internal stimulation that facilitates and maintains the proper connections between cells. It is known from studies of the sensory systems, especially vision, that stimulation of the growing brain is necessary for normal connections between its cells (Kalat, 1992). Facilitation of the proper connections occurs by eliminating those connections that do not contribute to normal functioning. In the absence of such stimulation during growth, the brain is permanently miswired, resulting in abnormal vision. This process is thought to be a representation of a general principle for all brain growth and development. But, external stimulation may not be enough. Or it may be too random and irregular. Or it may not be handled well enough by the immature nervous system to insure appropriate connections with other brain areas (Chase, 1986). An internal source of stimulation that is more controlled and more predictable is necessary to stimulate the growing nerve tissue appropriately and speed its structural growth and physiological maturation. It is proposed that REM does just this.

Experimental evidence supports this hypothesis. Using drugs to deprive rat pups of REM during critical weeks of brain growth results both in permanent changes in brain structure and adult behavior - especially emotional, sensory, and sleep functions (Corner, Mirmiram, Bour, Boer, van de Poll, van Oyen, & Uylings, 1980; Hilakivi, 1987;

Mirmiram, 1986). REM deprivation in kittens worsens adult visual deficits produced by abnormal early sensory input (Oskenberg, 1987). Also, if PGO spikes are surgically suppressed in kittens, functioning of the visual areas of the nervous system develops abnormally (Davenne & Adrien, 1987). Finally, preliminary results of experiments using self-induced suppression of REM in kittens seem to suggest a resulting lag in brain cell maturation (Chase, 1986). Additional support can be found in Anch et al (1988) and Horne (1988).

Under normal circumstances, REM decreases in the adult from what it had been during development but does not disappear (see Chapter 1). While it no longer facilitates proper brain growth and development, it may be necessary in brain maintenance. It is a predictable source of internal stimulation that maintains (self-corrects) the functional pathways of interaction between brain cells. Supportive observations (Oswald, 1980) include the decrease in REM during senility, less REM in mentally retarded individuals, an increase in REM following brain poisoning (presumably while the brain is trying to repair the damage), and a decline in REM in elderly with organic brain dysfunction (Kryger, Roth, & Dement, 1989). Other researchers have shown that the decrease in the amount of REM sleep is correlated with the decline in the level of cognitive ability in the elderly but not in young people (Prinz, 1980).

Cells in the pons that use norepinephrine, histamine, or serotonin as neurotransmitters have wide spread projections to other parts of the brain (see Chapter 2). During REM, there is a dramatic cessation of the activity of these cells that have been viewed as having functional significance (Hobson, 1989; Siegel, 1989; 1990). Unlike most brain cells, these cells are almost constantly active during wake. Since they are small cells, they are susceptible of running out of adequate supplies of their neurotransmitters unless turned off for a while. Alternatively, this sustained rate of firing may have an effect on the receptors. Over-stimulation of neural cell receptors causes a reduction in their sensitivity (Kalat, 1992) which could reduce their effectiveness in receiving signals carried by neurotransmitters. Drastic reduction of stimulation of these receptors during REM may be important in allowing them to maintain normal levels of sensitivity. Likewise, the dramatic reduction during REM of sympathetic nervous system activity (where the neurotransmitter is norepinephrine) may serve a similar function for the nervous system outside of the brain.

Maintianance of inherited behaviors. Jouvet (1980) (see also Hobson, 1989) speculates that REM provides an opportunity for the genetic codes for instinctive behaviors to be activated and then compared with the animal's recent experience. This comparison provides opportunity for corrections and adjustments - a type of reliable pattern and circuit check. REM is ideal for this, because normally during REM the brain mechanisms are exercised but the behaviors themselves are blocked by the muscle paralysis that accompany this state. This is shown in cats with brain lesions in or near the locus coeruleus that were observed by Jouvet to be behaving (see Chapter 2). These behaviors appeared to him to be genetically based, innate behavior patterns. According to ethologists (European experts in animal behavior), animals inherit basic behaviors necessary for their survival (feeding, fighting, bleeding) and reproduction (fornicating) (Alcock, 1975). Jouvet speculates that in intact animals, the brain mechanisms that produce these behavior patterns need to be regularly exercised when the animal is in isolation and safe from predators, and the body is prevented from carrying them out. They need this regular, periodic exercise in order to maintain their functional integrity in the face of irregularly unpredictable waking use and potentially dysfunctional modification by learned influences. Yet, some of these learned influences may be beneficial but need to be carefully integrated with the inherited behavior patterns. REM provides just such an opportunity.

Perhaps the erections in males during REM (and to a less obvious extent, changes in female external genitalia) are an outward manifestation of these brain circuit checks for innate behaviors. (The only other functional speculation for these phenomena appeared in a paper about the memory effects of REM, by Crick and Mitchison (1986) which mentioned erections in a section entitled "Side Effects of REM." They first point out that erections are not a result of the erotic content of dreams and then continue with:

> *There seems no obvious reason why erection should not also be inhibited in sleep. One may wonder whether this phenomenon might have selective advantage in evolution. It would not, after all, be too surprising if this particular state of male readiness for sexual intercourse contributed to the number of offspring fathered. However, this assumes that the female of the species will be in easy proximity to the male*

during or shortly after sleep. One wonders, therefore, if REM penile erection has been observed in animals such as tigers, which are solitary except for brief periods of sexual intercourse, as opposed to lions, which constantly sleep in close proximity to each other.(pp. 245)

Adrian Morrison (Horne, 1988; Morrison & Reiner, 1985; Morrison, Ball, Sanford, Mann, & Ross, 1990) has compared the features of REM to the components of the orienting response in awake animals. The orienting response is the name for behavioral and physiological responses made by an animal when alerted by unexpected or novel stimuli. During the orienting response, the animal freezes for a few moments in a state of heightened alertness. The muscle inhibition of REM may be similar to freezing of muscle activity during orientation and the low voltage fast brain activity with PGO spikes and hypocampal theta of REM may correspond to the heightened brain alertness of the orienting response. The low activity in the sympathetic nervous systems and the suppression of homeostatic responses (such as the restriction of body temperature regulation) that occur during REM seem to, likewise, occur during the orienting response. Consistent with this comparison between REM and the orienting response is the observation that waking up out of REM (compared to waking up from NREM) results in higher levels of arousal for 30 or more minutes (Lavie, 1989). The major difference between REM and the orienting response is the sustained duration of the former compared to the transient nature of the latter. Perhaps REM is a substitute for wake by maintaining brain activation while also maintaining sleep.

REM As Adaptive

Memory. The importance of REM sleep for memory has been the focus of much research and theorizing in dozens of published reports throughout this decade (Cohen, 1980; Dujardin, Guerrien, & Leconte, 1990; Smith, 1993; Tilley, Brown, Donald, Ferguson, Piccone, Plasto, & Statham, 1992). Part of the reason comes from the notion in psychology that something newly learned is in a vulnerable, labile form until it is "consolidated" into a relatively invulnerable and fixed memory trace. This consolidation process takes time and may occur well after the learning experience.

REM seems well suited to the job of memory consolidation (Dujardin et al, 1990). It is a time when the brain is very active yet isolated from external stimuli ("off-line" to use computer terminology [Hobson, 1991]). It occurs regularly every nychthemeron - soon enough to process any recent new learning. REM is found in higher animals that depend more on learning and memory but is absent in lower animals that depend on instinctive behaviors for their survival.

Three research strategies have been employed to test the importance of REM for memory consolidation (Cohen, 1980; Dujardin et al, 1990; Tilley et al, 1992). In general, most reviews of this research positively support the idea that REM is necessary for optimal memory consolidation. While there are some neutral findings, negative findings are rare. (Other authors reviewing these same experiments have come to similar, or more positive, or even more negative conclusions.)

First, subjects (both humans and other animals have been used) learn something new while awake, then subsequent sleep is monitored. Many studies (but not all) have shown increases in amount of REM, number of REM periods, and/or REM density. Positive results tend to be found where the newly learned material is complex, affectively significant, or is difficult to learn because the animal is not instinctively prepared to do so. Also, there was no increase in REM if the subject tried learning the material, but was unsuccessful.

An example of this research involved studying people in intensive language learning situations (DeKoninck et al, 1990). The more successful students had an increase in REM percent but no increase in total sleep time. These same subjects also dreamt in the language more and had more verbal communication in their dreams.

Second, subjects who learned something new were subsequently deprived of REM before being tested for retention. Overall, the results of such studies show REM-deprived subjects have poorer retention than subjects allowed to get REM sleep. Negative results occurred more often when the task was simple or was something for which the animal was instinctively prepared to learn easily. In human subjects, positive results tended to be obtained for tasks that required the learner to structure the material and use divergent thinking but negative results when the material was already structured and required convergent thinking. Also, tasks with effective importance to the person were more susceptible to negative effects of REM deprivation.

An example of this kind of research is a study by Pirolli and Smith (1989). Subjects learned a difficult logic task and a simpler paired word task. Subsequently, one group of subjects slept through the night, a second group was totally sleep deprived, a third REM deprived, and a fourth NREM deprived. One week later they were tested on both tasks. All groups performed equally well on the simple paired word task but only those subjects without REM (REM deprived and total sleep deprived) did worse on the difficult logic task.

The third research strategy is a bit more complicated. During the retention interval following new learning, some subjects are allowed to sleep (usually nap) when they would get a lot of one kind of sleep (REM or NREM) but little of the other kind. Other subjects remain awake. A problem for such research has been controlling successfully for time-of-day (e.g. circadian rhythm) confounds of when the sleep occurs. Nevertheless, some of this research has supported the notion that REM sleep is beneficial for memory consolidation, but a few studies have concluded that NREM is more beneficial.

For example, Scrima (1984) administered a complex associative memory task to narcoleptics. They were then allowed a 20 minute nap or were to remain awake for 20 minutes. Since narcoleptics have a high amount of REM napping (see Chapter 9), many of the naps were mostly REM. Recall was best after REM and worse after remaining awake, with recall after NREM intermediate between the two.

Carlyle Smith of Trent University of Peterborough, Ontario, Canada has developed the concept of REM windows (see for example Smith, 1993). These are periods of time (3-4 hour in length for several nycthemerons following complex cognitive learning) when the occurrence of REM sleep is crucial for the maximal retention of learning. That is, only some REM serves this function, but NREM never does. His research has shown the REM windows to be independent of circadian rhythms, to occur in humans as well as other animals, and to change with the nature of the task. It is during the REM window that an increase in REM following new learning can be observed. Also, he has shown that during critical REM windows, manipulations of brain chemistry interfere with retention. Similar manipulations of brain chemistry have no such effect during REM before or after the window.

The beneficial effects of REM sleep on retention in humans may be more significant for emotion-related material. For example, Cartwright (1984b) gave subjects crossword puzzles, word association tasks, and story completions to do. They ranged from neutral to emotional in character. Half of the subjects stayed awake, the other half obtained REM between the start and finish of the tasks. REM sleep was more beneficial the more emotion laden the problems. REM, but not wake, changed the way the subjects viewed the emotion-laden problems.

A number of theories have been advanced to explain why REM enhances memory consolidation (Tilley et al, 1992). Some of these maintain that REM adds or enhances something in the memory mechanism of the brain (Cohen, 1980; Scrima, 1984). The increase of protein synthesis during REM (which is blocked by REM deprivation) may be necessary to create and/or preserve memories (Anch et al, 1988; Drucker-Colin, 1979) by helping to create and maintain neural circuits (Cohen, 1980). REM may be necessary to relearn memories in view of the great molecular turnover in the brain (Davis, 1985). Or cells may need periodic, systematic stimulation before new memories become permanent (Davis, 1985), and the high level of neuron activation that occurs during REM may do just this (Dujardin et al, 1990). Or perhaps it is some aspect of the biochemistry of sleep that accounts for its memory enhancing effects, such as the relatively higher levels of acetylcholine activity relative to norepinephrine activity that occurs during REM (see Chapter 2) (Tilley et al, 1992).

Other theories suggest that REM subtracts something from the memory stores of the brain (see Chapter 7). A cleaning up of the memory banks occurs by the brain ridding itself of unwanted, useless, and even confusing associations. This leaves what remains clearer, cleaner, and more meaningful (Crick & Mitchison, 1986).

Others see the influence of REM on memory as being more selective. During REM new experiences from waking are selected, sorted, and consolidated, and linked with old experiences (Hobson, 1988; Koukkou & Lehmann, 1983). REM may reorganize memories by simultaneously activating old and new ones in the absence of distractions. Or it may integrate new information into the personality structure of the person (Webb, 1983). This might be viewed as a kind of off-line reprogramming that is both a consolidation of past learning and a preparation for future learning.

Finally, during wakefulness, the hippocampus "gates" short-term memory to long term memory. Consolidation may only be able to be completed during REM, because the hippocampus is freed from this gating function during this stage of sleep (Bootzen, Kihlstrom &

Schacter, 1990; Carskadon & Dement, 1989). Instead, the hippocampus may function to connect recently acquired long term memory in such a way as to actively help consolidation. The hippocampus may not be able to simultaneously perform its gating and consolidating functions. During REM, it shifts from gating to consolidation.

(A curious tangent to this research is the effects on memory for learning acquired soon *after* sleep [Tilley et al, 1992]. Sleep immediately prior to learning does not affect learning but may have a negative or positive affect on later memory. This may possibly be due to sleep-related biochemical processes in the brain or a decrease in the psychological process of proactive inhibition.)

Horne (1988), however, is not impressed with the evidence linking REM with memory functions, finding "only weak evidence from humans and questionable findings from animals" (p 282). The change in REM associated with learning are small in humans and only for difficult tasks. In animals, even long REM deprivation produces only small, if any, decrements in memory. Furthermore, it is not clear that decrements that do occur are caused directly by the lack of REM or by changes in drive caused by REM deprivation, and/or the stress of the deprivation procedure itself.

(A few studies have shown positive effects of NREM, not REM, sleep on memory. In one case, the occurrence of SWS (or SWS plus REM) during daytime naps had a beneficial effect on retention, whereas REM did not (Tilley et al, 1992). In another case, data on a performance task - human motor learning (pursuit rotor) - in contrast to the more frequently used mental tasks, showed retention disruption following various kinds of sleep deprivations that could only make sense if the reduction of stage 2 sleep was the only critical component (Smith & MacNeill, 1992a).)

Emotion. REM has also been postulated to play an important role in mood and emotions. It has been thought to result in "enhanced effective adjustment" and "greater interpersonal skill and inventiveness" (Cohen, 1980, p. 315). Included by some (see for example Webb, 1983) in this context, is Freud's discharge model (see Chapter 7) of dreams, which states that dreams act as a safety valve for repressed drive. Others see this emotional function as due to REM itself and not its accompanying dreams. For example, Vogel (1979) asserts that REM lessens wakening drive motivated behaviors. He infers this from the effects of REM deprivation on depressed individuals (Chapter 10). This occurs because REM deprivation increases many drive-motivated behaviors as a result of increasing excitability in many brain structures, including those important for drive. This brain excitation, hence anti-depressive effect, is easily and quickly reversed by even a little subsequent REM sleep because during REM sleep, neural excitability is increased, resulting in a corresponding decrease in neural excitation when awake. For what purpose might this occur? REM sleep may serve to modulate or tame the drives, leaving a person more flexible and adaptive when awake (Horne, 1988).

Other observations show an increase in REM sleep time after days of stress, worry, and intense learning (Greenberg, 1981; Hartmann, 1973). Generally, this will occur after a large variety of emotionally demanding events, both positive and negative, of the day. It can be seen in exaggerated form in variable length sleepers (see Chapter 1).

Other aspects of REM

What is the function of the eye movements of REM and the PGO spikes that accompany them? Speculations include (Drucker-Colin & Prospero-Garcia, 1990):

1) PGO spikes participate in generating alertness processes of REM.

2)They help develop (during growth) and maintain (during adulthood) proper functioning of the visual system.

3) PGO spikes mimic sensory inputs that cause cortical arousal as well as dream imagery.

4) PGO spikes help stimulate the forebrain to enhance the memory functions of REM.

Inclusive Theories

Some theories of sleep endeavor to include almost all of its functions. One of the better of these inclusive theories has been described by Horne (1983b; 1983c; 1988). He maintains that sleep has both restitutional and behavioral functions. However, each individual species may have a somewhat different, yet interacting, combination of these functions in their sleep which he calls core (obligatory) sleep and optional (facultative) sleep.

As its name implies, animals are obligated to obtain CORE sleep. It consists mainly of restorative and other, more internal, benefits for the animal, especially those involving brain mechanisms. Core sleep contains a high proportion of SWS that occurs earlier in the sleep period. The need for this kind of sleep builds with wakefulness and maybe waking brain effort. It is a "deeper sleep" necessary for normal functioning.

Optional sleep is more flexible. It can be extended or reduced a bit in accordance with environmental demands. It is more for safety, energy conservation, and efficiency kinds of functions. It can also function as relief from boredom and may accommodate brain restitution if necessary. Optional sleep contains a high proportion of REM sleep. It is on a circadian schedule but may also be governed by "behavioral drive." It may vary with the seasons (to act as a time occupier when the environment is less habitable).

These two kinds of sleep have different proportions in different animals - especially animals that occupy different branches of the phylogenetic tree. Core sleep is more important for animals higher up in the phylogenetic tree with their more advanced brains. Although these higher animals can and do engage in relaxed wakefulness, relaxed wakefulness can only relax the muscles, it cannot "relax" the brain; only sleep can to this. Optional sleep is more important in smaller, less advanced insectivores and rodents (that is, animals that tend to have high levels of activity when awake) in order to conserve energy. For them and others, the safety function may also be an important aspect of optional sleep. Other factors that determine the relative proportions of core and optional sleep include immaturity, safe sleeping habitat, and body size. For example, vulnerable animals have less AS (Meddis, 1983), a major component of optional sleep.

According to the theory, both core and optional mechanisms are operating at sleep onset in all animals. However, core sleep starts with greater strength early in the sleep period but has a rapid decline, leaving only optional sleep prevalent later in the sleep period. It is this rate of decline of core sleep that varies between animals. Figure 9-1 summarizes the factors affecting core and optional sleep in different kinds of animals.

Humans also appear to have both kinds of sleep. Sleep deprivation experiments show that human sleep does have an obligatory aspect to

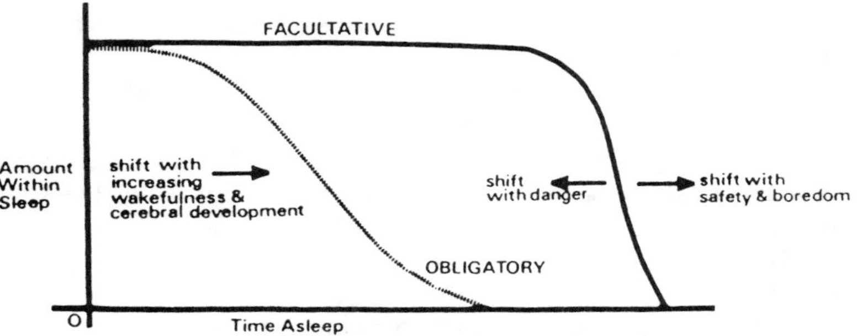

Figure 9-1. Hypothesized trends during sleep for core and optional sleep mechanisms, and the major influences seen to affect these trends. (From Horne [1983c]. Mammalian Sleep function with particular reference to man. In Mayes, A (Ed.) *Sleep and functions in humans and animals - an evolutionary perspective*. Birkshire, England: Van Nostrand Reinhold, with permission of Chapman and Hall, London.)

it (Mayes, 1983). Human core sleep appears to be three NREM/REM cycles (about 6 hours) but with a lot of individual variation (Benoit,1985). It is the minimum necessary sleep in adults (children need more). The optional component can be varied by 1-2 hours per nychthemeron via napping or lengthening the main sleep period (Horne, 1983c). According to this theory, human optional sleep probably originally developed to provide a time of safety, yet was flexible enough to enable humans to accommodate their daily sleep/wake schedule to the seasonal changing durations of daily light at the more extreme latitudes.

Others agree with Horne that there are these two kinds of sleep but do not agree that optional sleep is as optional as its name implies (Benoit, 1985; Stampi, Moffitt, & Hoffman, 1990). To some, optional sleep may more properly be described as "necessary but flexible" (Benoit, 1985, p 438). That is, it can be foregone for a while, but eventually it needs to be recovered. Other optional sleep may be a way of occupying time that is unproductive and does need not be recovered if missed (but may help us feel our absolute best). Or, perhaps, we can do without optional sleep in the short run, but not in the long run (Stampi et al, 1990).

The Functions of Dreams (and other mentation)

Why do we spend so much time dreaming? Why does our mind put forth the effort to create dream after dream night after night? Surely there must be good purpose for such an endeavor. Through the ages there have been many ideas about what dreams are (see Chapter 6). Some of these ideas are related to functions. Rather than review all of these ideas, we shall focus our attention here on theories that give primary importance to dream function and that are also in the forefront of current consideration.

One difficulty with attempting to discover the function of dreams is the difficulty of getting to the source of the data - the dreams themselves (see Chapter 6). This means that the theories of dreams tend to be even more speculative than theories involving other aspects of sleep. That is, the fact to assumption ratio is often quite low and the research attempting to test one or another of these theories have provided only weak support or contradictory results (Cartwright, 1989). Nevertheless, many of the contemporary theories are interesting, instructive, and seem to ring true. We will examine some of these.

Most contemporary theories emphasize an affective/emotional role for dreams. You dream about things that are important to you, in the sense of being emotionally arousing or effectively significant (Fiss, 1979). The process is adaptive since you focus on your problems and seek solutions (Cartwright, 1990). These solutions may subsequently be assimilated into existing memory structures (Cartwright, 1990). Dreams, then, are involved in the processes of self-regulation and self-reflectiveness (Moffitt, 1987). They function like a gyroscope to keep the self on a steady course in the face of the vicissitudes of daily life.

One way that they do this is by preserving our identity (Cartwright, 1977). They retell who we are. They act like an emotional thermostat (Kramer, 1987) making corrections to get us back toward an ideal. They bring a balance into our lives. They can also act like a safety valve allowing us to "let off" built up emotional pressure.

Dreams are best viewed as occurring between two periods of wake (Kramer, 1987; 1990; Fiss, 1979). The preceding period of wake affects the subsequent dream (or put another way, the dream reflects the preceding period of wake). But the dream then affects the subsequent period of wake as a kind of mood regulator.

Modern thinkers have seen the relationship of dreams to the dreamers waking life in one of two ways - complementary or continuous (Cartwright, 1977; 1978). Complementary dreams contain things that compensate or supplement what has recently occurred in waking life in an attempt to bring overall balance or harmony. For example, when Paul has been severely criticized for making an error at work which he felt may have jeopardized his chances for promotion, he subsequently dreamt that he was competing in pre-Olympic track trials and was doing quite well and was "still in the running." Jill during the day had been bragging about being selected as one of 10 finalists in a contest by a popular teen magazine for a modeling feature in a future issue. That night her dreams contained an image of a group of strangers pruning rose bushes ("cutting them down to size").

Continuous dreams, on the other hand, are those in which the themes, concerns, and events of waking life are continued in our dreams. Jerry had recently been working nights and weekends at his job, hoping to make a good impression and be rapidly promoted. After an argument with his wife about his "never being home," he had a dream that he was in a hot air balloon race in which he was "rising fast but on a collision course with a house that looked like mine."

Which is correct? Do our dreams take an active role in attempting to compensate for our waking lives in an effort to bring balance to our psyche? Or is the focus of our dreams continuous with the cares and events of our waking lives? Probably, both are correct. Our mind may choose one or the other depending on current need or perhaps the created dream may contain an element of each. The choice seems to depend on where the greatest need, exists in a person's life at the moment.

Defense of Self

What are the kinds of needs dreams meet, and how do they endeavor to meet those needs? There seem to be several answers (Cartwright, 1977). First and foremost, our dreams can defend the self in the face of attack. They may take the form of retrenchment, or perhaps of giving oneself reassurance, or a reconciliation of the self with unavoidable, objective information. In any case, the dream is endeavoring to build and preserve a unity of the personality that is whole and reasonably healthy. The following dream that Bill had demonstrates this well.

Before the dream, it had been one of those weeks where nothing was going well. I had a lot of tests and a paper due. Yet, this was the week when the guys down the hall decided to see who had the most powerful stereo. That went on for about three nights. Then my roommate was having problems with his parents and needed to talk to me for a couple of hours. I knew I wasn't doing a good job on any of my tests and papers, and I was beginning to have thoughts of quitting school. Things were out of my control, and I just couldn't keep up. I was depressed.

Then I had this dream. Some men - they looked like CIA or FBI or something - were looking for a guy to do an important, complex mission. They came to my dorm room and told me that I had all the characteristics needed to get the job done. I kept trying to tell them that I wasn't good enough, but they kept insisting that I was. They had a big briefcase full of papers they kept showing me. They said that they were about me. Each one had a big gold star on it. Another briefcase was full of cash which they said would be mine for completing the task. Again and again they urged me to go on and do it. I woke up feeling pretty good.

Dealing with Emotions

Of next, and nearly equal, importance is the effort of dreams to deal with emotion-laden issues from our personal current life which need attending to. If the issue is particularly strong or complex, the dreams of several nights may be devoted to it until it is reasonably well resolved. There is an advantage in dealing with emotions in dreams, for there is an absence of inhibition from logic and no fear of ridicule while dreaming. We can relate our waking stresses to past memories of a similar nature without being disturbed by interruptions that are frequent when we are awake. We are then freer to try out different solutions because we are free from the consequences and social constraints of waking life (Koulack, 1991). We are also freer to mix ideas than when we are awake. So, unlike when awake, our mind can work more directly on the emotional problem on its own terms. This is often more successful than trying to deal with them than when in the waking mode of thought. The end result is that we can assimilate the emotional problem into our psyche in a way that promotes overall well being. Mark's dreams two nights before his piano recital are an example of this.

> *On May 9, I dreamt that I could see myself practicing my part. I could see my hands on the keyboard the way one would, seated at a piano, but every once in a while I would switch and be someone at the door looking in at myself through a window in the door.*
>
> *On May 10, I dreamt a vague and indistinct dream. I don't remember seeing much except clouds and a bust of Mozart (who wrote the piece), but I heard the entire piece (actual playing time: 35 minutes) from beginning to end with all instruments present.*
>
> *I woke up feeling much more confident and relaxed.*

Laboratory studies show that there is a measurable change in certain aspects of mood after dreaming compared to before (Kramer, 1993). There is a lower average mood and less variability following dreaming. Furthermore, behavior is changed as a result. These studies have also shown that it is the dream content, especially the characters in the dream, that is related to the mood change. And some of these mood changes are not just due to the physiology of sleep. While some aspects of mood are affected by sleep physiology, such as "clear thinking," others are affected by the dreaming, such as "unhappiness" (see above).

Others, like Freud, see the function of dreams as gratification and release of pent up unconscious impulses while maintaining sleep (see Chapter 7). Koulack (1991) (reminiscent of Freud) maintains that we also have "avoidance dreams" that occur to protect the consolidation of sleep from (1) disturbing material in our minds that may awaken us (we may either not dream about the disturbing subject or have compensatory dreams) and (2) external stimuli by incorporating them into our dreams.

It has been hypothesized that during dreaming memories are reorganized by associations as a way of integrating the past with the present (Hobson, 1989). This helps keep our own memories more efficiently organized. A related idea is that dreams are important for reprocessing waking experiences and important for their survival into our memories (Winson, 1990) (see Chapter 7). For animals, the survival value of dreams involves memories for things like where to obtain food or where to escape from predators. In this way, dreams are biologically relevant. For humans, the survival value is more involved with the complex interrelationships of humans and the complexities of human personality.

Foulkes (1983) also focuses on a memory function of dreaming. He was struck by the parallel between Piagetan cognitive development in children and the development of their dreams (see Chapter 6). As a result he developed a theory that states that dreams help integrate our knowledge - especially that knowledge available to conscious recall. This integration occurs both within types of memory and between types of memory (such as semantic and episodic, recent and distant, verbal and visual-spatial). The integration occurs even though we do not remember much of our dreams. As a result, we are left with: 1) an increase in the range of our experiences that even includes unrealistic things; 2) greater reality testing since when we awaken we know that much of what we dreamed was not real, and thus we can more easily recognize that our minds are capable of creating things that are not real; 3) better self-knowledge because of combining motor memories with recognition memories giving us more flexibility.

Cartwright (1989) incorporates some of these ideas about dream functions into the current understanding of how the brain works. The result is her Parallel Distributed Processing Model of dreaming. Our mind is composed of patterns of cognitions resulting from experiences while trying to meet our biological and psychological (such as self esteem) needs. Affect accompanies these experiences concerning how successful we are in getting our needs met. All of these factors are stored in different places in the brain (distributed) at about the same time (i.e., in parallel) with interconnections of varying strengths. The result is different from what might occur when awake because of a different brain organization when asleep. Other related memories and past associations may also be stimulated in the process. The end result is the dream that we are aware of.

Creativity

The next level at which we may use our dreams is to create. Dreams by their very nature are creative, so it is not surprising that they can offer solutions to practical problems or yield artistic inspirations (see chapter 6). Your dreams may also have a similar function, although in a more subtle way, by suggesting solutions to your everyday problems (Koulack, 1987). They do this by providing access to our recent and remote memories tying them to alternate cognitive strategies, followed by assimilation or accommodation into our existing memories and/or personality (Cartwright, 1990). But, there seems to be natural constraints on this. First, you must be working on the problem or, in some other way, have the need for such a dream during your waking life. Second, you need to be able to recognize that the dream is offering a solution. Third, such dreams appear to be rather unpredictable, meaning that you cannot pick and choose when they will occur and that you have to be ready to record and use them when they do come. The following excerpt from a dream that Tom had shows these things.

> *Before this dream, I'd been having trouble deciding how to work out a color scheme on a particular woodcut for art class. In my dream, consequently, I somehow worked out an idea and woke up knowing what I was planning to do next. I also had short conversations with the class professor in my dream, although I don't remember exactly what was discussed. This class, where I work with my hands and tools a lot, is often included in my dreams.*

Watt's lead shot dream presented in Chapter 6 is another excellent example of all of the factors involved with creative dreams. It was an important problem that he had been working on during his waking life, yet he had to have the dream several times before he recognized what it was saying to him. (I can only wonder what new discoveries have been lost because dreamers did not pay attention to what their dream might have been trying to tell them).

Play

Finally, in the absence of any of the above needs, it seems that we are free to escape and play in our dreams (Hobson, 1988). Carefree, purposeless frolic, seemingly devoid of any purpose appears to be possible. The following dream excerpt seems to be one of pure play. The mood is light and enjoyable. None of the objects, characters, or locations seemed to Jack to have much meaning other than that of light-hearted frolic.

We were in Jim's blue convertible driving to the beach or something. Jim and I and a couple of our friends. It was a bright, sunny, warm, but not hot, day. We were as free and as light as the breeze. Some really great song was playing loud on the radio and we were kinda singing along. I couldn't tell you the song now - in fact, I don't think I ever heard it before.

Suddenly, we arrived, only it was a ski resort. There was snow on the ground, yet it wasn't cold. I began skiing down the mountain - beautifully, smoothly making wide parallel turns...then I kinda glided off the ground and was flying in the air. I didn't have skis on - I don't think I ever did. It was beautiful; I just started going up and up till I could look down and see the whole ski area. Then the alarm went off, darn it. I would have liked to have stayed and flown some more.

This, like the other functions, can be important. Dreams may keep the cerebrum entertained during sleep (Horne, 1988). Or they can provide respite from our problems. In such cases, we dream of pleasant things or unrelated stressful experiences (Koulack, 1987).

A Common Function

Careful analysis of all of these functions shows the central importance of emotions in dreams. Even the creative and play dreams can be said to involve emotions. The creative dreams involve things that are important or necessary to the dreamer - things in which the dreamer has invested much of his/her recent waking life. Even the play that occurs in dreams can be said to have an emotional basis and benefit, just as awake play does. This is an important point in understanding dreams; that regardless of whatever else they may be, they have an emotional focus or core.

If the dreams are successful in fulfilling any of these purposes, the dreamer awakens better able to cope and be more productive. If, however, the dream was unsuccessful or provided only partial success, subsequent dreams may deal with the subject matter again or the actual dream may be repeated again.

But, not all dreams successfully accomplish what they were intended to do; (Cartwright, 1991) some fail, some are trivial, and some are noxious. "Just as not all sleep is physiologically restorative, so not all dreams are necessarily psychologically restorative" (Fiss, 1979, p.64).

In contrast to this view of the functions of dreams, there have been numerous statements made minimizing the functions of dreams (see Cartwright, 1990 for a review) including Crick and Mitchison (1983) and interpretations of the Hobson and McCarley Activation-Synthesis hypothesis (1977) (see Chapter 7). Dreams are thought to be meaningless epiphenomona of what occurs in the brain during sleep (Antrobus, 1987). When a lawnmower cuts grass it makes noise. The noise does not have a function; it does not help cut the grass. It is a by-product (or epiphenomon) of the activity of the lawnmower. Similarly, dreams are seen as a by-product of the activity of the brain as it goes about its other (real) functions during sleep.

Summary

My own view (which is similar to that of Feinberg & Floyd, 1982) of the functions of sleep, including dreams, incorporates most of the ideas presented in this chapter. Yet, I am struck by evidence that sleep does not seem to be absolutely necessary for anything. People and animals can do without it for long periods of time. Only work from Rechtschaffen's lab (reviewed above) has shown that sleep deprivation can have serious physical consequences in rats, but this was only after a few weeks of continuous sleeplessness. In most other cases, things that occur during sleep can occur when we are awake or we can do without them. Aspects of sleep brain waves, muscle inhibition, PGO waves, and so on have been found to occur outside of sleep in narcoleptics, sleep-walkers, and in people who are severely sleep deprived. Likewise, the following have been demonstrated regarding REM and its components (Sakai, 1985):

- REM without PGO waves (in animals with lesions in the dorsal ponto-mesencephalic tegmentum);
- REM without muscle paralysis (in humans with REM behavior disorder);
- REM without its characteristic brain waves (following administration of the drug atropine);

Each of the aspects thus appears to be an independent process for which sleep is not necessary and, therefore, not the cause (Fiss, 1979). Yet, each instance of such a dissociation is caused by a deviation from the optimal, normal level of functioning. In short, we do not do as well without sleep. Perhaps sleep has no function other than to orchestrate the various aspects and provide a convenient time when they can occur most easily and most efficiently (Adam & Oswald, 1983; McGaugh et al, 1979). This is not to belittle this function; efficiency is important and in the long run may even be essential, as the Rechtschaffen research shows. But, in the short run, it can be sacrificed for other, more pressing needs.

Sleep has a rhythmic character (Chapter 4). In this respect it is no different from many other rhythms seen in life on our planet. It may have evolved out of a simple rest/activity cycle seen in other animals (Chapter 5) primarily as a behavioral strategy to keep its practitioner out of harms way and to conserve a little energy at the same time. As warm blooded animals evolved, sleep may have become more important in the regulation of body temperature. Still later, with the evolution of bigger and more complex brains, sleep also assumed importance in the development and maintenance of this very delicate, yet complex structure. Likewise, sleep, thus evolved, could be a convenient time to perform some cognitive and emotional housekeeping, thus dreams were added. Remnants of this evolutionary history are evident today in present species that have different places on the evolutionary tree (Horne, 1988). Remnants are also evident within individual higher species since, during evolution, existing functions of sleep were not simply replaced but new functions were also added on. Later, these add-ons may have gained primary importance, with the others becoming secondary but still remaining present.

Sleep may be likened to an American university. There are many aspects and functions of universities - education, research, extension services, athletics, to name a few. Each helps define the university and make it what it is, yet each can exist apart from it. The assemblage of these various potentially autonomous entities not only defines the university but also lends a certain efficiency to each of its parts. Yet, the university can be recognized even if some of its parts are absent. So too with sleep. It may in the end just be the "recruitment and coupling" of potentially independent elements (McGinty, 1985), including dreams.

Just as at the university teaching may be considered a primary function and athletics a secondary function, some of the functions of sleep may be more primary and others secondary (Meddis, 1979). Also, the function of the university may differ at different times in history (at one time the primary function of many universities was to produce teachers and preachers) just as the function of sleep has differed throughout evolution (Horne, 1983c).

Also, the function of the university may differ for different students depending on their attributes and needs. The more musically gifted may value the music courses and organizations more than the academic and athletic functions. In contrast, another student with intellectual abilities may value the classroom and library much more. All of these students may also participate in other things while at the university because they are available and convenient, but they are of more or less secondary importance. So too with sleep, the extent to which sleep is for safety, energy conservation, restoration, or whatever may depend on such interrelated things such as the size of the body, degree of cerebral development, and constituents of the diet (Horne, 1988). This is certainly true of other characteristics of animals. Some animals have claws, others hooves, and still others fingers. Some have fins and others have no appendages at all. Behaviorally, we can also see differences between animals. Some rely heavily on fixed inherited instincts, while others rely on learned behaviors. Some animals live in very structured social groups, while others are mostly solitary. Likewise, different types of animals may have different functions for sleep according to their own unique needs.

Finally, just as the function of the university may change for an individual student during the course of their stay there (it is not unusual for students to change majors or perhaps they were attracted to the university primarily because of its social and extracurricular activities but discovered the joy of serious study by the time they graduated), so too the function of sleep may change during the course of its nightly duration (Horne, 1988). The greater amounts of SWS early in the night followed by more REM later certainly support such a notion.

In the end, then, the function of sleep may be to provide optimal circumstances for many diverse functions. Its function may be summed up in one word - EFFICIENCY.

This does not mean that sleep is unimportant. As Webb has said very well (1979, P 31):

My position views sleep as a process which evolved to aid us to adapt our behavior to an environment of eons ago. The sleep of Babylon is the sleep of today. For those times and places it functioned effectively as a biological system. But, modern times have brought the Edison Age of electric lights and is abolishing the natural rhythm of night and day, the jet aircraft tosses sleep across multiple time zones, and drugs have given promises of bending sleep to our momentary demands. Pervasively, we raise our strident cries and push our self-centered demands that sleep be subservient to our whimsy, bend to our needs, pressures and terrors. We ominously move toward viewing our failures of sleep to be "illnesses" to be "cured."

My view point is to the contrary. In a reasonably natural and stable environment sleep will serve its function as a silent and well-trained servant. It is rather our "misbehaviors" in relation to sleep, goaded by a changed environment and a thoroughly anthropomorphic arrogance about "nature", which "fails" sleep as it is pushed beyond its natural limits. From my perspective, anchored in my adaptive theory of sleep, we must rather than learn the proximal causes of sleep, learn the laws of sleep. In turn we must teach ourselves to act in accord with these laws. I agree with Francis Bacon of 500 years ago: "Nature cannot be commanded except by being obeyed."

Epilog

We have come to the end of our exploration sleep, dreaming, and sleep disorders. I hope that I have covered these topics well for you. However, you may still have some questions unanswered or perhaps comments or suggestions about this book. If you do, I encourage you to write me. I will try to answer the questions and incorporate the suggestions in the next edition of this book. My address is:

Bill Moorcroft, Ph.D.
Director, Sleep Laboratory
Luther College
Decorah, Iowa
52101.

I look forward to hearing from you.

References

(The numbers in parenthesis at the end of each reference refer to the chapter in which the reference is cited.)

Acebo C, Davis S S, Herman K B, & Carshadon M A (1991). Undergraduate sleep patterns: evidence of adaptation over time. *Sleep Research, 20,* 111. (1)

Achermann P & Borbély A A (1990). Modeling the ultradian dynamics of EEG slow-wave activity and REM sleep. *Sleep research, 19,* 127. (4)

Achermann P & Borbély A A (1990). Simulation of human sleep: ultradian dynamics of electroencephalographic slow-wave activity. *Journal of biological rhythms, 5,* 141-157. (4)

Adam K (1980). Dietary habits and sleep after bedtime food drinks. *Sleep, 5,* 47-58. (2,11)

Adam K & Oswald I (1983). Protein synthesis, bodily renewal and the sleep-wake cycle. *Clinical Science, 65,* 561-567. (11)

Addison R G, Thorpy M J, & Roth T (1987). A survey of the United States public concerning the quality of sleep. *Sleep Research, 16,* 244. (3)

Agnew H W, Webb W K, & Williams R L (1967). Comparison of stage 4 and 1-REM sleep deprivation. *Perception and Motivation Skills, 24,* 851-858.(3)

Åkerstedt A (1984). Work schedules and sleep. *Experientia, 40,* 417-422. (4)

Alcock J (1975). *Animal Behavior: an Evolutionary Approach.* Sunderland, Mass.: Sinauer Associates, Inc. (11)

Allen R & Mirabile J (1989). Self-reported sleep-wake patterns for students during the school year from two different senior high schools. *Sleep Research, 18,* 132. (1)

Allison T & Van Twyver H (1970). The evolution of sleep. *Natural History, 79*, 56-65. (3,5,10)

Allison T, Van Twyver H, & Goff W (1972). Electrophysiological studies of the echidna. *Archives of Italalian Biology, 110*, 145-184. (5)

American Sleep Disorders Association (1990). *The international classification of sleep disorders.* First edition, prepared by the Sleep Disorders Classification Committee, M Thorpy, Chairman. Kailey: Kansas. (2)

Anch A M, Browman C P, Mitler M M, & Walsh J K (1988). *Sleep: a scientific perspective.* Englewood Cliffs, New Jersey: Prentice Hall. (1,2,3,4,9,10,11)

Anders T, Emde R, & Parmelee (Eds.) (1971). *A manual of standardized terminology, techniques, and criteria for scoring states of sleep and wakefulness in newborn infants.* Los Angeles: UCLA Brain Information Service/Brain Research Institute. (1)

Anders T & Roffwarg H P (1968). The relationship between infant and maternal sleep. *Psychophysiology, 5*, 227-228. (2)

Anonymous (1991). *Basic sleep research.* Washington: Institute of medicine. (2)

Antrobus J (1987 June-July). *Is there a function for REM sleep mentation?.* Presented at the Fifth International Congress of Sleep Research, Copenhagen, Denmark. (11)

Antrobus J (1990). The neurocognition of sleep mentation: rapid eye movements, visual imagery, and dreaming. In R R Bootzin, J F Kihlstrom, & D L Schacter (Eds.), *Sleep and Cognition* (pp. 1-24). Washington: American Psychological Association. (6)

Arkin A M (1981). *Sleeptalking: Psychology and Psycholphysiology* Hillsdale, NJ: L. Erlbaum Associates. (9)

Armitage R, Bell I, Campbell K, & Stelmack R (1990). Asymmetrical auditory probe evoked potentials during REM and NREM sleep. *Sleep, 13*, 69-78. (6)

Aserinsky E & Kleitman W (1953). Regularly occurring periods of eye motility and concommitant phenomena during sleep. *Science, 118*, 273-274. (6)

Association of Sleep Disorders Centers (1979). *Diagnostic classification of sleep and arousal disorders* (1st ed.). Prepared by the Sleep Disorders Classification Committee, H P Roffwarg, Chairman, *Sleep, 2*, 1-137. (6,9)

Atkinson R L, Atkinson R C, Smith E E, & Hilgard E R (1987). *Introduction to psychology, 9th ed.* New York: Harcourt, Brace, Jovanovich. (10)

Badia P (1990). Memories in sleep: Old and new. In R R Bootzin, J F Kihlstrom, & D L Schachter (Eds.), *Sleep and cognition* (pp. 67-76). Washington: American Psychological Association. (5) (5,10)

Ball N J, Shaffery J P, Opp M R, Schmidt, D F, & Amlaner, C J (1987 June-July). *Homeostatic control of sleep in birds.* Presented at the Fifth International Congress of Sleep Research, Copenhagen, Denmark. (5)

Beare D J, Roehrs T A, Battle D, Waller P, Zorick F, & Roth T (1992). Sleepiness and ethanol effects on simulated driving performance. *Sleep Research, 21*, 99. (2)

Benington J H & Heller H C (1991). Cholinergic and monoaminergic modulation of sleep cycling in the rat: a new analysis based on REM sleep transition. *Sleep Research, 20*, 59. (2)

Benoit O (1985). Homeostatic and adaptive roles of human sleep. *Experientia, 40*, 437-440.(3,11)

Berlin R M & Qayyum U (1986). Sleepwalking: Diagnosis and treatment through the life cycle. *Psychosomatics, 27*, 755-760. (9)

Bigler P J & Carskadon M A (1990). Sleep/wake patterns of college students across a smester. *Sleep Rerearch, 19,* 113. (1)

Billiard M & Passouant P (1973). Sleep study in women. Influence of menstrual cycle, pregnancy and hypothalamic amenorrhea on night sleep. In W P Koella and P L Basel (Ed.), *Sleep* (pp. 395-399). Basel: Karger. (2)

Bixler E O, Kales A, Jacoby J A, Soldatos C R, & Vela-Bueno A (1984). Nocturnal sleep and wakelfulness: Effects of age and sex in normal sleepers. *International Journal of Neuroscience, 23*, 33-42. (1)

Bonnet M H (1986). Performance and sleepiness as a function of frequency and placement of sleep disruption. *Psychophysiology, 23*, 263-271. (3)

Bonnett M (1990). The perception of sleep onset in insomniacs and normal sleepers. In R R Bootzin, J F Kihlstrom, & N S Schacter (Eds.), *Sleep and Cognition* (pp 148-158). Washington, D.C.: American Psychological Association. (3)

Bonnet M H & Johnson L C (1978). The relationship of depth of sleep (arousal threshold) to subjective depth and quality of sleep. *Sleep Research, 7*, 156. (3)

Bootzen R R, Kihlstrom J F, & Schacter N S (Eds.) (1990). *Sleep and Cognition*. Washington, D.C.: American Psychological Association. (11)

Borbély A A (1982). A two process model of sleep regulation. *Human Physiology, 1,* 195-204. (4)

Borbély A A (1984). Sleep regulation: outline of a model and its implications for depression. In A A Borbély & J L Valatx (Eds.), *Sleep mechanisms* (pp. 272-284). Berlin: Springer-Verlag (4,5)

Borbély A A (1986). *The secrets of sleep*. New York: Basic Books. (2,3,4,5,6,10,11)

Borbély A A & Tobler I(1989) Endogenous sleep-producing substances and sleep regulation. *Physiology Review, 69*, 605-669. (2)

Branchey M & Petre-Quadens O (1968). A comparative study of sleep parameters during pregnancy. *Acta Neurologica, 68*, 453-459a. (2)

Bridgeman B (1988). *The Biology of Behavior and Mind*. New York: Wiley (6)

Broughton R J (1968). Sleep disorders: disorders of arousal? *Science, 159,* 1070-1078. (6)

Broughton R (1982). Human consciousness and sleep/waking rhythms: A review and some neuropsychological considerations. *Journal of Clinical Neuropsychology, 4,* 193-218. (6)

Broughton R (1987 June-July). *Subjective and performance aspects of daytime sleepiness.* Presented at the Fifth International Congress of Sleep Research, Copenhagen, Denmark. (3)

Browman C (1980). Sleep following susutained exercise. *Psychophysiology, 17*, 577-580. (2)

Browman C & Cartwright R (1980b). The first night effect on sleep and dreams. *Biological Psychiatry, 15*, 809-812. (10)

Brown R, Price R J, King M G, & Husband, R T (1988). Autochthonous intestinal bacteria and coprophagy: a possible contribution to the ontogeny and rhythmicity of slow wave sleep in mammals. *Medical Hypothese, 26,* 171-175. (2)

Bunnell D E, Phillips N H, & Berger R J (1991). Effects of carbohydrate ingestion on tympanic temperature and slow-wave sleep. *Sleep Research, 20*, 40. (2)

Campbell S S & Tobler I (1984). Animal sleep: A review of sleep duration across phylogeny. *Neuroscience and Behavioral Reviews, 8*, 269-300. (5)

Carskadon M A (1982). The second decade. In C Guilleminault (Ed.), *Sleeping and waking disorders: Indications and techniques* (pp. 99-125). Menlo Park, California: Addison-Wesley. (1)

Carskadon M A (1990a). (presentation as a part of a symposium on Daytime sleepiness in children) Presented at the fourth annual meeting of the Association of Professional Sleep Societies, Minneapolis. (1)

Carskadon M A (1990b). Patterns of sleep and sleepiness in adolescents. *Pediatrician, 17*, 5-12. (1)

Carskadon M A (1991). Yawning elicited by reading: is an open mouth a sufficient stimulus? *Sleep Research, 20*, 116. (10)

Carskadon M A (Ed.) (1993). *Encyclopedia of Sleep and Dreaming*. New York: Macmillian. (4,5,6,11)

Carskadon M A & Davis S S (1989). Sleep-wake patterns in the high-school-to-college transition: preliminary data. *Sleep Research, 18*, 113. (1)

Carskadon M A & Dement W C (1981). Cumulative effects of sleep restriction on daytime sleepiness. *Psychophysiology, 18*, 107-113. (1,3)

Carskadon M A & Dement W C (1982). The multiple sleep latency test: what does it measure? *Sleep, 5 (suppl 2)*, s67-s72. (1)

Carskadon M A & Dement W C (1987). Sleepiness in the normal adolescent. In C Guilleminault (Ed.), *Sleep and its disorders in children* (pp. 53-66). New York: Raven Press. (1)

Carskadon M A & Dement W C (1989). Normal human sleep: an overview. In M H Kryger, T Roth, & W C Dement (Eds.), *Principles and practice of sleep medicine* (pp. 3- 13). Philadelphia: Saunders. (1,3,11)

Carskadon M A, Seifer R, Davis S S, & Acelo C (1991). Sleep, Sleepiness, and mood in college-bound high school seniors. *Sleep Research, 20*, 464. (1)

Cartwright R D (1974). Problem solving: waking and dreaming. *journal of abnormal psychology, 83*, 451-455.

Cartwright R D (1977). *Night life: Explorations in dreaming*. Englewood Cliffs, New Jersey: Prentice-Hall. (3,6,8,11)

Cartwright R D (1978). *A primer on sleep and dreaming*. Reading, Mass: Addison-Wesley. (3,6,8,11)

Cartwright R D (1979). The nature and function of repetitive dreams: A survey and speculation. *Psychiatry, 42*, 131-137. (6,7,11)

Cartwright R D (1989). Dreams and their meaning. In Kryger M H, Roth T, & Dement W C (Eds.). *Principles and practice of sleep medicine.*(pp. 184 - 190). Philadelphia: Saunders. (6,11)

Cartwright R (1990). A network model of dreams. In R R Bootzin, J F Kihlstrom, & D L Schacter (Eds.), *Sleep and Cognition* (pp. 179-189). Washington: American Psychological Association. (11)

Cartwright R D (1991). *Who needs dreams?* Presented at The Upper Midwest Sleep Society Meeting, St Paul, Minnesota. (11)

Cartwright R D, Kravitz H M, Eastman CI, & Wood E (1991). REM latency and the recovery from depression: getting over divorce. *American Journal of Psychiatry, 148,* 1530-1535. (6)

Cartwright R D & Lamberg L (1992) *Crisis Dreaming*. New York: Harper Collins. (6)

Cartwright R D, Lloyd S, Knight S, & Trenholme I (1984). Broken dreams: A study of the effects of divorce and depression dream content. *Psychiatry, 47,* 251-259. (6)

Chase M H (Ed.) (1986). Overview of sleep research, circa 1985. *Sleep, 9,* 452-457. (11)

Chase M H & Roth T (Eds.) (1990). *Slow Wave Sleep: Its Measurement and Functional Significance.* Los Angeles: Brain Information Service/Brain Research Institute. (2,11)

Cipolli C, Baroncini P, Fagioli I, Fumai A, & Salzarulo P (1987). The thematic continuity of mental sleep experience in the same night. *Sleep, 10,* 473-479. (6)

Clodore M, Foret J, & Benoit O (1987). Diurnal patterns of alertness, sleep schedules and morningness/eveningness factor. *Sleep Research, 16,* 600. (4)

Cohen D B (1979). *Sleep and dreaming: Origins, nature, and functioning.* New York: Pergamon Press. (3,6)

Cohen D B (1980) The cognitive activity of sleep. *Progress in Brain Research, 53,* 307-324. (11)

Coleman R M (1986). *Wide awake at 3:00am: By choice or by chance?* New York: Freeman. (3,4,10,11)

Colligan D (1982). Lucid dreams. *Omni, 4,*68-72,115. (6)

Connell L J, Dinges D F, Rosekind M R, Gregory K B, Roundtree M S, & Graeber R L (1991). Preplanned cockpit rest: changes in aircrew subjective alertness during long-haul flights. *Sleep Research, 20*, 119. (3)

Coons S (1987). Development of sleep and wakefulness during the first six months of life. In C Guilleminault (Ed.), *Sleep and its disorders in children* (pp. 17-27). New York: Raven Press. (1)

Corner M A, Mirmiran M, Bour H L M G, Boer N E , van de Poll H G, van Oyen M A, & Uylings H B M (1980). Does rapid-eye-movement sleep play a role in brain development. In P S McConnel, G J Boer, H J Romijn, N E van de Poll, & M A Corner (Eds.), *Adaptive Capabilities of the Nervous System* (pp. 347-356). Amsterdam:Elsevier. (11)

Coxhead D & Hiller S (1976). *Dreams: Vision of Night.* London: Thames & Hudson. (6)

Crick F & Mitchison G (1983). The function of dream sleep. *Nature, 30*, 111-114. (5,6,8,11)

Crick F & Mitchison G (1986). REM sleep and neural nets. In R E Hasbell (Ed.). *The Journal of Mind and Behavior, Vol 7, Cognition and Dream Research*, 229-249. (6,7)

Czeisler C A & Allan J S (1988). Pathologies of the Sleep - Wake Schedule. In R L Williams, I K Karacan, & C A Moore (Eds). *Sleep Disorders: Diagnosis and Treatment 2nd ed.* (Pp. 109-129). New York: Wiley. (2,4)

Daan S,Beersma D G M, & Borbely A A (1984). Timing of human sleep: recovery process gated by a circadian pacemaker. *American Journal of Physiology, 1984*, R161-183. (4)

Danguir, J. (1988), Internal Milieu and Sleep homeostasis. In Inoué S & Schneider-Helmert D (1988). *Sleep Peptides: Basic and Clinical Approaches*(pp. 53-72). New York: Springer-Verlag. (5)

Danguir J & Nicoloides S (1985). Feeding, metabolism, and sleep: Peripheral and central mechanisms of their interaction. In D J McGinty,R Drucker-Colin,A Morrison, & P L Parmeggiani (Eds.). *Brain Mechanisms of Sleep* (Pp. 361-340). New York: Raven Press. (2)

Davenne D & Adrien J (1987). Lesion of the ponto-geniculo-occipital pathways in kittens. I. Effects on sleep and on unitary discharge of the lateral geniculate nucleus. *Brain research, 409*, 1-9. (11)

Davenne D, Dugovic C, Franc B & Adrien J (1989). Ontogeny of slow-wave sleep. In Wauquier A, Dugovic C, & Radulovacki M (Eds.). *Slow wave sleep: Physiological, pathophysiological, and functional aspects* (pp. 21-30). New York: Raven Press. (5)

Davis B D (1985). Sleep and the maintenance of memory. *Perspectives in Biology and Medicine, 28*, 457-464. (11)

DeKoninck J, Christ G, Hébert G, & Rinfret, N (1990) Language learning, dreams and REM sleep: converging findings. *Sleep Research, 19*, 134. (11)

Delaney G (1988). *Living your dreams:Revised Edition*. New York: Harper & Row. (8)

Delaney, G (1991). *Breakthrough Dreaming*. New York: Bantam Books. (6)

Dement W C (1978). *Some must watch while some must sleep.* New York: Norton. (1,3,6,10)

Dement W C & Carshadon M A (1981). An essay on sleepiness. In M Maldy-Moulinier (Ed), *Actualités en Medecine Experimentate, en Hommage au Professeur P. Passovant* (pp. 47-71). Montpellier: Euromed. (3)

Dement W C & Mitler M M (1974). An introduction to sleep. In O Petre-Quadens & J D Schlag (Eds.), *Basic sleep mechanisms* (pp. 271-296). New York: Academic Press. (3)

Deming (1972). *Sleep, our unknown life.* New York: Thomas Nelson Inc. (6)

Dinges D (1987 June-July). *The expression of sleepiness in mood and behavior: A contextual-dependence hypothesis*. Presented at the Fifth International Congress of Sleep Research, Copenhagen, Denmark. (3)

Dinges D F (1989). The nature of sleepiness: causes, contexts, and consequences. In Stunkard A J & Baum A (Eds.), *Eating, sleeping, and sex* (pp. 147-180). Hillsdale, New Jersey: Erlbaum. (3,4,10)

Dinges D (1992). Probing the limits of functional capability: The effects of sleep loss on short - duration tasks. In R J Broughton & R D Ogilvie (Eds). *Sleep, Arousal, and Performance* (pp 176-188). Boston: Birkanser. (3)

Dinges D F, Orne M T, & Orne E C (1985). Sleep depth and other factors associated with performance upon abrubt awakening. *Sleep Research, 14*, 92. (10)

Dinges D F, Orne M T, Whitehouse W G, & Orne E C (1987). Temporal placement of a nap for alertness: Contributions of circadian phase and prior wakefulness. *Sleep, 10*, 313-329. (3)

Dinges P F & Powell J W (1989). Sleepiness impaires optimum response capability - it's time to move beyond the lapse hypothesis. *Sleep Research, 18*, 366. (3)

Dortland (1977) *Pocket medical dictionary, twenty-second edition.* Totonto: Saunders. (1)

Downey R & Bonnet M H (1987). Performance during frequent sleep disruption. *Sleep, 10,* 354-63. (3)

Drucker-Colin R (1979). Protein molecules and the regulation of REM sleep: Possible implications for function. In R Drucker-Colin, M Shkurovich, & M B Sterman (Eds.), *The functions of sleep* (pp. 99-111). New York: Academic Press. (11)

Drucker-Colin R (1981). Endogenous sleep peptides. In D Wheatley (Ed.), *Psychopharmacology of sleep* (pp. 53-72). New York: Raven Press. (2)

Drucker-Colin R & Prospero-Garcia O (1990) Neurophysiology of sleep. In M J Thorpy (Ed.). *Handbook of Sleep Disorders.* (Pp. 33-53). New York: Marcel Dekker, Inc. (2,11)

Dujardin K, Guerrien A, & Leconte P (1990). Sleep, brain activation and cognition. *Physiology and behavior, 47,* 1271-1278. (11)

Dunham D W, Broughton R J, & Hoffman R F (1991). In-home ambulant polysomnographic monitoring and the "first night effect." *Sleep Research, 20,* 425. (10)

Durie D J B (1981). Sleep in animals. In D Wheatley (Ed.), *Psychopharmacology of sleep* (pp. 1-18). New York: Raven Press. (5)

Ehret C F & Scanlon L W (1983). *Overcomming jetlag.* New York: Berkley. (4)

Eich E (1990). Learning during sleep. In R R Bootzin, J F Kihlstrom, & D L Schachter (Eds.), *Sleep and cognition* (pp. 88-108). Washington: American Psychological Association. (5,10)

Elgar M A, Pagel M D, & Harvey PH (1988). Sleep in mammals. *Animal Behavior, 36,* 1407-1419. (5)

Fagioli I, Baroncini P, Ricour C, & Salzarulo P (1989). Decrease of slow-wave sleep in children with prolonged absence of essential lipids intake. *Sleep, 12,* 495-499. (2)

Faraday A (1972). *Dream power.* New York: Coward, McCann & Geoghegan. (1,6,8)

Faraday A (1974). *The dream game.* New York: Afar. (8)

Fein G, Floyd T C, & Feinberg I (1981). Computer measures of sleep EEG reliably sort visual stage 2 epochs by NREM period of origin. *Psychophysiology, 18,* 686-693. (6)

Feinberg I (1976). Functional implications of changes in sleep physiology with age. In R D Terry & S Gershon (Eds.), *Neurobiology of aging* (pp. 23-41). New York: Raven Press. (11)

Feinberg I (1987). Delta increase after total and partial sleep loss is limited to NREMP1. *Sleep research, 16,* 522. (2)

Feinberg I (1989). Effects of maturation and aging on the slow wave sleep in man: Implications for Neurology. In Wauquier A, Dugovic C, & Radulovacki M (Eds.). *Slow wave sleep: Physiological, pathophysiological, and functional aspects.* (pp. 31-48) New York: Raven Press. (4)

Feinberg I, Koresko R L, & Heller N (1967). EEG sleep patterns as a function of normal and pathological aging in man. *Journal of Psychiatric Research, 5,* 107-144. (11)

Feinberg I & Floyd T C (1982). The regulation of human sleep. *Human Neurobiology, 1,* 185-194. (11)

Fiss H (1979). Current dream research: A psychobiological perspective. In B F Wolman (Ed.), *Handbook of dreams* (pp. 20-75). New York: Van Nostrand Reinhold. (6,11)

Fiss H (1983). Toward a classically relevant experimental psychology of dreaming. *Hillside Journal of Clinical Psychiatry, 5.* 147-159. (6)

Flanigan W F (1973a). Sleep and wakefulness in chelonian reptiles: The eastern box turtle. *Sleep Research, 2,* 83. (5)

Flanigan W F (1973b). Sleep and wakefulness in chelonian reptiles: The red tortoise. *Sleep Research, 2,* 82. (5)

Foret J & Petit C (1987). Influence of rising time on alertness indices. *Sleep Research, 16,* 610. (4)

Foret J, Toaron N, Benoit O, & Bouard G (1985). Sleep and body temperature in "Morning" and "Evening" people. *Sleep, 8,* 311-318. (4)

Foulkes D (1966). *The Psychology of sleep.* New York: Scribner. (6)

Foulkes D (1982). *Children's dreams: Longitudinal studies.* New York: John Wiley & Sons. (6)

Foulkes D (1983). Cognitive processes during sleep: Evolutionary aspects. In A Mayes (Ed.), *Sleep mechanisms and functions in humans and animals - an evolutionary prespective* (pp. 313-337). Berkshire, England: Van Nostrand Reinhold. (5,10,11)

Foulkes D (1985). *Dreaming: A cognitive-psychological analysis.* Hillsdale, New Jersey: Lawrence Erlbaum. (6)

Freeman F R (1972) *Sleep research: A critical review.* Springfield, Ill.: Charles C. Thomas.(3)

Freud S (1900). *Interpretations of dreams.* New York: Modern Library. (6,7)

Freud S (1901/1980). *On dreams.* New York: Norton.(6)

Freud S (1958). *The standard edition of the complete psychological works of Sigmund Freud, Vol. 12.* London: Hogarth. (7)

Fromm E & Shor R E (1979). *Hypnosis: Developments in research and new perspectives.* New York: Aldine. (10)

Gackenbach J & Bosveld J (1989). *Control Your Dreams.* New York: Harper and Row. (6)

Gaillard J M (1990). Neurotransmitters and sleep pharmacology. In M J Thorpy (Ed.), *Handbook of Sleep Disorders* (Pp. 55-76). New York: Marcel Dekker, Inc. (2)

Gaillard A W K, & Steyvers F J J M (1989. Sleep loss and sustained performance. In A Coblentz (Ed.), *Vigilance and performance in automatized systmes* (pp. 241-250). Boston: Kluwer Academic Publishers. (3)

Garma L & Anbin H (1989). Yawning: A vigilance-enhancing factor? *Sleep Research, 18,* 4. (10)

Gillberg M, Anderzén I, & Åkerstedt T (1991). Recovery within day-time slow wave sleep suppression. *Electroencephalography and clinical Neurophysiology, 78,* 267-273.(3)

Glenn L L (1985). Brainstem and Spinal Control of Lower Limb Motoneurons with Special Reference to Phasic Events and Startle. In D J McGinty, R Drucker-Colin, A Morrison, & P L Parmeggiani, (Eds.). *Brain Mechanisms of Sleep* (pp. 81-95). New York: Raven Press. (2)

Greenberg R (1981). Dreams and REM sleep: An intergrative approach. In W Fishbein (Ed.), *Sleep, Dreams, and Memory (pp. 125-133).*New York: Spectrum. (11)

Griffith R M, Miyago O & Togo A (1958). The universality of typical dreams: Japanese vs. Americans. *American Anthropologist, 60,* 1173-1179. (6)

Grunstein R R & Sullivan C E (1990). Neural control of respiration during sleep. In M J Thorpy (Ed.). *Handbook of Sleep Disorders.* 77-102. New York: Marcel Dekker. (2)

Guilleminault C (1980). Sleep and respiration in infants. In L Popovicin, B Asgian, & G Bodin (Eds.), *Sleep 1978* (pp. 133-137). New York: Karger. (9)

Guilleminault C (Ed) (1982). *Sleeping and waking disorders: Indications and techniques*. Menlo Park, California: Addison-Wesley. (9)

Guilleminault C & Lugaresi E (1983). *Sleep-wake disorders: Natural history, epidemiology, and long-term evaluation*. New York: Raven Press.(9)

Guyton (1976). *Textbook of medical physiology*. Philadelphia: Saunders (2)

Hall C (1953). A cognitive theory of dreams. *Journal of General Psychology, 49*, 273-282. (6)

Hall C (1966). *The meaning of dreams*. New York: McGraw-Hill (7)

Hall C & VandeCastle R (1966). *The content analysis of dreams.* Appleton-Century-Crofts. (6)

Hansel C E M (1980). *ESP and parapsychology: a critical reevaluation.* Buffalo: Prometheus Books. (6)

Harsh J & Badia P (1990). Stimulus control and sleep. In R R Bootzin, J F Kihlstrom, & D L Schachter (Eds.), *Sleep and cognition* (pp. 58-66). Washington: American Psychological Association. (5)

Hartmann E (1984). *The Nightmare: The psychology and biology of terrifying dreams.* New York: Basic Books. (6)

Hartmann E (1989). Normal and abnormal dreams. In Kryger M H, Roth T, & Dement W C (Eds.), *Principles and practive of sleep medicine* (pp. 191-195). Philadelphia: Saunders. (6)

Hartmann E L (1973). *The functions of sleep*. New Haven: Yale University Press. (3,11)

Harvey A & Moldofsky H (1991). The epidemiology of sleep: a canadian time diary perspective. *Sleep Research, 20*, 121. (1)

Hauri P (1979). What can insomniacs teach us about the functions of sleep? In R Drucker-Colin, M Shkurovich, & M B Sterman (Eds.), *The functions of sleep* (pp. 251-271). New York: Academic Press. (3,11)

Hauri P (1982). *The sleep disorders*. Kalamazoo, Michigan: Upjohn. (2,4,6,9)

Hauri P & Linde A (1990). *No more sleepless nights.* New York: Wiley. (1,2,9)

Hayaishi O (1988). Sleep-wake regulation by prostaglandins D_2 and E_2. *Journal of Biological Chemistry, 263,* 14593-14596. (2)

Hayaishi O (1989 June). Invited Address. Presented at the Third Annual Meeting of the Assocation of Professional Sleep Societes, Washington, D.C. (2)

Hayaishi O (1991). Molecular mechanisms of sleep-wake regulatioin: roles of prostaglandins D_2 and E_2. *FASEB J, 5,* 2575-2581. (2)

Hediger H (1983). Natural sleep behavior in vertebrates. In M Monnier & M Meulders (Eds.), *Functions of the nervous system, Vol 4.* (pp. 105-128). New York: Elsevier (5,10)

Heller, H C. (1979). Hibernation: neural aspects. *Annual Review of Physiology, 41,* 305-21. (10)

Hennager K M, Griggs A J, & Moorcroft W H (1991). Cognition during sleep: Prevalence of awakening at a predetermined time without using an alarm. *Sleep Research, 20,* 123. (4)

Herman J H, Erman M, Boys R, Peiser L, Taylor M E, & Roffwarg H P (1984). Evidence for a directional correspondence between eye movements and dream imagery in REM sleep. *Sleep, 7,* 52-63. (6)

Herman J H, Rampy P, Hirshkowitz M, Thorpe G, Bliss K & Roffwarg H (1987). EEG asymmetry during REM sleep waking imagery, and mentation. *Sleep Research, 16,* 232. (6)

Herman J H, Laljiani K, Polokof R, Armitage R, Roffwarg H, & Hirshkowitz M (1992). Human vigilance and the visual evoked potential. *Sleep research, 21,* 24. (1)

Hertz G, Fast A, Feinsilver S H, Albertario C, & Schulman H (1991). Sleep patterns in late pregnancy. *Sleep Research, 20,* 257. (2)

Hicks R A & Pellegrini R J (1977). Anxiety levels of short and long sleepers. *Psychological reports, 41,* 569-570. (3)

Hilakivi L (1987 June-July). *Sleep and sleep function in mammalian development.* Presented at the Fifth International Congress of Sleep Research, Copenhagen, Denmark. (11)

Hirshkowitz M & Howell J W (1988). Advances and methodology in the study of dreaming. In R L Williams, I Karacan, & C A Moore (Eds.), *Sleep disorders: diagnosis and treatment.* New York: Wiley. (6)

Hobson A (1988). *The Dreaming Brain.* New York: Basic Books. (11)

Hobson J A (1989). Dream theory: A new view of the brain mind. *The Harvard Medical School Mental Health Letter, 5,* 3-5. (7,11)

Hobson J A (1991). Of symbols, metaphors, dreaming, and the brain: A scientific view. Forward to G Delaney, *Breakthrough Dreaming*(pp. xiii-xx). New York: Bantam Books.(7,11)

Hobson J A, Lydic R, & Baghogan H A (1986). Evolving concepts of sleep cycle generation: from brain centers to neuronal populations. *Behavioral and Brain Sciences, 9*, 371-400. (4)

Hobson A & McCarley R (1977). The brain as a dream state generator: an activation-synthesis hypothesis of the dream process. *American Journal of Psychiatry, 134,* 1335-1348. (7,11)

Hoppenbrouwers T (1987). Sleep in infants. In C Guilleminault (Ed.), *Sleep and its disorders in children* (pp. 1-15). New York: Raven Press. (1)

Hoppenbrouwers T, Ugartechea J C, Combs D, Hodgman J E, Harper R M & Sterman M D (1978). Studies of maternal-fetal interaction during the last trimester of pregnancy: Ontogenesis of the basic rest-activity cycle. *Experimental Neurology*, *61*, 136-153. (2)

Horne J A (1983a). Human sleep and tissue restitution: Some qualifications and doubts. *Clinical Science, 65*, 569-578. (11)

Horne J A (1983b). Interacting functions of mammalian sleep. In W P Koella (Ed.), *Sleep 1982*(pp. 130-134). Basel: Karger. (4,5,11)

Horne J A (1983c). Mammalian sleep function with particular reference to man. In A Mayes (Ed.), *Sleep mechanisms and functions in humans and animals - an evolutionary perspective* (pp. 262-312). Birkshire, England: Van Nostrand Reinhold. (3,11)

Horne J A (1987 June-July). *Exercise and SWS - is a hot brain the answer?* Presented at the Fifth International Congress of Sleep Research, Copenhagen, Denmark. (2)

Horne J A (1988). *Why we sleep.* New York: Oxford University Press. (1,2,3,4,5,10,11)

Horne J A (1989). Aspirin and nonfebrile waking oral temperature in healthy men and women: links with SWS changes? *Sleep, 12*, 516-512. (11)

Horne J A (1992). "Core" and "optional" sleepiness. In R J Broughton & R D Ogilvie (Eds). *Sleep, Arousal, and Performance* (pp 27-44). Boston: Birkanser. (11)

Horne J A & Östberg O (1976). A self-assessment questionnaire to determine morningness-eveningness in human circadian rhythms. *International Journal of Chronobiology, 4,* 97-110. (4)

Hume I (1983). The rhythmical nature of sleep. In A Mayes (Ed.), *Sleep mechanisms and functions in humans and animals - an evolutionary prespective* (pp. 18-56). Berkshire, England: Van Nostrand Reinhold. (4)

Hunt H H (1989). *The Multiplicity of Dreams: Memory, Imagination, and Consciousness*. New Haven: Yale University Press. (6,7,8)

ICSD - Diagnostic Classification Steering Committee, M J Thorpy (Ed.) (1990). International classification of sleep disorders: Diagnostic and coding manual. Rochester, Minnesota: American Sleep Disorders Association. (3,9)

Inoué S (1989). *The biology of sleep substances.* Boca Raton: CRC Press. (2)

Ishihara K, Miyasita A, Inugami M, Fukuda K, & Miyata R (1987). Differences in sleep-wake habits and EEG sleep variables between active morning and evening subjects. *Sleep, 10,* 330-342. (4)

Johnson L C, Church M W, Seales D M & Rossiter V S (1978). Mood and performance in good and poor sleepers and the effect of Flurazepam on mood and performance. *Sleep Research, 7,* 101. (3)

Johnson, L C & Spinweber C L (1983). Quality of Sleep and Performance in the Navy: a longitudinal study of good and poor sleepers. In C Guilleminault & E Lugaresi (Eds), *Sleep/wake Disorders: Natural history, Epidemiology, and Long-term Evolution*, (13-28). New York: Raven Press. (3)

Jones B E (1985). Neuroanatomical and Neurochemical Substrates of Mechanisms Underlying Paradoxical Sleep. In D J McGinty, R Drucker-Colin, A Morrison, & P L Parmeggiani (Eds.). *Brain Mechanisms of Sleep.* New York: Raven Press, (Pp. 139-156). (2)

Jones B E (1989). Basic mechanisms of sleep-wake states. In Kryger M H, Roth T, & Dement W C (Eds.), *Principles and practice of sleep medicine*(pp. 121-138). Philadelphia: Saunders. (2)

Jones B E (1990). What are the chemical mediators and modulators of slow wave sleep: overview. In M H Chase & T Roth (Eds.), *Slow Wave Sleep: Its Measurement and Functional Significance.* (pp 41-44). Los Angeles: Brain Information Service/Brain Research Institute. (2)

Jouvet M (1980). Paradoxical sleep and the nature - nuture controversy. *Progress in Brain Research, 53*, 331-346. (2,11)

Jouvet M (1984). Indolamines and sleep-inducing factors. In Borbély A & Valatx J L (Eds.), *Sleep mechanisms.* Berlin: Springer-Verlag. (2)

Jouvet M (1989). The regulation of paradoxical sleep by the hypothalamo-hypophysis. *Archives of Itallian biology, 126,* 259-274. (2)

Jung C G (1933). *Modern Man in Search of a Soul.* New York: Harcourt, Brace and World. (7)

Jung C G (1964). *Man and His Symbols.* New York: Dell. (7)

Jung C G (1974). *Dreams.* Princeton, NJ: Princeton University Press. (7)

Kahn E, Fisher C, & Edwards A (1978). Night terrors and anxiety dreams. In A Arkin, J S Antrobus & S J Ellman, *The mind in sleep: Psychology and psychophysiology* (pp. 533-542). Hillsdale, NJ: Erlbaum. (6)

Kaiser W & Steiner-Kaiser J (1983). Neuronal correlates of sleep, wakefulness and arousal in a diurnal insect. *Nature, 301*, 707-709. (5)

Kalat J W (1992). *Biological psychology, Second edition.* Belmont, California: Wadsworth. (4,6,7,10,11)

Karacan I (1968). Sleep patterns in pregnancy and postpartum. *Psychophysiology*, *5*, 229-230. (2)

Karacan I, Heine W, Agnew H W, Williams R L, Webb W B & Ross J J (1968). Characteristics of sleep patterns during late pregnancy and the postpartum periods. *American Journal of Obstetrics & Gynecology, 101*, 579-586. (2)

Karacan I & Moore C (1985). Physiology and neurochemistry of sleep. In R E Hales & A J Frances (Eds.), *American Psychiatric Association Annual Review, Vol 4.* Washington: American Psychiatric Press. (2)

Karacan I & Williams R L (1970a). Current advances in theory and practice relating to postpartum syndromes. *Psychiatry in Medicine, 1*, 307-328. (2)

Karacan I & Williams R L (1970b). Sleep patterns in pregnancy and postpartun. *Psychophysiology, 5*, 229-230, (abst.). (2)

Karacan I, Williams R L, Hursch C J, McCaulley M & Heine M W (1969). Some implications of the sleep patterns for postpartum emotional disturbances. *Brittish Journal of Psychiatry, 115*, 925-929. (2)

Karmanova I G (1982). *Evolution of sleep: Stages of the formulation of the 'wakefulness-sleep' cycle in vertebrates.* New York: Karger. (5)

Kelly P D (1981). Physiology of sleep and dreaming. In E R Kandel & J D Schwartz (Eds.), *Principles of Neural Science* (pp. 472-485). New York: Elsevier. (2)

Kilduff T S, Bennington J H, Bickler P E, Bartholomew G A, & Heller H C (1989). Sleepin' lizards! A 2-deoxyglucose study in Dipsosaurus Dorsalis. *Sleep Research, 18*, 15. (5)

Kimura-Takeuchi M, Kovalzon V, & Inoué S (1990). Delta-sleep-inducing peptide and its analogues: structure-activity relationship for sleep modulation in rats. *Sleep Research, 19*, 68. (2)

Kleitman N (1972). *Sleep and wakefulness*. Chicago: U of Chicago Press. (1,3,4,10)

Kleitman N (1982). Basic rest-activity cycle - 22 years later. *Sleep, 5*, 311-317. (4).

Knox M, Roehrs T A, Claiborne D, Stepanski E J, & Roth T (1991). Duration of residual sedation after ethanol. *Sleep Research, 20*, 66. (2)

Koukkou M & Lehman D (1983). REM sleep dreams and the activation-synthesis hypothesis. *Brittish Journal of Psychiatry, 142*, 221-231. (6,11)

Koulack D (1987 June-July). *Dreams and adaptation to contemporary stress.* Presented at the Fifth International Congress of Sleep Research, Copenhagen, Denmark. (11)

Koulack D (1991). *To Catch a Dream: Explorations of Dreaming*. Albany, New York: State University of New York Press. (1,2,3,6,11)

Krakow B & Neidhardt J (1992). *Conquering bad dreams and nightmares.* New York: Berkley Books. (9)

Kramer M (1987 June-July). *The mood regulatory function of dreaming: The dream as selective affective modulator.* Presented at the Fifth International Congress of Sleep Research, Copenhagen, Denmark. (11)

Kramer M (1990). Nightmares (dream disturbances) in posttraumatic stress disorder: Implications for a theory of dreaming. In R F Bootzin, J F Kihlstrom, & D L Schacter (Eds.), *Sleep and Cognition* (pp. 190-202). Washington; American Psychological Association. (9,11)

Kramer M (1993). The selective mood regulatory function of dreaming: and update and revision. In A Moffitt, M Kramer, & R Hoffmann (Eds.), *The functions of dreaming* (pp. 139-195). New York: State University of New York Press (11)

Kramer M, & Kinney L (1988). Sleep patterns in trauma victims with disturbed dreaming. *Psychiatric Journal of the University of Ottawa, 13*, 12-16. (6)

Kramer M, Kinney L, & Scharf M (1983). Social change in dreams ofmen and women. In W P Koella (Ed), *Sleep, 1982* (pp. 359-361). New York: Karger. (6)

Krilewiez (1991). (presentation as a part of a symposium on Sleep and Mammalian Hibernation: Homologous Adaptations & Homologous Mechanisms). Presented at the Fifth annual meeting of the Association of Professional Sleep Societies, Toronto.(10)

Kripke D F, Simons R N, Garfinkel L, & Hammond E C (1979). Short and long sleep and sleeping pills: Is increased mortality associated? *Archives of General Psychiatry, 36*, 103-116. (3)

Krueger, J M, Obal F, Johansson L, Cady A B & Foth L Kruege (1989). Endogenous slow wave sleep substance: A review. In A Wauquier, Dugovic, & M Radulovacki (Eds.). *Slow wave sleep: Physiological, Pathophysiological, and functional aspects* (pp. 75-90). New York: Raven Press. (2)

Krueger J M, Obál F, Opp M, Cady A B, Johannsen L, Toth L, & Majde J (1990a). Putative sleep neuromodulators. In J Montplaisir & R Godbout (Eds.). *Sleep and biological rhythms* (Pp. 163-185). New York: Oxford University Press. (2)

Krueger J M, Obal F, Opp M, Cady A B, Johannsen, L Toth L, & Majde J (1990b). Putative sleep neuromodulators. In J Montplaisir & R Godbout (Eds.), *Sleep and biological rhythms* (pp. 163-185). New York: Oxford . (2)

Krueger J M, Toth L A, Cody A B, Johannsen L & Obal F Jr. (1988). Immunomodulation and Sleep. In S Inoué & D Schneider-Helmert (Eds.), *Sleep peptides: biological basis and clinical approaches* (pp. 95-129). New York: Springer-Verlag. (2)

Krueger J M, Toth L A, Johannsen L, & Opp M R (1990). Infectious disease and sleep: involvement of neuroendocrine-neuroimmune mechanisms. *Intern. J. Neuroscience, 51*, 359-362. (2)

Kryger M H, Roth T, & Dement W C (Eds.) (1989). *Principles and practice of sleep medicine.* Philadelphia: Saunders. (1,2,3,4,6,5,9,11)

Kupfer D J & Reynolds C F (1989). Slow-wave Sleep and Protective Factor. In Stunkard A J & Baum A (Eds.), *Eating, Drinking, and Sex* (pp. 131-145). Hillsdale, New Jersey: Erlbaum. (2)

LaBerge S P (1981). Lucid dreaming: directing action as it happens. *Psychology Today,15,* 48-57. (6)

Lahmeyer H W (1988). Sleep in craniopagus twins. *Sleep, 11*, 301-306. (2)

Lamberg L (1984). *The AMA guide to better sleep.* New York: Random House. (4)

Lamberg L (1985). Newly awakened interest in sleep research spans many specialities. *Journal of the American Medical Association, 254*, 1275-7, 1281, 1284. (4,9)

Landis C A, Bergmann B M, Ismail M M, & Recktschaffen A, 1992). Sleep deprivation in the rat: ambbient temperature choice in paradoxical sleep-deprived rats. *Sleep, 15,* 13-20. (11)

Lapierre O, Montplaisir J, Lamarre M, & Bedard M A (1990). The effect of gamma-hydroxybutyrate on nocturnal diurnal sleep in normal subjects: further consideration on REM sleep-triggering mechanisms. *Sleep, 13*, 24-30. (2)

Lauber J K & Kayten P J (1988). Sleepiness, circadian dysrhythmia, and fatigue in transportation system accidents. *Sleep, 11*, 503-512. (3,4)

Lavie P (1986). Ultrashort sleep-waking schedule. III. 'Gates' and 'forbidden zones' for sleep. *Electroencephalography and Clinical Neurophysiology, 63*, 414-425. (4)

Lavie P (1989). To nap, Perchance to Sleep - Ultradian Aspects of Napping. In D F Dinges & R J Broughton, *Sleep and Alertness: Chronobiological, Behavioral, and Medical Aspects of Napping* (pp. 99-120). New York: Raven Press. (3,4,11)

Lavie P & Segal J (1989). Twenty-four-hour structure of Sleepiness in morning and evening persons inverstigated by ultrashort sleep-wake cycle. *Sleep, 12*, 522-528.(3)

Lehmann, H E (1979). Yawning: a homeostatic reflex and its psychological significance. *Bulletin of the Menninger Clinic, 43*, 123-36. (10)

Lendrem D W (1983). Sleeping and vigilance in birds. In W P Koella (Ed), *Sleep (1982)* (pp. 134-138). Basel: Karger. (5)

Levine B, Lumely M, Roehrs T, Zorick R, & Roth T (1988). The effects of sleep restriction and extension on sleep and efficiency. *International Journal of Neuroscience, 43*, 139-43. (1)

Lloyd (1987). The collection of home and laboratory dreams by means of an instrumental response technique. *Sleep Research, 16*,234. (6)

Loftus E F (1979). The malleability of human memory. *American Scientist, 67*, 312-320. (5)

Lyon J (1990). Making brain waves. *Chicago Tribune Magazine*, January 7, 1990, 10-12,14,16,25. (6)

MacLean A W, Reiz W A, Austin P, Coulter M, Brunet D B, & Knowles J B (1990). Psychophysiological correlates of lapses: Power spectral analysis of the EEG. *Sleep Research, 19*, 120. (3)

Mahoney, M F (1966). *The meaning in Dreams and Dreaming: The Jungian Viewpoint*. Seacaucus, NJ: The Citadel Press. (7)

Mahowold M W & Ettinger M G (1990). Things that go bump in the night: the parasomnias revisited. *Journal of Clinical Neurophysiology*, *1*, 119-143. (6,9)

Mahowold M W & Rosen G M(1990) Parasomnias in children. P*ediatrician, 17,* 21-31. (9)

Manson P (1898). *Tropical diseases.* London: Cassell. (10)

Mauri, M (1990). Sleep and the reproductive cycle: A review. *Health Care for women, international, 11*, 409-421. (2)

Maybruck P (1986). Contents of dreams of pregnant women. *Association for the Study of Dreams Newsletter, 3* **(1)**, 8-9. (6)

Mayes A (1983). Overview: Comments on general themes and a discussion of sleep pathology. In A Mayes (Ed.), *Sleep mechanisms and functions in humans and animals - an evolutionary perspective* (pp. 338-351). Birkshire, England: Van Nostrand Reinhold. (5,11)

McCarley R W (1978). Where dreams come from: a new theory. *Psychology Today, 12,* 54-56,60,62,65,141. (7)

McCarley R (1981). Mind-body isomorphism and the study of dreams. In W Fishbein (Ed.), *Advances in Sleep Research, Vol. 4* (pp. 205-238). New York: Spectrum Publications. **(7)**

McCarley R W (1990). Brainstem cholinergic systems and models of REM sleep production. In J Montplaisir & R Bodbout (Eds). *Sleep and Biological Rhythms* (pp 131-147). New York: Oxford University Press. (2)

McCarley R (1991). (presentation as a part of a symposium on the Neurochemistry of REM sleep). Presented at the Fifth annual meeting of the Association of Professional Sleep Societies, Toronto.(2)

McCarley R W & Hobson J A (1975). Neuronal excitability modulation over the sleep cycle: a structural and mathematical model, *Science*, *189*, 58-60. (2)

McCarley R W & Hobson J A (1979). The form of dreams and the biology of sleep. In B B Wolman (Ed). *Handbook of dreams: Research, theories and applications* (pp. 76-130). New York: Van Nostrand Reinhold. (7)

McCarley R W & Massaquoi S G (1986). A limit cycle mathematical model of the REM sleep oscillator system. *American Journal of Physiology, 257,* R1011-R1029. (2)

McCarley R W & Massaquoi S G (1992). Neurobiological structure of the revised limit cycle reciprocal interaction model of REM cycle control. *J. Sleep Research, 1,* 132-137. (2)

McGaugh J L, Jensen R A, & Martinez J L Jr. (1979). Sleep, brain state, and memory. In R Drucker-Colin, M Shkurovich, & M B Sterman (Eds.), *The functions of sleep* (pp. 295-301). New York: Academic Press. (3,11)

McGinty D J (1985). Physiological equilibrium and the control of sleep states. In McGinty D J, Drucker-Colin R, Morrison A, & Parmeggiani P L. *Brain Mechanisms of Sleep* (Pp. 361-384). New York: Raven Press. (11)

McGinty D J & Drucker-Colin R R (1982). Sleep mechanisms: Biology and control of REM sleep. *International Review of Neurobiology, 23,* 391-436. (4)

McGinty D J, Drucker-Colin R, Morrison, A, & Parmeggiani P L (1985). *Brain mechanisms of sleep.* New York: Raven Press. (2)

McGinty D J & Szymusiak R (1987 June-July). *Physiological role of the basal froebrain hypnogenic mechanism.* Presented at the Fifth International Congress of Sleep Research, Copenhagen, Denmark. (11)

McGinty D J & Szymusiak R (1989). The basal forebrain and slow wave sleep: Mechanistic and functional aspects. In A Wauquier, C Dugovic, & M Radulovacki (Eds.). *Slow wave sleep: Physiological, pathophysiological, and functional aspects.* (pp. 61-73). New York: Raven Press. (2)

McGinty D J & Szymusiak R (1990). Hypothalamic thermoregulatory control of slow wave sleep. In Mancia M & Marini G (Eds.), The diencephalon and sleep (pp. 97-110). New York: Raven Press. (2)

McGinty D J & Szymusiak R (1990b). Keeping cool: a hypothesis about the mechanisms and functions of slow-wave sleep. *Trends in neuroscience, 13,* 480-487. (11)

McGrath M J & Cohen D B (1978). REM sleep facilitation of adaptive waking behavior: A review of the literature. *Psychological Bulletin, 85,* 24-57. (11)

Meddis R (1975). On the function of sleep. *Animal Behavior, 23,* 676-601. (5)

Meddis R (1979). The evolution and function of sleep. In D A Oakley & H C Plotkin (Eds.), *Brain, behavior, & evolution* (pp. 99-125). London: Methuen. (3,5,11)

Meddis R (1983). The evolution of sleep. In A Mayes (Ed.), *Sleep mechanisms and functions in humans and animals - an evolutionary prespective* (pp. 57-106). Berkshire, England: Van Nostrand Reinhold. (5,11)

Mendelson W B (1987). *Human Sleep: Research and Clinical Care.* New York: Plenum. (2,4)

Meyers D (1992). *Psychology, third edition.* New York: Worth. (6)

Mikulincer M, Babkoff H, Caspy T, & Sing H. (1989). The effects of 72 hours of sleep loss on psychological variables. *Brittish Journal of Psychology, 80*, 145-162. (3)

Mirmiram, M (1986). The importance of fetal/neonatal REM sleep. *European Journal of Obstetrics, Gynecology and Reproductive Biology, 21* 283-291. (11)

Mirmiran M & Bos N P (1990). Hypothalamic regulation of sleep-wae circadian rhythms. In M Mancia & G Marini (Eds). *The Diencephalon and Sleep* (pp 125-132). New York: Raven Press. (2)

Mitler M M, Geyavarty K S & Browman C P (1982). Maintenance of wakefulness test: a polysomnographic technique for evaluating treatment in patients with excessive somnolence. *Electroencephalography and Clinical Neurophysiology, 53*, 658-61. (3)

Moffitt (1987 June-July). *Experimental studies of indicidual differences in dream recall and the question of dream function.* Presented at the Fifth International Congress on Sleep Research, Copenhagen, Denmark. (11)

Moldofsky H, Lue F A, Eisen J, Keystone E, & Gorczynski R M (1986). The relationship of interleukin and immune functions to sleep in humans. *Psychosomatic Medicine, 8*, 309-18. (2)

Monk T (1989). Circadian rhythms in subjective activation, mood, and performance efficiency. In Kryger M H, Roth T, & Dement W C (Eds.) (1989). *Principles and practice of sleep medicine* (pp. 163-172). Philadelphia: Saunders. (4)

Monk T H & Moline M L (1988). Removal of temporal constraints in the middle-aged and elderly: effects on sleep and sleepiness. *Sleep, 11,* 513-520. (4)

Monnier M (1983). Rest, sleep, and waking in vertebrates (and EEG correlates). In M Monnier & M Meulders (Eds.), *Function of the nervous system, Vol 4* (pp. 131-139). New York: Elsevier. (5)

Monnier M, Dudler L, Cachter R, Maier P F, Tobler H J, & Schoenenberger G A (1977). The delta sleep inducing peptide (DSIP). Comparative properties of the original and systhetic nonapeptide. *Experimentia, 34,* 548-552. (2)

Montgomery I, Trinder J, Paxton S, & Fraser G (1987). Aerobic exercise and fitness: effect on the sleep of young and older subjects. *Sleep Research, 16,* 254. (2)

Monti J M, Piñeyro, G, Orellana C, Boussard M, Jantos H, Labraga P, Olivera S, & Alvariño F (1990). 5-HT receptor agonists 1-(2,5-dimethoxy-4-iodophenyl)-2-aminopropane (doi) and 8-oh-dpat increase wakefulness in the rat. *Sleep Research, 19,* 81.

Moorcroft W H & Clothier J (1987). An overview of the body and the brain in sleep. In J Gackenbach (Ed), *Sleep and dreams: A sourcebook* (pp. 30-16). New York: Garland. (1,2,4)

Morgane P J, Stern W C, & Bronzino J D (1977). Experimental studies of sleep in animals. In R D Myers (Ed), *Methods in psychobiology, Vol 3* (pp. 189-239). New York: Academic Press. (5)

Morris H H & Estes M L (1987). Traveler's amnesia: Transient global amnesia secondary to tiazolam. *Journal of the American Medical Association, 258,* 945-946. (4)

Morris M, Lack L, & Dawson D (1990). Sleep-onset insomniacs have delayed temperature rhythms. *Sleep, 13,* 1-14. (4)

Morrison A R & Reiner P B (1985). A dissection of paradoxical sleep. In D J McGinty, R Drucker-Colin, A Morrison, & P L Parmeggiani P L (Eds). *Brain Mechanisms of Sleep.* (pp. 97-110) New York: Raven Press. (2,11)

Morrison A R, Ball L D, Sanford G L, Mann G L, & Ross R J (1990). Orienting can be elicited by tones in paradoxical sleep without atonia. *Sleep Research, 19,* 23. (11)

Moruzzi G (1966). The functional significance of sleep with particular regard to the brain mechanisms underlying consciousness. In J C Eccles (Ed), *Brain mechanisms and conscious experience.* New York: Springer-Verlag. (5)

Muehlbach M J, Schweitzer P K, Stuchey M L, & Walsh J K (1991). The Effect of Caffeine on continuous performance at night. *Sleep Research, 20,* 464. (2)

Mukhametov L M (1984). Sleep in marine mammals. In A A Borbely & J L Valat, *Sleep mechanisms* (pp. 227-238). New York: Springer-Verlag. (5)

Mukhametov L (1992). *Sleep and sleep deprivation in aquatic mammals.* Invited address presented at the 6th annual meeting of the Association of Professional Sleep Societies, May 29-June 3, 1992. Phoenix, Arizona. (5)

Muller F M (1974). Dreaming an intermediate state. In R L Woods & H B Greenhouse (Eds.), *The new world of dreams* (pp. 125-126). New York: MacMillan. (6)

Murray H A & Wheeler D R (1937). A note on the possible clairvoyance of dreams. *Journal of Psychology, 3*, 309-313. (6)

Nakagawa Y (1987). Sleep disturbances due to exposure to tone pulses throughout the night. *Sleep, 10*, 463-472. (3)

Neidhardt E J, Krakow B , Kellner R, & Pathak D (1992). A single treatment session for chronic nightmare sufferers. *Sleep Research, 21, 137. (9)*

Obal F Jr (1984). Thermoregulation and sleep. In A A Borbely & J L Valat (Eds.), *Sleep mechanisms* (pp. 157-172). New York: Springer-Verlag. (11)

Ogilivie F D, Simons, I A, Kuderian R H , MacDonald T & Rustenburg J (1991). Behavioral, event-related potential, and EEG/FFT. In *Psychophysiology, 28*, 54-64. (1)

Oleksenko A I, Mukhametov L M, Polyakova I G, Supin A Y, & Kovalzon V M (1992). Unihemispheric sleep deprivation in bottlenose dolphins. *J. Sleep Research, 1*, 40-44. (5)

Opp M R & Krueger J M (1991). Effects of an interleukin-1 receptor antagonist on recovery sleep of rabbits after total sleep deprivation. *Sleep research, 20,* 416. **(2)**

Orem JM (1985). Behavior of respiratory cells during NREM sleep. In McGinty D J, Drucker-Colin R, Morrison A, & Parmeggiani P L. *Brain Mechanisms of Sleep* (Pp. 341-359). New York: Raven Press.

Orem J & Barnes C D (1980). *Physiology in sleep.* New York: Springer-Verlag. (1)

Osborn T & Moorcroft W H (1981). Sleep patterns in undergraduates. Unpublished manuscript.

Oskenberg A (1987). *Sleep and sleep function in mammalian development: REM sleep and CNS development in the visual system of the kitten.* Presented at the Fifth International Congress on Sleep Research, Copenhagen, Denmark. (11)

Oswald I (1974). *Sleep.* Baltimore, Maryland: Penguin. (5, 10)

Oswald I (1980). Sleep as a restorative process: Human clues. *Progress in Brain Research, 53*, 279-288. (11)

Palmblad J, Petrini B, Wasserman J, & Åkerstedt, T (1979). Lymphocyte and granulocyte reactions during sleep deprivations. *Psychosomatic Medicine, 4*, 273-278. (2)

Pappenheimer J R, Miller T B, & Goodrich C A (1967). Sleep promoting effects of cerebral spinal fluid from sleep deprived goats. *Proceedings of the National Academy of Sciences, 58*, 513-518. (2)

Parmeggiani P L (1987). Interaction between sleep and thermoregulation: an aspect of the control of behavioral states. *Sleep, 10*, 426-435. (2)

Parmeggiani, P L (1991). Physiologica risks during sleep. In J H Peter, T Penzel, T Podszus, & P von Wichert (Eds.), *Sleep and health risks* (pp. 119-123). New York: Springer-Verlag. (2)

Parmeggiani P L, Morrison A, Drucker-Colin, R R, & McGinty D (1985). Brain Mechanisms of Sleep: An Overview of Methodological Issues. In P L Parmeggiani, A Morrison, R R Drucker-Colin, & D McGinty (Eds.), *Brain Mechanisms of Sleep.* New York: Raven Press, 1-33. (2)

Partinen M, Kaprio J, Koskenvuo M, Putkonen P, & Langinvainio H (1983). Genetic and environmental determination of human sleep. *Sleep, 6*, 179-185. (3)

Penetar D, Redmond D & Belenky G (1989). Characterization of sleep during U.S. Army Ranger training. *Sleep Research, 18*, 373. (3)

Penn P E, Bootzin R R, Wood J M (1991). Nightmare frequency in sexual abuse survivors. *Sleep Research, 20*, 313. (6)

Perls F (1969). *Gestalt therapy verbatim.* Moab, Utah: Real People Press. (8)

Persinger M A (1980). *The weather matrix and human behavior.* New York: Praeger. (2)

Petre-Quadens O, DeBarsy A M, Devos J & Sfaello A (1967). Sleep in pregnancy: Evidence of fetal sleep characteristics. *Journal of Neurolgical Science, 4*, 600-605. (2)

Petre-Quadens O, & DeLee C (1974). Sleep-cycle alterations during pregnancy, postpartum, and the menstrual cycle. In M Ferin, F Halberg, R M Richart & R L VendeWiele (Eds.) *Biorhythms and Human Reproduction* (pp. 335-352). New York: Wiley. (2)

Petre-Quadens O, Hardy J L & DeLee C (1969). Comparative study of sleep in pregnancy and in the newborn. In R J Robinson (Ed.), *Brain and Early Behavior* (pp. 177-192). New York: Academic Press. (2)

Pirolli A & Smith C(1989). REM sleep deprivation in humans impairs learning of a complex task. *Sleep Research, 18,* 375. (11)

Pivik T, Azumi K & Dement W (1969). Sleep patterns during pregnancy. *Psychophysiology*, *6*, 236 (abstr). (2)

Plath D, Roehrs T A, Zwyghuizen-Doorenbos A, Sidlesteel J, Wittig R M & Roth T (1989). The alerting effects of caffine after sleep restriction. *Sleep Research, 18.* 124. (2)

Poceta J S, Ho S, Jeong D, & Mitler M M (1990). The maintenance of wakefulness test in obstructive sleep apnea syndrome. *Sleep Research, 19,* 268. (3)

Prinz P N (1980). Sleep changes with aging. In C Eisdorfer & W E Fann (Eds.), *Psychopharmacology of aging* (pp. 1-12) (3). Jamaica, NY: S P Medical & Scientific Books. (1,11)

Prinz P & Raskin M (1978). Aging and sleep disorders. In R Williams & I Karacan (1978). *Sleep disorders: Diagnosis and treatment* (pp. 303-321). New York: Wiley. (1)

Provine R R (1989). Faces as releasers of contagious yawning: an approach to face detection using normal human subjects. *Bulletin of the Psychonomic Society*, *27*, 211-4. (10)

Provine R R & Hamernik H B (1986). Yawning: effects of stimulus interest. *Bulletin of the Psychonomic Society*, *24*, 437-8. (10)

Radulovacki M, Virus R M, Djuricic-Nedelson M, Baglajewski T, Meyer E, & Green R D (1985). Adenosine and adenosine analogs: Effects on sleep in rats. In D J McGinty, R Drucker-Colin, A Morrison, & P L Parmeggiani (Eds.). *Brain Mechanisms of Sleep* (Pp. 235-252). New York: Raven Press. (2)

Rattray R S (1974). Sex dreams of the African ashantis. In R L Woods & H B Greenhouse (Eds.), *The new world of dreams* (pp. 117-118). New York: MacMillan. (6)

Rechtschaffen A (1971). The control of sleep. In W A Hunt (Ed.), *Human behavior and its control* (pp. 75-92). Cambridge, Mass: Schenkman. (11)

Rechtschaffen A (1979). The function of sleep: methodological issues. In R Drucker-Colin, M. Shkurovich, & M B Sterman (Eds.), *The functions of sleep* (pp. 1-17). New York: Academic Press. (3)

Rechtschaffen A (1983). Dream Psychophysiology and the Mind-Body Problem. In M Chase and E D Weitzman (Eds.), *Advances in sleep research, vol. 8, Sleep Disorders: Basic and Clinical Research.* New York: S P Medical and Scientific Books. (7)

Rechtschaffen A & Kales A (1968). *A manual of standardized terminology, techniques and scoring system for sleep stages of human subjects.* Los Angeles: BIS/BRI UCLA. (1)

Rechtschaffen A, Bliwise D, Litchman J, & Pivik R T (1978). Phasic EMG in human sleep: IV. Comparison of good and poor sleepers. *Sleep Research, 1*, 59. (3)

Reynolds C F and Shipley J E (1985). Sleep in depressive disorders. In R E Hales & A J Frances (Eds.), *American Psychiatric Association annual review* (pp. 341-351). Washington, D.C.: American Psychiatric Press, Inc. (3)

Roehrs T A, Vogel G, Claiborue D, Lamphere J, Bohannon M, & Roth T (1990). Sleepy versus alert subjects in a phase advance. *Sleep Research, 19*, 123. (3)

Roehrs T A, Zwyghuizen-Doorenbos A, Zwyghuizen H, Timms V, Fortier J, & Roth T (1989). Sedating effects of alcohol and time of drinking. *Sleep Research, 18*, 71. (2)

Roffwarg H, Muzio J & Dement W (1966). Ontogenetic development of human sleep-dream cycle. *Science, 152*, 604-18. (5,11)

Rojas-Ramirez J A & Drucker-Colin R R (1977). Phylogenetic correlations between sleep and memory. In R R Drucker-Colin & J L McGaugh (Eds.), *Neurobiology of sleep and memory* (pp. 57-74). New York: Academic Press. (5)

Rosa R R (1990). Napping at home and alertness on the job: results from two worksites on rotating 8-hr and 12-hr shifts. *Sleep Research, 19,* 402. (3)

Rosa R R & Bonnet M H (1991). Predicting nighttime alertness following prophylactic naps or, "How long should I nap before that all-nighter?", *Sleep Research, 20*, 417. (3)

Röschke J & Aldenhoff J B (1992). A nonlinear approach to brain function: deterministic chaos and sleep EEG. *Sleep, 15*, 95-101. (6)

Rosen J (1990). (presentation as a part of a symposium on Daytime sleepiness in children) Presented at the fourth annual meeting of the Association of Professional Sleep Societies, Minneapolis. (1)

Rosenthal L D, Krstevska S, Roehrs T A, Kontich D, Fortier J, & Roth T (1992). Nocturnal sleep latenicies and TST is sleepy, sleep deprived and alert subjects. *Sleep Research, 21*, 110.(3)

Rosenthal L D, Merlotti L, Rosen A, Jast R G, Roehrs T A, & Roth T (1991). Total sleep time and level of sleepiness following partial and total sleep deprivation. *Sleep Research, 20*, 418. (3)

Rosenthal L D, Roehrs T A, Krstevska S, Rosen A, Sicklesteel J, & Roth T (1992). Auditory awakening thresholds in sleepy, alert, and sleep deprived subjects. *Sleep Research, 21*, 111. (3)

Ross R J, Ball W A, Sullivan K A, & Caroff S N (1989). Sleep disturbance as the hallmark of posttraumatic stress disorder. *American Journal of Psychiatry, 146,* 697-707. (6)

Roth T (1990). (presentation as a part of a symposium on Ethanol and sleep/wake function: basic and clinical issues) Presented at the fourth annual meeting of the Association of Professional Sleep Societies, Minneapolis. (2)

Ruckebusch Y (1972). The relevance of drowsiness in the circadian cycle of farm animals. *Animal Behavior, 20,* 637-43. (5)

Sakai K (1985). Anatomical and Physiological Basis of Paradoxical Sleep. In D J McGinty,R Drucker-Colin,A Morrison, & P L Parmeggiani, (Eds.). *Brain Mechanisms of Sleep.* New York: Raven Press, (Pp. 111-137). (2,11)

Sakai K (1986). Central mechanisms of paradoxical sleep. *Brain development, 8,* 402-407. (2)p

Sanchez R & Bootzin R R (1985). A comparison of white noise and music: Effects of predictable and unpredictable sounds on sleep. *Sleep Research, 14*, 121. (10)

Sangal R B, Thomas L, & Mitler M M (1992). Disorders of excessive sleepiness: treatment improves ability to stay awake but does not reduce sleepiness. *Sleep research, 21,* 255. (3)

Sastre P J-P & Jouvet M (1979). Le Comportenment Onirique Du Chat. *Physiology and Behavior, 22,* 979-989. (2)

Schenck C H, Bundlie S R, Patterson A L, & Mahowold M W (1987). Rapid eye movement sleep behavior disorder: A treatable parasomnia affecting older adults. *Journal of the American Medical Association, 257,* 1786-1789. (9)

Schubert F C (1977). Personality traits and polygraphic sleep patterns: correlations between personality factors and polygraphically recorded sleep in healthy subjects. *Waking and sleeping, 1,* 165-170.

Schulz H & Lavie P (Eds.) (1985). *Ultradian rhythms in physiology and behavior.* Berlin: Springer-Verlag (4)

Schweiger M S (1972). Sleep disturbance in pregnancy - a subjective survey. *American Journal of Obstetrics & Gynecology , 114,* 879-882. (2)

Scrima, L (1984). Dream sleep and memory: New findings with diverse implications. *Integrative Psychiatry,* 211-216. (11)

Segalowitz S J, Ogilvie R D, Janicki M, Simons I, & Buetow C (1991). ERP evidence for the paradox of REM sleep: attention and distraction while awake and while asleep. *Sleep Research, 20,* 40. (1)

Seligman M E P & Yellen A (1987). What is a dream? *Behavior Research and Therapy, 25,* 1-24. (1,2,7)

Shapiro C M, Bortz R, Mitchell D, Bartel P, & Jooste P (1981). Slow-wave sleep: A recovery period after exercise. *Science, 214,* 1253-1254. (2)

Shiromani P J, Gillin J C, & Henriksen S J (1987). Acetylcholine and the regulation of REM sleep: basic mechanisms and clinical implications for affective illness and narcolepsy. *Ann Rev Pharmacol Toxicol, 27,* 137-156. (2)

Siegel A (1983). Expectant father's dreams. *Dream Craft,* **2**, 5-7. (6)

Siegel J M (1989). Brainstem mechanisms generating REM sleep. In Kryger M H, Roth T, & Dement W C (Eds.) (1989). *Principles and practice of sleep medicine* (pp. 104-120). Philadelphia: Saunders. (2,11)

Siegel J M (1990). Mechanisms of sleep control. *J Chn Neurophysiol, 7,* 49-65. (2,11)

Siegel J (1992). *Brainstem control of muscle tone; basic and clinical implications.* Invited address presented at the 6th annual meeting of the Association of Professional Sleep Societies, May 29-June 3, 1992. Phoenix, Arizona. (2)

Smith A (1992). Sleep, colds, and performance. In Broughton R J & Ogilvie R D (Eds.), *Sleep, arousal, and performance* (pp. 233-242). Boston: Birkhäuser. (2)

Smith C (1993). REM sleep anb learning: some recent findings. In A Moffitt, M Kramer, & R Hoffmann (Eds.), *The functions of dreaming* (pp. 341-362). New York: State University of New York Press(11)

Smith C & MacNeill C (1992a). Memory for a motor task is impaired by stage 2 sleep loss. *Sleep Research, 21,* 139. (11)

Smith C S, Reilly C, Midkiff K (1989). Evaluation of three circadian rhythm questionnaires with suggestion for an improved measure of morningness. *Journal of Applied Psychology, 74,* 728-38. (4,9)

Snyder F (1966). Toward an evolutionary theory of dreaming. *American Journal of Psychiatry, 123,* 121-136. (6)

Spiegel R (1981). *Advanced in sleep research, Volume 5: Sleep and sleeplessness in advanced age.* New York: SP Medical and Scientific Books. (1,3,6)

Spiegel R, Koferle S, & Allen S R (1986). Significance of slow wave sleep: Considerations from a clinical viewpoint. *Sleep, 9,* 66-79. (11)

Stampi C, Broughton R, Mullington J, & Rivers M (1989). Short-memory performance is impaired by sleep inertia after 80- or 50-, but not after 20-min naps during polyphasic sleep schedules. *Sleep Research, 18,* 446. (3)

Stampi C, Moffitt A, & Hoffman R (1990). Leonardo Da Vinci's polyphasic ultrashort sleep: a strategy for sleep reduction? *Sleep research, 19,* 408. (11)

Stepanski E, Lamphere J, Bodin P, Zorich F & Roth T (1984). Sleep fragmentation and daytime sleepiness. *Sleep, 7,* 18-26. (3)

Steriade M (1990). [No title]. In M H Chase & T Roth (Eds.), *Slow Wave Sleep: Its Measurement and Functional Significance.* (pp 51-53). Los Angeles: Brain Information service/Brain Research Institute. (2)

Steriade M & Pare D. (1990). Brainstem genesis and thalamic transfer of internal signals during dreaming sleep; cellular data and hypotheses. In J Montplaisir & R Bodbout (Eds). *Sleep and Biological Rhythms* (p 148-162). New York: Oxford University Press. (2)

Sterman M D (1967). Relationship of intrauterine fetal activity to maternal sleep stage. *Experimental Neurology, supplement Q,* 98-106. (2)

Sterman M B & Shouse M N (1985). Sleep "Centers" in the Brain: The Preoptic Basal Forebrain Area Revisited. In McGinty D J, Drucker-Colin R, Morrison A, & Parmeggiani P L. *Brain Mechanisms of Sleep* (Pp. 277-299). New York: Raven Press. (3)

Sterman M G, Symusiak R S & McGinty D J (1990). Integrative Funcions of the basal forebrain area in sleep regulation. In M Mancia and G Marini (Eds.), *The Diencephalon and Sleep,* (pp 147-170). New York: Raven Press. (2)

Strogatz S H (1986). *The mathematical structure of the human sleep-wake cycle*. New York: Springer-Verlag. (4)

Strumwasser F (1971). The cellular basis of behavior in aplysia. *Journal of Psychiatric Research, 8*, 237-257. (5)

Stukane E (1985). *The dream worlds of pregnancy*. New York: Quill.(6)

Stuss D & Broughton R (1978). Extreme short sleep: Personality profiles and a case study of sleep requirement. *Waking and sleeping, 2*, 101-105. (3)

Szymusiak R & Satinoff E (1985). Thermal influence on basal forebrain hyprogenic mechanisms. In D J McGinty, R Drucker-Colin,A Morrison, & P L Parmeggiani (Eds.). *Brain Mechanisms of Sleep* (Pp. 301-319). New York: Raven Press.

Tangel D J, Mezzanotte W S, Wheatly J R, & White D P (1992). Palatal muscle activity: Influence of respiratory route and NREM sleep. *Sleep Research, 21*, 45. (2)

Tauber E S (1974). Phylogeny of sleep. In E D Weitzman (Ed.), *Advances in sleep research, Vol. 1* (pp. 133-172). Flushing, NY: Spectrum Publications, Inc. (5)

Tedlock B. (ed.) (1987). *Dreaming: anthropological and psychological interpretations*. Cambridge: Cambridge University Press. (6)

Thomas M L, Sing H C, Belenky G, Shepanek N, Thorne D R, McCann U D, Penetar D M, Fertig J, & Redmond D P (1990). EEG changes following 48 hours of sleep deprivation in humans. *Sleep Research, 19*, 358. (3)

Tilley A J, Brown S, Donald M, Ferguson S, Piccone J, Plasto K, & Statham D (1992). Human sleep and memory processes. In R J Broughton & R D Ogilvie (Eds). *Sleep, Arousal, and Performance* (pp. 117-130). Boston: Birkanser. (11)

Tobler I (1982). Phylogenetic approaches to the functions of sleep: Introduction. In *Sleep 1982* (pp. 126-130). Basel: Karger. (5)

Tobler I (1983). Introduction. In W P Koella (Ed.), *Sleep 1982* (pp. 126-130). Basel: Karger. (5)

Tobler I (1984). Evolution of the sleep process: a phylogenetic approach. In A A Borbely & J L Valatx, *Sleep mechanisms* (pp. 207-226). New York:Springer-Verlag. (5)

Tobler I (1987 June-July). *Sleep and sleep regulation in various species*. Presented at the Fifth International Congress of Sleep Research, Copenhagen, Denmark. (5)

Tobler, I (1992). Behavioral Sleep in the Asian Elephant in captivity. *Sleep, 1*, 1-12. (5)

Tobler I & Borbely A (1985). Effect of rest deprivation on motor activity of fish. *Journal of Comparative Physiology (A)*, **157**, 817-22. (5)

Tobler I & Stalder J (1987). Rest in the scorpion - a sleep-like state?. *Sleep Research, 16*,196. (5)

Toth L & Krueger J M (1992). Clinical correlates of sleep patterns after bacterial challange. *Sleep research, 21*, 315. (2)

Trenholme I, Cartwright R, & Greenberg G (1984). Dream dimension differences during a life change. *Psychiatry research, 12*, 35-45. (6)

Trinder J, Montgomery I, & Paxton S (1987 June-July). *The effect of physical fitness on sleep*. Presented at the Fifth International Congress of Sleep Research, Copenhagen, Denmark. (2)

Ullman M, Krippner S, & Vaughan A (1989). *Dream telepathy: experiments in nocturnal ESP*. Jefferson, N.C.: McFarland. (6)

Ullman M & Zimmerman N (1979). *Working with dreams*. New York: Dell. (6,8)

VandeCastle R L (1971). *The psychology of dreaming*. Morristown, NJ: General Learning Press. (6)

Vanderwolf C H (1990). (Untitled). In M H Chase & T Roth (Eds.), *Slow Wave Sleep: Its Measurement and Functional Significance*. (pp 38-40). Los Angeles: Brain Information Service/Brain Research Institute. (2)

Vaughan C J (1963). The development and use of an operant techinique to provide evidence for visual imagery in rhesus mankey under 'sensory deprivation.' Unpublished PhD dissertation, University of Pittsburg.

Viot-Blanc V, Benoit O, Pailhous E, & Bouard G (1987). Sleep length, sleep schedule and day activity level comparison between poor and good sleepers. *Sleep research, 16*, 450. (3)

Vitiello M V & Prinz P N (1990). Sleep and sleep disorders in normal aging. In M J Thorpy (Ed.), *Handbook of sleep disorders* (139-154). New York: Marcel Deker. (1)

Vogel G W (1979). A motivational function of REM sleep. In R Drucker-Colin, M Shkurovich, & M B Sterman (Eds.), *The functions of sleep* (pp. 233-250). New York: Academic Press. (3,11)

Walker J M & Berger R J (1980). Sleep as an adaptation for energy conservation functionally related to hibernation and shallow torpor. *Progress in Brain Research*, *53*, 255-78. (2,5,10,11)

Walsh J K, Muehlbach M J, Humm T M, Dickins Q S, Sugerman J L, & Schweitzer P K (1990). Effect of caffeine on physiological sleep tendency and ability to sustain wakefulness at night. *Psychoparmocology*, *101*, 271-3. (2,3)

Walsh J K, Muehlbach M J, Humm T, Stokes Dickins Q & Schweitzer P K. (1989). Effect of caffine on physiological sleep tendency and ability to sustain wakefulness at night. *Sleep Research, 18,* 82. (2)

Ward C D (1986). Encephalitis lehtargica and the development of neuropsychiatry. *The Psychiatric Clinics of North America, 9*, 215-218. (10)

Ware J C (1988). Sleep and Anxiety. In R L Williams, I K Karacan, & C A Moore(Eds.). *Sleep Disorders: Diagnosis and Treatment 2nd ed.* (Pp. 189-214). New York: Wiley. (3)

Warner B F & Huggins S E (1978). An electroencephalographic study of sleep in young cainans in a colony. *Comp. Biochem. Physiol, 59A*, 139-144. (5)

Wauquier A, Dugovic C, & Radulovacki M (Eds.) (1989). *Slow wave sleep: Physiological, pathophysiological, and functional aspects*. New York: Raven Press. (11)

Webb W B(1973). Sleep research past and present. In W B Webb (Ed.), *Sleep: An active process* (pp. 1-10). Glenview, Ill.: Charles C Thomas. (3)

Webb W B (1975). *Sleep: The gentle tyrant*. Englewood Cliffs, NJ: Prentice-Hall. (1,3,5,6)

Webb W B (1979). Theories of sleep functions and some clinical implications. In R Drucker-Colin, M Shkurovich, & M B Sterman (Eds.), *The functions of sleep* (pp. 19-35). New York: Academic Press. (11)

Webb W B (1981). *The nature of naps: A discussion.* Presented at the Annual Meeting of the Association for the Psychophysiological Study of Sleep, Hyannis, Mass. (3)

Webb W B (1983). Theories in modern sleep research. In A Mayes (Ed.), *Sleep mechanisms and functions in humans and animals - an evolutionary prespective* (pp. 1-17). Berkshire, England: Van Nostrand Reinhold. (11)

Webb W B (1987). REM cycling revisited: Fixed and free running. *Sleep Research, 16*, 253. (4)

Webb W B (1992). *Sleep: The gentle tyrant.* Boston: Anker. (4,6)

Webb W B & Agnew H W (1975). Are we chronically sleep-deprived? *Bulletin of the Psychonomic Society, 6*, 47-8. (3)

Webb W B & Cartwright R D (1978). Sleep and dreams. *Annual Review of Psychology, 29*, 223-252. (3)

Weber S, Bergan D, Golden H, Moorcroft W H, & Hansen G (1983 July). *Alpha delta sleep in fibrositis patients*. Paper presented at the Fourth InternationalCongress of Sleep Research, Balogna, Italy. (9)

Wehr T A (1990). Effects of wakefulness and sleep on depression and mania. In J Montplaisir & R Godbout (Eds.), *Sleep and biological rhythms* (pp. 42-86). New York: Oxford. (2)

Whitton J L, Kramer P, & Eastwood R (1982). Weather and infradian rhythms in self-reports of health, sleep and mood measures. *J. of Psychosomatic Res, 26*, 231-235. (2)

Williams R L & Karacan I (1978). *Sleep disorders: Diagnosis and treatment.* New York: Wiley. (9)

Williams R L, Karacan I & Hursch C J (1974). *Electroencephalography (EEG) of human sleep: Clinical applications*, New York: John Wiley and Sons. (1,2,3)

Willich S N, Tobler G H, & Muller J E (1987 June-July). *Morning peak in the incidence of sudden cardiac death: association with increase in platelet aggregability.* Presented at the Fifth International Congress of Sleep Research, Copenhagen, Denmark.(2)

Winson, J (1990). The meaning of dreams. *Scientific American, 263,* 86-96. (11)

Wolff G & Money J (1973). Relationship between sleep and growth in patients with reversible somatotropin deficiency (Psychosocial dwarfism). *Psychological Medicine, 3*, 18-27.(3)

Yehuda S, Carasso R L (1988) DSIP - a tool for investigating the sleep onset mechanism: a review. *International Journal of Neuroscience, 38*, 345-353. (2)

Zarcone V (1990). (presentation as a part of a symposium on Ethanol and sleep/wake function: basic and clinical issues) Presented at the fourth annual meeting of the Association of Professional Sleep Societies, Minneapolis. (2)

Zepelin H (1983). A life span perspective on sleep. In A Mayes (Ed.), *Sleep mechanisms and functions in humans and animals - an evolutionary prespective* (pp. 126-160). Berkshire, England: Van Nostrand Reinhold. (11)

Zepelin H (1989). Mammalian sleep. In Kryger M H, Roth T, & Dement W C (Eds.) (1989). *Principles and practice of sleep medicine* (pp. 30-49). Philadelphia: Saunders. (5)

Zepelin H & Rechtschaffen A (1974). Mammalian sleep, longevity and energy metabolism. *Brain, Behavior, and Evolution, 10*, 425-470. (5,11)

Zulley J, Wever R, & Aschoff J (1981). The dependence of onset and duration of sleep on the circadian rhythm of rectal temperature. *Pflugers Archiv (European Journal of Physiology), 391*, 314-318. (4)

Zwyghurizen-Doorenbos A, Roehrs T A, Russo L, Buzenski R, Wittig R M, Lomphere J & Roth T (1989). Continued sedation and decline in drug concentrations. *Sleep Research, 19*, 84. (2)

Index

About the Author

"Everyone in the lab is going to the international sleep meeting in Europe. Why don't you come along. The round trip charter cost is only $180.00."

I was told this when I was doing postdoctoral research on the maturation of brain waves in baby rats at the University of Nebraska Medical School shortly after receiving a Ph.D. in psychology (psychobiology) from Princeton University. I went. I admit that the main reason was to spend a month in Europe. However, what I learned at the meeting, held in the summer of 1971, fascinated me. It was the start of a continuing interest in sleep and all of its ramifications.

Shortly after my return from Europe, I began to teach at Luther College and found myself reading and lecturing frequently about sleep. Within a few years, my research interests shifted away from baby rat brains to sleep. Soon I started a sleep research laboratory at Luther College in which I have studied various aspects of sleep and dreaming. I also kept on attending the meetings (some again in Europe, others in places like Cap Cod and San Antonio) of what was to become the Sleep Research Society. Later I joined the Association for the Study of Dreams and attended its first meeting (in San Francisco). In 1980, I learned about sleep disorders and did some research in that area while on sabbatical at the Sleep Disorders Center of Rush Medical School in Chicago. Most recently, I was on another sabbatical at the Mayo Medical Center's Sleep Disorders Center in Rochester Minnesota. While at Mayo, I again did some sleep disorders research but mainly worked on completing this book.

In the future, I intend to keep on studying, researching, lecturing, and writing about sleep, dreaming, and sleep disorders. And of course, I intend to continue to attend those wonderful meetings.